Thyroid Disease: Clinical Diagnosis and Therapy

Thyroid Disease: Clinical Diagnosis and Therapy

Edited by Joaquin Noah

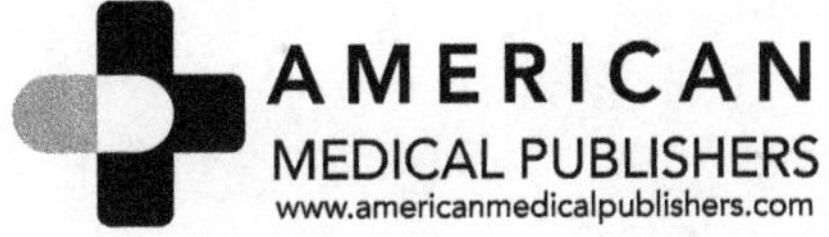

American Medical Publishers,
41 Flatbush Avenue,
1st Floor, New York,
NY 11217, USA

Visit us on the World Wide Web at:
www.americanmedicalpublishers.com

ISBN: 978-1-63927-126-9

Cataloging-in-Publication Data

Thyroid disease : clinical diagnosis and therapy / edited by Joaquin Noah.
p. cm.
Includes bibliographical references and index.
ISBN 978-1-63927-126-9
1. Thyroid gland--Diseases. 2. Thyroid gland--Diseases--Diagnosis.
3. Thyroid gland--Diseases--Treatment. I. Noah, Joaquin.
RC655 .T49 2022
616.44--dc23

Table of Contents

Preface

The medical condition that affects the function of the thyroid gland is referred to as thyroid disease. The thyroid gland produces thyroid hormones. These hormones help in regulating energy use, infant development and childhood development. Thyroid diseases are classified into five groups. These are hypothyroidism, hyperthyroidism, structural abnormalities, tumors and abnormal thyroid. The symptoms of hypothyroidism are tiredness, slow movement, muscle cramps, etc. Common symptoms of hyperthyroidism are insomnia, anxiety, palpitations, etc. The diagnosis of this disease is based on these symptoms. Its further diagnosis can be done through ultrasound, biopsy and radioiodine scanning. The treatment of thyroid involves the intake of medications like thioamide drugs, or through surgery such as thyroidectomy, and radioiodine therapy. Different approaches, evaluations and advanced studies on thyroid disease have been included in this book. It will also provide interesting topics for research which interested readers can take up. The extensive content of this book offer the readers new insights into this field.

After months of intensive research and writing, this book is the end result of all who devoted their time and efforts in the initiation and progress of this book. It will surely be a source of reference in enhancing the required knowledge of the new developments in the area. During the course of developing this book, certain measures such as accuracy, authenticity and research focused analytical studies were given preference in order to produce a comprehensive book in the area of study.

This book would not have been possible without the efforts of the authors and the publisher. I extend my sincere thanks to them. Secondly, I express my gratitude to my family and well-wishers. And most importantly, I thank my students for constantly expressing their willingness and curiosity in enhancing their knowledge in the field, which encourages me to take up further research projects for the advancement of the area.

Editor

1

Hypothyroidism among military infants born in countries of varied iodine nutrition status

Marcus M Cranston[1], Margaret AK Ryan[2], Tyler C Smith[3*], Carter J Sevick[3], Stephanie K Brodine[4]

Abstract

Background: Iodine deficiency is a global problem representing the most common preventable cause of mental retardation. Recently, the impact of subtle deficiencies in iodine intake on children and pregnant women has been questioned. This study was designed to compare hypothyroidism among infants born to US military families in countries of varied iodine nutrition status.

Methods: A cohort design was used to analyze data from the Department of Defense Birth and Infant Health Registry for infants born in 2000-04 (n = 447,691). Hypothyroidism was defined using ICD-9-CM codes from the first year of life (n = 698). The impact of birth location on hypothyroidism was assessed by comparing rates in Germany, Japan, and US territories with the United States, while controlling for infant gender, plurality, gestational age, maternal age, maternal military status, and military parent's race/ethnicity.

Results: Hypothyroidism did not vary by birth location with adjusted odds ratios (OR) as follows: Germany (OR 0.82, [95% CI 0.50, 1.35]), Japan (OR 0.67, [95% CI 0.37, 1.22]), and US territories (OR 1.29, [95% CI 0.57, 2.89]). Hypothyroidism was strongly associated with preterm birth (OR 5.44, [95% CI 4.60, 6.42]). Hypothyroidism was also increased among infants with civilian mothers (OR 1.24, [95% CI 1.00, 1.54]), and older mothers, especially ages 40 years and older (OR 2.09, [95% CI 1.33, 3.30]).

Conclusions: In this study, hypothyroidism in military-dependent infants did not vary by birth location, but was associated with other risk factors, including preterm birth, civilian maternal status, and advanced maternal age.

Background

Over 1.9 billion people, 31% of the world's population, live in areas of iodine deficiency [1]. Iodine deficiency disorders affect over 200 million people and are the most common preventable cause of brain damage and mental retardation worldwide [2]. Iodine deficiency exists primarily in areas of low soil iodine content, and although strategies exist to combat iodine deficiency, they are not employed uniformly throughout the world [3]. As a result, iodine nutrition varies between countries.

Early public health efforts focused on severe iodine deficiency with the goal of preventing goiter and cretinism. More recently, concerns have been raised regarding the effects of lesser degrees of iodine deficiency in vulnerable populations, such as pregnant women and children. When iodine deficiency is present during the fetal stage to the third month after birth, even mild to moderate deficiency may lead to abnormalities of psychoneuromotor and intellectual development [4,5].

Iodine deficiency disorders were a significant problem in the United States until the 1920s, when the general use of iodized salt was initiated [6]. Based on the National Health and Nutrition Examination Survey (NHANES) III, performed from 1988 to 1994, the World Health Organization (WHO) has classified US iodine intake as "more than adequate" [3]. However, the adequacy of iodine intake during pregnancy has been questioned, as changes in thyroid hormone metabolism and renal iodine handling increase maternal iodine needs [4,7]. It has been proposed that a median urinary iodine (UI) concentration of 150-245 ug/l during pregnancy be used to define a population with sufficient iodine intake [8]. NHANES III and the 2001-2002 NHANES reported median UI concentrations at the lower limit of these recommendations for pregnancy, 141 and 173 ug/l, respectively [7,9].

* Correspondence: tyler.c.smith@med.navy.mil
[3]Naval Health Research Center, San Diego, California, USA

The overwhelming majority of hypothyroidism during infancy is due to congenital hypothyroidism with etiologies including a variety of environmental and genetic factors, but the major determinant of prevalence worldwide is iodine intake. In areas of iodine sufficiency, congenital hypothyroidism may be as rare as 1:4000, while transient thyrotropin elevations may be seen in up to 40% of neonates in areas of severe iodine deficiency [1,10]. The impact of more subtle differences in iodine intake on hypothyroidism is unclear.

Families of US military members often reside in countries with varied iodine nutrition status. The majority of military-dependent births outside of the United States occur in Germany where iodine intake in the host-nation population is lower than the United States, Japan where iodine intake is higher than the United States and US territories in which little data regarding iodine intake is available [3,11]. No prior studies have examined iodine intake, iodine nutrition status or iodine-dependent outcomes in US military families residing in these different geographic locations. However, all infants sponsored by the Department of Defense (DoD) undergo hypothyroidism screening at birth, and diagnostic data for these children are captured in the DoD Birth and Infant Health Registry, previously titled the DoD Birth Defects Registry. As a result, this registry provides a unique opportunity to compare rates of hypothyroidism during infancy and gain insight into the relative iodine nutrition of military families living in these areas. In addition, the DoD Birth and Infant Health Registry is positioned to examine other potential risk factors for hypothyroidism during infancy, an area in which prior studies have focused on congenital hypothyroidism and are somewhat limited. Therefore, this study was designed to compare hypothyroidism among infants born to US military families in countries where the host populations have varied iodine nutrition status.

Methods

Study population

This cohort study used the DoD Birth and Infant Health Registry to identify all infants born to US military members during 2000-2004. Potential subjects were excluded for incomplete gender data (n = 26) and maternal age (n = 8), as well as the inability to reliably link diagnosis data (n = 22). In addition, only infants born in the United States, Germany, Japan, or US territories, the locations with numbers of births sufficient for comparison, were included in this study (n = 447,691). This research has been conducted in compliance with all applicable federal regulations governing the protection of human subjects in research (Protocol NHRC.2007.0026).

Identification of hypothyroidism

All military-sponsored infants undergo hypothyroidism screening, regardless of birth location, and the DoD Birth and Infant Health Registry captures all hospitalization and outpatient encounter data for military-dependent children during the first year of life using International Classification of Diseases, Clinical Modification (ICD-9-CM)-coded diagnoses. Further details regarding the registry have been previously published [12]. For this study, infant records were searched for ICD-9-CM codes 243, congenital hypothyroidism, and 244, acquired hypothyroidism [13]. To avoid inclusion of screening encounters in the outcome, cases of hypothyroidism were defined as those infants with the ICD-9-CM code 243 or 244 on at least two separate health care encounter dates, or at least one inpatient encounter.

Hypothyroidism risk factors

The independent variable of interest was birth location, and the United States, Germany, Japan, and US territories represented the location of 96.8% of all military-dependent births. Births in the current and former US territories of American Samoa, Federated States of Micronesia, Guam, Marshall Islands, Northern Mariana Islands, Palau, Puerto Rico, US Virgin Islands, and other outlying islands were categorized as US territory. Variables previously shown to be associated with congenital hypothyroidism were also assessed, including maternal age, infant gender, infant plurality, and estimated gestational age [14-16]. The estimated gestational age in this study was classified as full-term (≥37 weeks) or preterm (<37 weeks), based on ICD-9-CM codes in 765 series. Infant race/ethnicity, which has been reported to be associated with congenital hypothyroidism, was not available [16]. However, the race/ethnicity of the military sponsor, the parent to whom health care eligibility is linked, was analyzed. This was the only independent variable with missing data and an unknown category was used where the race/ethnicity data for the military sponsor were not available (n = 14,786). White, non-Hispanic race/ethnicity was designated as the reference due to the previously reported lower rates of congenital hypothyroidism for infants in this category [16]. Maternal military status was categorized as active-duty military or civilian.

Statistical methods

Univariate analyses were performed to explore the unadjusted associations of hypothyroidism, location of birth, and demographic characteristics. The impact of independent variables on hypothyroidism was estimated as crude and adjusted odds ratios with 95% confidence intervals by applying a multivariable logistic regression model. Regression diagnostics and multicollinearity investigations were completed. All independent variables were included in the final logistic regression model due to either significant unadjusted odds ratios or previously reported associations with congenital hypothyroidism. Computer analyses were performed using SAS version 9.1 (SAS Institute, Inc., Cary, North Carolina).

Results

The characteristics of the study population of infants from the DoD Birth and Infant Health Registry born in 2000-2004 (n = 447,691) are illustrated in Table 1. These infants were predominately born in the United States to civilian mothers, who were married to active-duty military members. The majority of military sponsors self-reported their race/ethnicity to be white, non-Hispanic. The rate of preterm births was 8.8%, while 2.8% were multiple births.

Odds ratios for the associations of hypothyroidism with birth location and other independent characteristics are shown in Table 2. Hypothyroidism did not differ for infants born in Germany (OR 0.82, [95% CI 0.50, 1.35]), Japan (OR 0.67, [95% CI 0.37, 1.22]) or US territories (OR 1.29, [95% CI 0.57, 2.89]) when compared with infants born in the United States. Hypothyroidism was associated with preterm birth (OR 5.44, [95% CI 4.60, 6.42]). In addition, hypothyroidism was more frequent among infants born to older mothers, women aged 25-29 years (OR 1.32, [95% CI 1.09, 1.59]) and women aged 40 years and older OR 2.09, [95% CI 1.33, 3.30]) when compared with infants with younger mothers, aged 20-24 years. Hypothyroidism was also slightly more common in infants born to civilian mothers (OR 1.24, [95% CI 1.00, 1.54]), than for those born to active-duty military mothers. Infant gender, plurality, and military sponsor race/ethnicity were not found to be associated with hypothyroidism. Of note, there was no significant change in odds ratio measures for birth locations when infants with missing data for military sponsor race/ethnicity were excluded from the analysis.

Table 1 Characteristics of infants in the DoD Birth and Infant Health Registry, born 2000-2004 (*N* = 447 691)

Characteristic	*n* (%)	
Birth location		
United States	419 756	(93.8)
Germany	13 685	(3.1)
Japan	10 994	(2.5)
US territory	3256	(0.7)
Sex of infant		
Male	229 530	(51.3)
Female	218 161	(48.7)
Infant plurality		
Singleton	435 021	(97.2)
Multiple birth	12 670	(2.8)
Estimated gestational age (weeks)		
Full-term (≥37)	408 224	(91.2)
Preterm (<37)	39 467	(8.8)
Maternal age (years)		
≤19	27 951	(6.2)
20-24	164 066	(36.6)
25-29	129 000	(28.8)
30-34	85 433	(19.1)
35-39	34 742	(7.8)
≥40	6499	(1.5)
Maternal military status		
Civilian	365 953	(81.7)
Military	81 738	(18.3)
Military sponsor race/ethnicity		
White, non-Hispanic	287 834	(64.3)
Black, non-Hispanic	76 529	(17.1)
Hispanic	42 382	(9.5)
Asian/Pacific Islander	16 044	(3.6)
American Indian/Alaska Native	5510	(1.2)
Other	4606	(1.0)
Unknown	14 786	(3.3)

DoD, US Department of Defense

Discussion

In this study of infants born to US military families, our data did not demonstrate differences in hypothyroidism for the birth locations examined. Iodine intake has never been studied in these military family populations and the application of practices that may increase iodine intake, such as consuming US-based food products on military bases or iodine-containing prenatal vitamins, is unknown. For example, the Department of Defense uses multiple US-based sources for prenatal vitamins and during the period of this study, some of the sources contained iodine and others did not. With the lack of information regarding iodine intake among US military families, the findings of this study are reassuring given the historical differences in iodine intake and iodine deficiency disorders in the host nation populations in these regions of the world. In the 1980s, estimates of transient neonatal hypothyroidism in Belgium were as high as 1:100 compared with 1:50 000 in the United States [17]. Over the past two decades iodine intake has decreased in the United States and increased in Europe, but differences in iodine nutrition still exist and the WHO classification of iodine nutrition is lower for Germany than the United States [3,7]. In Japan there is an absence of nationally representative data, but available data suggest iodine intake is much higher than in the United States [11]. Specific iodine nutrition data are also lacking for the current and former US territories examined in this study, but WHO regional data would

Table 2 Adjusted odds of congenital hypothyroidism for infants in DoD Birth and Infant Health Registry, born 2000-2004 (*N* = 447 691)

Variable	No Hypothyroidism (*N* = 446 993)	Hypothyroidism (*N* = 698)	OR[a] [95% CI]
Birth location			
United States	419 091	665	1.00 Reference
Germany	13 669	16	0.82 [0.50, 1.35]
Japan	10 983	11	0.67 [0.37, 1.22]
US territory	3250	6	1.29 [0.57, 2.89]
Sex of infant			
Male	229 163	367	1.00 Reference
Female	217 830	331	0.97 [0.84, 1.13]
Infant plurality			
Singleton	434 375	646	1.00 Reference
Multiple Birth	12 618	52	0.91 [0.67, 1.23]
Estimated gestational age (weeks)			
Full-term (≥37)	407 765	459	1.00 Reference
Preterm (<37)	39 228	239	**5.44 [4.60, 6.42]**
Maternal age (years)			
≤19	27 911	40	1.04 [0.74, 1.45]
20-24	163 852	214	1.00 Reference
25-29	128 777	223	**1.32 [1.09, 1.59]**
30-34	85 298	135	1.16 [0.93, 1.44]
35-39	34 678	64	1.27 [0.95, 1.69]
≥40	6477	22	**2.09 [1.33, 3.30]**
Maternal military status			
Military	81 633	105	1.00 Reference
Civilian	365 360	593	**1.24 [1.00, 1.54]**
Military sponsor race/ethnicity			
White, non-Hispanic	287 401	433	1.00 Reference
Black, non-Hispanic	76 402	127	1.09 [0.89, 1.33]
Hispanic	42 321	61	1.01 [0.77, 1.33]
Asian/Pacific Islander	16 018	26	1.12 [0.75, 1.66]
American Indian/Alaska Native	5498	12	1.55 [0.87, 2.76]
Other	4600	6	0.88 [0.39, 1.98]
Unknown	14 753	33	1.26 [0.87, 1.81]

DoD, US Department of Defense; OR, adjusted odds ratio; CI, confidence interval.
[a]Model adjusted for birth location, sex of infant, infant plurality, estimated gestational age, maternal age, maternal military status, and military sponsor race/ethnicity.

suggest that intake in these areas is significantly less than that of the United States [3]. The influence of host nation practices on the nutritional status of military families is not known and iodine-dependent outcomes have not previously been assessed in these populations, highlighting the importance of the findings of this study.

Given universal screening for congenital hypothyroidism at birth, along with the rare clinical recognition of acquired hypothyroidism due to indolent onset and non-specific symptoms during infancy, the majority of cases of hypothyroidism in our study likely represent congenital hypothyroidism, despite provider use of both ICD-9-CM codes 243, congenital hypothyroidism, and 244, acquired hypothyroidism. This is supported by the fact that 76.1% of those with ICD-9-CM code 243 and 58.8% of those with ICD-9 code 244 had diagnostic codes entered within the first 10 weeks of life. Iodine deficiency is responsible for the majority of transient congenital hypothyroidism, while permanent congenital hypothyroidism causes include thyroid dysgenesis, dyshormonogenesis, and central hypothyroidism and is relatively rare, with incidence estimates for each etiology ranging from 1:4500 to 1:100 000 [18]. With the exception of inborn errors of thyroid hormone synthesis, the etiologic mechanism in most cases is unknown, thus contributing to the interest in identifying risk factors for congenital hypothyroidism [19].

In our study, the factor most strongly association with hypothyroidism was preterm birth. This is consistent with previous descriptive studies of congenital hypothyroidism and is thought to represent transient hypothyroxinemia, due to incomplete thyroid gland development [20,21]. We also found hypothyroidism during infancy to be associated with increased maternal age, with the greatest risk for those aged 40 years and older. Previously, a registry-based study of congenital hypothyroidism in California found no linear trend across maternal age categories, while an Italian case-control study found higher rates of permanent congenital hypothyroidism for maternal age ≥40 years [15,16]. Our study also found hypothyroidism to be slightly more common in infants born to civilian mothers. These associations between maternal factors and hypothyroidism may represent differences in the health of the maternal populations. It is possible that younger age and the military entrance screening process reduce the prevalence of maternal disorders, such as autoimmune diseases, and decrease the risk for genetic disorders, leading to lower rates of hypothyroidism among infants born to these maternal groups.

Interestingly, we did not find hypothyroidism to be associated with infant gender, while most prior studies of congenital hypothyroidism have shown a female predominance [15,16,20,22-24]. However, studies isolating permanent and transient causes have found a gender influence only among permanent cases of congenital hypothyroidism [15,20]. Given our use of ICD-9-CM codes to define cases, it is likely that many transient cases were captured. This is suggested by our relatively high overall prevalence and may explain the lack of a gender relationship in our study. Congenital hypothyroidism rates have been reported to be higher for Hispanic, Native American, and Asian infants and lower for black infants when compared to white infants [16,23,24]. However, we did not see an association with the ethnicity/race of the military sponsor, which may be due to an absence of data regarding the spouse.

While the DoD Birth and Infant Health Registry provides many advantages, certain limitations must be considered. Defining cases by ICD-9-CM code alone raises concern regarding the accuracy of the outcome measure. However, given that screening is universal, health care encounter data are captured electronically, the number of hypothyroidism codes is limited, and hypothyroidism care requires multiple clinic visits for the infant, unidentified cases of hypothyroidism should be rare in this study. In addition, we required diagnostic codes from two separate health care encounter dates to improve specificity, primarily by excluding visits to perform screening tests. The use of birth location as a measure of the geographically-defined iodine nutrition exposure also has potential limitations. However, given that thyroid function adapts to changes in iodine intake within weeks and travel during the final weeks of pregnancy is uncommon, birth location likely corresponds well with the location of iodine exposure that would impact thyroid function at the time of birth. Finally, the birth locations examined in this study were limited to those with the largest sample sizes and the possibility of the presence of locations of greater risk must be considered.

Conclusions

Military families and other mobile populations assume health risks associated with their varied environments. Therefore, ongoing surveillance and studies are needed to detect adverse outcomes and determine the need for intervention. In this study, the DoD Birth and Infant Health Registry allowed for the first-ever investigation of an iodine-dependent outcome in a mobile population across different locations. While the assessment of other potential risk factors contributes to the overall understanding of hypothyroidism in infancy, the lack of differences in hypothyroidism rates for the geographic areas studied provides much-needed reassurance for military families and medical providers.

Acknowledgements

We thank Scott L. Seggerman and Greg D. Boyd from the Defense Manpower Data Center, Monterey Bay, California, for providing the demographic data. We thank Michelle Stoia, from the Naval Health Research Center, San Diego, California, for editorial assistance. We appreciate the support of the Henry M. Jackson Foundation for the Advancement of Military Medicine, Rockville, Maryland.

This represents report 08-16, supported by the Department of Defense, under work unit no. 60504. The views expressed in this article are those of the authors and do not reflect the official policy or position of the Department of the Navy, Department of the Army, Department of the Air Force, Department of Defense, or the US Government. This research has been conducted in compliance with all applicable federal regulations governing the protection of human subjects in research (Protocol NHRC.2007.0026).

Author details

[1]Keesler Medical Center, Keesler AFB, Mississippi, USA. [2]Naval Hospital, Camp Pendleton, California, USA. [3]Naval Health Research Center, San Diego, California, USA. [4]San Diego State University, San Diego, California, USA.

Authors' contributions

MC, MR, TS, CS, and SB all helped conceive the study, participated in its design and coordination, and helped to draft the manuscript. All authors read and approved the final manuscript.

Competing interests

The authors declare that they have no competing interests.

References

1. WHO, UNICEF, ICCIDD: **Assessment of iodine deficiency disorders and monitoring their elimination: a guide for programme managers.** Geneva: World Health Organization 2007.
2. WHO, UNICEF, ICCIDD: **Indicators for assessment of iodine deficiency disorders and the control programme report of a joint WHO/UNICEF/ICCIDD consultation.** Geneva: World Health Organization 1993.
3. WHO (ed.): **Iodine status worldwide: WHO Global Database on Iodine Deficiency.** Geneva: World Health Organization 2004.
4. Glinoer D: **Pregnancy and iodine.** *Thyroid* 2001, **11(5)**:471-481.
5. Glinoer D, de Nayer P, Bourdoux P, Lemone M, Robyn C, van Steirteghem A, Kinthaert J, Lejeune B: **Regulation of maternal thyroid during pregnancy.** *J Clin Endocrinol Metab* 1990, **71(2)**:276-287.
6. Wu T, Liu GJ, Li P, Clar C: **Iodised salt for preventing iodine deficiency disorders.** *Cochrane Database Syst Rev* 2002, , **3**: CD003204.
7. Hollowell JG, Staehling NW, Hannon WH, Flanders DW, Gunter EW, Maberly GF, Braverman LE, Pino S, Miller DT, Garbe PL, *et al*: **Iodine nutrition in the United States. Trends and public health implications: iodine excretion data from National Health and Nutrition Examination Surveys I and III (1971-1974 and 1988-1994).** *J Clin Endocrinol Metab* 1998, **83(10)**:3401-3408.
8. Becker DV, Braverman LE, Delange F, Dunn JT, Franklyn JA, Hollowell JG, Lamm SH, Mitchell ML, Pearce E, Robbins J, *et al*: **Iodine supplementation for pregnancy and lactation-United States and Canada: recommendations of the American Thyroid Association.** *Thyroid* 2006, **16(10)**:949-951.
9. Caldwell KL, Jones R, Hollowell JG: **Urinary iodine concentration: United States National Health And Nutrition Examination Survey 2001-2002.** *Thyroid* 2005, **15(7)**:692-699.
10. Delange F, Benker G, Caron P, Eber O, Ott W, Peter F, Podoba J, Simescu M, Szybinsky Z, Vertongen F, *et al*: **Thyroid volume and urinary iodine in European schoolchildren: standardization of values for assessment of iodine deficiency.** *Eur J Endocrinol* 1997, **136(2)**:180-187.
11. Ishigaki K, Namba H, Takamura N, Saiwai H, Parshin V, Ohashi T, Kanematsu T, Yamashita S: **Urinary iodine levels and thyroid diseases in children; comparison between Nagasaki and Chernobyl.** *Endocr J* 2001, **48(5)**:591-595.
12. Ryan MA, Pershyn-Kisor MA, Honner WK, Smith TC, Reed RJ, Gray GC: **The Department of Defense Birth Defects Registry: overview of a new surveillance system.** *Teratology* 2001, **64(1)**:S26-29.
13. American Medical Association: *Physician ICD-9-CM 2008. Chicago* 2008.
14. McElduff A, McElduff P, Wiley V, Wilcken B: **Neonatal thyrotropin as measured in a congenital hypothyroidism screening program: influence of the mode of delivery.** *J Clin Endocrinol Metab* 2005, **90(12)**:6361-6363.
15. Medda E, Olivieri A, Stazi MA, Grandolfo ME, Fazzini C, Baserga M, Burroni M, Cacciari E, Calaciura F, Cassio A, *et al*: **Risk factors for congenital hypothyroidism: results of a population case-control study (1997-2003).** *Eur J Endocrinol* 2005, **153(6)**:765-773.
16. Waller DK, Anderson JL, Lorey F, Cunningham GC: **Risk factors for congenital hypothyroidism: an investigation of infant's birth weight, ethnicity, and gender in California, 1990-1998.** *Teratology* 2000, **62(1)**:36-41.
17. Fisher DA: **Effectiveness of newborn screening programs for congenital hypothyroidism: prevalence of missed cases.** *Pediatr Clin North Am* 1987, **34(4)**:881-890.
18. La Franchi S: **Congenital Hypothyroidism: Etiologies, Diagnosis, and Management.** *Thyroid* 1999, **9(7)**:735-740.
19. Park SM, Chatterjee VK: **Genetics of congenital hypothyroidism.** *J Med Genet* 2005, **42(5)**:379-389.
20. Ray M: **Audit of screening programme for congenital hypothyroidism in Scotland 1979-93.** *Arch Dis Child* 1997, **76**:411-415.
21. Sobel EH, Saenger P: **Hypothyroidism in the newborn.** *Pediatr Rev* 1989, **11(1)**:15-20.
22. Law WY, Bradley DM, Lazarus JH, John R, Gregory JW: **Congenital hypothyroidism in Wales (1982-1993): demographic features, clinical presentation and effects on early neurodevelopment.** *Clin Endocrinol (Oxf)* 1998, **48(2)**:201-207.
23. Lorey FW, Cunningham GC: **Birth prevalence of primary congenital hypothyroidism by sex and ethnicity.** *Hum Biol* 1992, **64(4)**:531-538.
24. Harris KB, Pass KA: **Increase in congenital hypothyroidism in New York State and in the United States.** *Mol Gen Met* 2007, **91**:268-277.

2

Identification of a novel pax8 gene sequence variant in four members of the same family: from congenital hypothyroidism with thyroid hypoplasia to mild subclinical hypothyroidism

Monica Vincenzi[1], Marta Camilot[1,2], Eleonora Ferrarini[3], Francesca Teofoli[1,2], Giacomo Venturi[1], Rossella Gaudino[1,2], Paolo Cavarzere[2*], Giuseppina De Marco[3], Patrizia Agretti[3], Antonio Dimida[3], Massimo Tonacchera[3], Attilio Boner[1,2] and Franco Antoniazzi[1,2]

Abstract

Background: Congenital hypothyroidism is often secondary to thyroid dysgenesis, including thyroid agenesis, hypoplasia, ectopic thyroid tissue or cysts. Loss of function mutations in TSHR, PAX8, NKX2.1, NKX2.5 and FOXE1 genes are responsible for some forms of inherited congenital hypothyroidism, with or without hypoplastic thyroid. The aim of this study was to analyse the PAX8 gene sequence in several members of the same family in order to understand whether the variable phenotypic expression, ranging from congenital hypothyroidism with thyroid hypoplasia to mild subclinical hypothyroidism, could be associated to the genetic variant in the PAX8 gene, detected in the proband.

Methods: We screened a hypothyroid child with thyroid hypoplasia for mutations in PAX8, TSHR, NKX2.1, NKX2.5 and FOXE1 genes. We studied the inheritance of the new variant R133W detected in the PAX8 gene in the proband's family, and we looked for the same substitution in 115 Caucasian European subjects and in 26 hypothyroid children. Functional studies were performed to assess the *in vitro* effect of the newly identified PAX8 gene variant.

Results: A new heterozygous nucleotide substitution was detected in the PAX8 DNA-binding motif (c.397C/T, R133W) in the proband, affected by congenital hypothyroidism with thyroid hypoplasia, in his older sister, displaying a subclinical hypothyroidism associated with thyroid hypoplasia and thyroid nodules, in his father, affected by hypothyroidism with thyroid hypoplasia and thyroid nodules, and his first cousin as well, who revealed only a subclinical hypothyroidism. Functional studies of R133W-PAX8 in the HEK293 cells showed activation of the TG promoter comparable to the wild-type PAX8.

Conclusions: *In vitro* data do not prove that R133W-PAX8 is directly involved in the development of the thyroid phenotypes reported for family members carrying the substitution. However, it is reasonable to conceive that, in the cases of transcriptions factors, such as Pax8, which establish several interactions in different protein complexes, genetic variants could have an impact *in vivo*.

Keywords: PAX8 gene, Thyroid, Congenital hypothyroidism, Variable phenotypic expressivity, R133W-PAX8

* Correspondence: paolocavarzere@yahoo.it
[2]Azienda Ospedaliera Universitaria Integrata di Verona, Verona, Italy
Full list of author information is available at the end of the article

Background

Congenital hypothyroidism (CH) is a common disease with a worldwide incidence of 1 in 3,000-4,000 newborns [1]. In 85% of the cases, CH is secondary to thyroid dysgenesis, including thyroid agenesis, hypoplasia, ectopic thyroid tissue or cysts [2].

Loss of function mutations of the thyrotropin receptor (TSHR) are responsible for some forms of recessively inherited congenital hypothyroidism, either with normal or hypoplastic glands [3]. Other cases of thyroid dysgenesis may result from mutations in some of the transcription factors genes involved in thyroid development, such as PAX8, NKX2.1 (also known as TTF1), FOXE1 and NKX2.5 [2,4-6].

Pax8 is a member of the large mammalian Pax protein family, a group of important developmental regulators defined by the presence of a highly conserved DNA-binding motif of 128 amino acids, the so-called "paired-box domain". This element is well conserved during evolution and consists of two distinct structurally independent subdomains, each containing a helix-turn-helix motif, joined by a linker region [7]. The N- and C- terminal subdomains are called PAI and RED, respectively [8].

During mouse embryogenesis, PAX8 gene is expressed in the developing thyroid, in the kidney and in several areas of central nervous system [9-11]. In addition to its role in thyroid development, Pax8 is an important regulator of thyroid differentiation through the activation of specific genes expression, namely thyroid peroxidase (TPO) and thyroglobulin (TG) [12,13].

In humans, PAX8 gene maps to chromosome 2q12-q14 and consists of at least ten exons [14]. So far, several PAX8 mutations and a rare sequence variant have been reported [2,15-27]. They have been mostly detected in patients with normally located but hypoplastic thyroid gland, often associated with renal anomalies, and in a few patients with complete athyreosis [2,16-19,21]. The aim of this report is to analyse PAX8 gene in members of the same family with variable phenotypic expressivity: from congenital hypothyroidism with thyroid hypoplasia, to mild subclinical hypothyroidism, in order to establish whether a correlation between variants in the PAX8 gene and different phenotypes is present.

Methods

Subjects

In this study we analysed 9 members of a family with history of hypothyroidism, 26 patients with congenital hypothyroidism and 115 healthy subjects.

Patient III-2 (Figure 1), the proband, a male subject, was born in 1983 after an uneventful pregnancy. The patient was diagnosed as hypothyroid in the reference centre for newborn screening programs of North-Eastern Italy. TSH and total T4 values, assayed in dried blood spot collected at 3–5 days of life by radioimmunoassay, were 281 mIU/L (controls <10 mIU/L) and 18 nmol/L (controls >60 nmol/L), respectively.

Serum investigations confirmed the diagnosis of congenital hypothyroidism (TSH 93 mIU/L and free T4 17 pmol/L, normal values 0.4-4.0 mIU/L and 10.3-24.5 pmol/L respectively), and substitution therapy with L-thyroxine 37 μg daily was started at three weeks of life. The dose was adjusted to 50 μg/d at four months of life, and was stabilized at 75 μg/d when the infant was ten months old. He is now assuming 125 μg daily. The ultrasound examination demonstrated a hypoplastic but normally located thyroid gland. Abdomen ultrasound investigation showed no abnormalities. His growth, renal function (at blood tests), neuropsychological development and IQ (measured several times and with different test depending on the age) were normal. During one of the follow-up examinations and after obtaining written informed

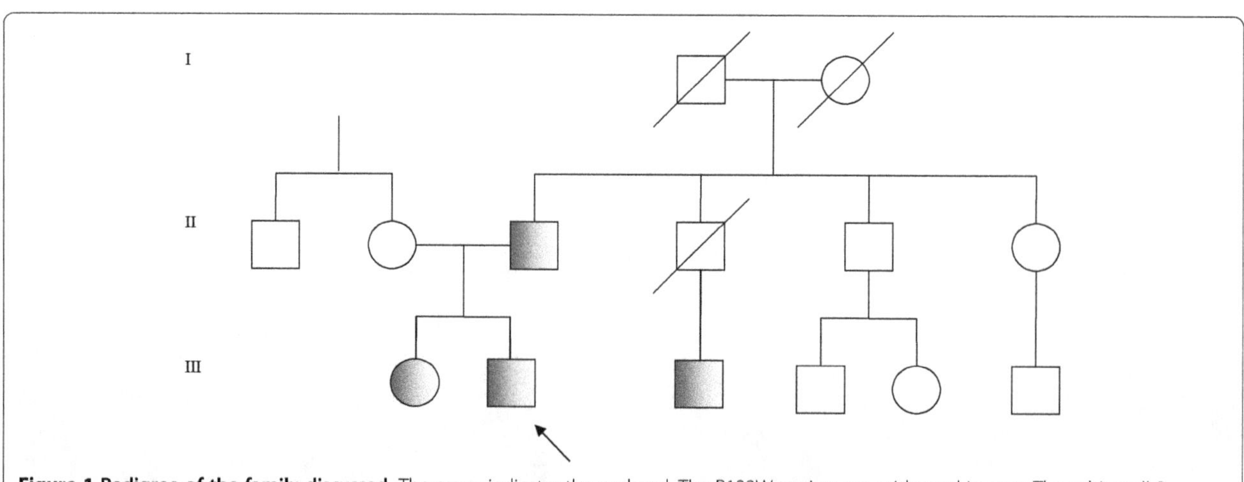

Figure 1 Pedigree of the family discussed. The arrow indicates the proband. The R133W carriers are evidenced in grey. The subjects II-2, II-5, II-6, III-4, and III-5 were subject to DNA analysis and they did not carry the R133W variant.

consent, peripheral blood samples in EDTA were collected from the patient and his parents in order to screen for mutation in the PAX8, TSHR, FOXE1, NKX2.1, NKX2.5 genes.

Upon detection of the same PAX8 sequence variant detected in the index case, subject II-3, father of the proband, was submitted to endocrinological examination; at that time he was 60 years old. Serum determinations evidenced TSH concentration of 20.5 mIU/L (normal values 0.4-4.0 mIU/L) and free T4 level of 9.4 pmol/L (n.v. 10.3-24.5 pmol/L). Thyroid autoantibodies were negative and serum thyroglobulin was in the normal range. Substitutive therapy with L-thyroxine 50 μg daily was promptly started. After four months of therapy, plasma TSH decreased to 7.39 mIU/L (n.v. 0.35-5.50 mIU/L) and free T4 raised to 14.7 pmol/L (n.v. 11.5-22.7 pmol/L). Substitutive therapy was changed to 50–75 μg every other day, and both serum TSH and free T4 returned within the corresponding ranges of the reference population. Despite the lack of substitutive therapy until the age of 60, the physical and intellectual development was normal. He did not present neurological alterations. Renal function was in the normal range for age. Ultrasound examination revealed a normally located thyroid gland with hypoplasia of the left lobe (measuring 10 × 5 mm), and the presence of three nodules with calcifications (measuring 15 × 16 mm) in the right one. A fine needle aspiration biopsy was performed on the right lobe. A moderate colloid amount and some aggregates of thyroid cells with hypertrophic nucleus were detected. Malignant cells search was negative. Thyroid scintigraphy revealed poor uptake. The presence of the isthmus was not reported on ultrasound examination, and it was not on uptake scan.

Seven members of the same family (subjects II-2, II-5, II-6, III-1, III-3, III-4, III-5) were asked to send us capillary blood samples absorbed on paper (Schleicher & Schuell 903 paper), in order to search for the same PAX8 variant. Subject III-1, the proband's sister, aged 30 years, revealed to be a carrier of the PAX8 sequence variant. Her serum TSH was 6.85 mIU/L (n.v. 0.25-3.50 mIU/L) and serum free T4 was 16.9 pmol/L (n.v. 10.3-24.4 pmol/L). Thyroid autoantibodies were negative. Serum thyroglobulin was 244.00 ng/mL (upper limit 60.00 ng/mL). The ultrasound investigation evidenced a thyroid gland located in the normal position, with isthmus agenesis, hypoplastic left lobe and right one with three nodules. A fine needle aspiration biopsy was performed on the right lobe. No abnormalities were reported at the cytological analysis. Abdomen echography showed no anomalies. No neurological or renal dysfunctions were evidenced. Her condition was periodically monitored and L-thyroxine therapy was no indicated, since her hypothyroidism remained subclinical. As for the father (subject II-3), the daughter (III-1) came to our attention undetected from birth, because at the time of their birth newborn screening for congenital hypothyroidism still had to be instituted.

Patient III-3, cousin of the proband, showed to be a carrier of the PAX8 sequence variant too. His serum TSH value is mildly elevated (4.66 mIU/L, n.v. 0.27-4.20 mIU/L) with a fT4 in the normal range. Thyroid autoantibodies were negative and serum thyroglobulin was 95.70 ng/mL (upper limit 60.00 ng/mL). His thyroid function was periodically checked, evidencing a persistent subclinical hypothyroidism. At the moment he takes no therapy. He was submitted to thyroid ultrasound that evidenced a normally located thyroid gland with both the lobes slightly reduced in size. No other clinical abnormalities were found. Notably, he reported that his father (patient II-4, proband's uncle) was treated with L-thyroxine for one year before cardiac surgery. He died of heart failure.

In all the other relatives reported in Figure 1 thyroid function was evaluated and TSH, fT4 and fT3 values were in the normal range. No relevant clinical alterations were described for them. Given the family history, we recommended to these unaffected family members a periodic follow-up. At the moment, we have no information of alterations in their thyroid function.

In order to exclude the occurrence of the new PAX8 genetic variant as a common polymorphism, 115 healthy Caucasian European subjects have been screened for the same substitution. They signed written informed consent for the genetic analysis.

In addition, 26 patients with congenital hypothyroidism followed at Pediatric Endocrinology Division of Verona Hospital during 2011, were screened for the same substitution, after their parents' written consents were obtained. All of them were older than fourteen and were in L-thyroxine treatment from birth. Thirty-one per cent of them did not present echographic alterations, 25% showed thyroid hypoplasia, 31% ectopia and the remaining 13% agenesis of the gland.

The study was conducted in compliance with the terms of the Helsinki II Declaration and written informed consent for the enrolment and for the publication of individual clinical details was obtained from patients or, whenever participants were children, from their parents or guardians.

In our country, namely Italy, this type of clinical study does not require Institutional Review Board/Institutional Ethics Committee approval to publish the results.

Genetic analysis

Genomic DNA was extracted from peripheral venous blood on EDTA by means of the Gentra Puregene Blood kit (QIAGEN S.p.A, Milan, Italy), following the manufacturer's instructions.

Genomic DNA was extracted from the blood spot paper cards by means of the QIAamp® DNA Micro kit (QIAGEN

S.p.A., Milan, Italy), according to the manufacturer's instructions.

We amplified by PCR all the exons of PAX8, TSHR, FOXE1, NKX2.1, NKX2.5 genes by means of intronic primers. Fragments were first analyzed by Denaturing High Performance Liquid Chromatography on a WAVE DNA Fragment Analysis System (Transgenomic, Omaha, NE), and sequenced on an automated CEQ 8800 Genetic Analysis System (Beckman Coulter GmbH, Germany) whenever a sequence variation was suspected. PCR conditions, partial denaturing temperature (t_{pd}) for DHPLC analysis and sequencing conditions for TSHR and PAX8 genes have been previously described [28]. For FOXE1, NKX2.1 and NKX2.5 genes, sequencing conditions are available upon request.

Polyphen prediction

PolyPhen (=*Poly*morphism *Pheno*typing) is an automatic tool for prediction of possible impact of an amino acid substitution on the structure and function of a human protein. This prediction is based on straightforward empirical rules which are applied to the sequence, phylogenetic and structural information characterizing the substitution [29]. PolyPhen-2 is a new development of the popular PolyPhen tool and is available as freeware at http://genetics.bwh.harvard.edu/pph2/ web site.

Construction of the expression vector and functional analysis

The wild-type PAX8 protein (WT-PAX8) was expressed in the vector pcDNA3 as already described [20].

Human thyroglobulin promoter was cloned in the pGL3 luciferase report vector (TG prom-pGL3), designed to provide enhanced reporter gene expression. TTF1-pcDNA3 and pCMV-HA-p300 expression vectors have been previously described [20]. pRL-TK, expressing Renilla luciferase activity, (Promega Corporation, Madison, WI) was used as internal control vector.

Mutant harbouring the single nucleotide missense substitution (R133W) was generated by site-directed mutagenesis using the GeneTailor site-directed mutagenesis system (Invitrogen Life Technologies, Carlsbad, CA). The accuracy of the recombinant construct was verified by direct sequencing.

HEK293 cells were grown in DMEM supplemented with 2 mM L-glutamine, 25 mM D-glucose, 50 U/mL Penicillin, 50 µg/mL Streptomycin and 10% FBS (Invitrogen Life Technologies, Carlsbad, CA) and plated in 12-well plates (2×10 [5] cells for well) for 24 h before transfection. Transfection was carried out with FuGENE 6 reagent, following the manufacturer's instructions (Roche Diagnostic Corporation, Indianapolis, IN, USA), with a total amount of plasmid DNA of 1170 ng per well.

Cells were harvested 48 h later and analysed sequentially for firefly and *Renilla* luciferase activities by Dual-Luciferse Reporter Assay System (Promega Corporation, Madison,WI). The luminescence production in cell extracts was assayed using the Lumino luminometer (Stratec Electronic; GMBH, Birkenfeld, Germany). Light intensity was quantified using a pre-produced standard curve and was reported in relative light units (RLUs). The assay was performed in triplicate.

Statistical analysis

Values of transcriptional activity of R133W mutant were compared with respect to the values obtained for wild type Pax8 using the Student two tails t-test. To test the significance, the risk level (p) was set at 0.05.

Results

Genetic analysis

DHPLC analysis and direct sequencing of TSHR, FOXE1, NKX2.1 and NKX2.5 genes in genomic DNA of the patient III-2 revealed no variation compared to the NCBI Reference Sequences NM_000369.2, NC_000009.11, NC_000014.8 and NG_013340.1, respectively.

During DHPLC analysis, a nucleotide substitution was suspected in the PAX8 fifth exon and its direct sequencing revealed the presence of a heterozygous transition of cytosine to thymine (C → T) at position 397 of the coding sequence (NCBI Reference Sequence NM_003466.3), leading to a change of a conserved arginine at codon 133 to tryptophan (c.397C/T, R133W) (Figure 2). The mutation was detected in the paired domain, the highly conserved PAX8 DNA-binding motif, at the end of the third alpha helix of the RED subdomain. This sequence variant was first detected in the propositus, affected by congenital hypothyroidism with a hypoplastic thyroid. The same substitution was present at the heterozygous state in his father, in his sister and in his first cousin, who evidenced mild hypothyroidism the first, and subclinical hypothyroidism the other two. In both the father and sister on the index case, the morphology of the thyroid showed hypoplasia and the presence of thyroid nodules.

We accessed the NCBI Single Nucleotide Polymorphism database and R133W was not found as a common variant. Moreover, the R133W variant was not present in a screen of 115 Caucasian European subjects (230 control chromosomes), reducing the likelihood that this substitution could represent a neutral common variant.

In addition, the PAX8 fifth exons of 26 hypothyroid children were analysed and none carried the R133W variant.

PolyPhen prediction

The Polyphen Tool forecasted for the R133W variant a hydrophobicity change at buried site. Accordingly, R133W was predicted to be a pathogenic variant.

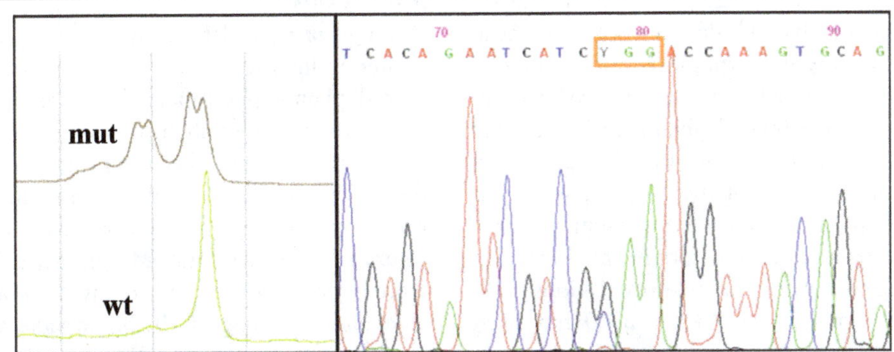

Figure 2 ***In the left side:*** **DHPLC profiles of wild type (green) and mutated (brown) PAX8 exon 5.** The partial denaturing temperature was set at 61.3°C and the chromatographic parameters were obtained by means of the WAVEMaker software (Transgenomic, Omaha, NE), based on the amplicon sequence [23]. *In the right side:* Sequencing electropherogram of exon 5. A heterozygous C→T transition is shown where a Y is reported, corresponding to nucleotide 397 of the PAX8 coding sequence (NCBI Reference Sequence NM_003466.3). The mutation replaces a conserved arginine at position 133 with a tryptophan residue (R133W).

Activation of TGprom-pGL3 by WT-PAX8 and R133W-PAX8

pCMV-HA-p300 was cotransfected with expression vector carrying WT-PAX8 or R133W-PAX8, together with an internal control (pRL-TK *Renilla*) and the TG prom-pGL3 (Firefly). The firefly to Renilla luminescence activity ratios were calculated and compared between groups. The transfection of WT-PAX8 together with 500 ng pCMV-HA-p300 revealed a significant increase in the TG promoter activity compared to WT-PAX8 alone ($p < 0.01$, Figure 3, columns 2–3), and this in accordance to literature [20,30]. R133W-PAX8, when transfected with pCMV-HA-p300, showed a significant increased TG promoter activity, to the same extent of WT-PAX8 ($p < 0.01$, Figure 3, columns 5–6 compared to 2–3). Cotransfection of TTF1-pcDNA3 resulted in a synergistic effect of p300 and the R133W-PAX8 or WT-PAX8 on the TG promoter (Figure 3 columns 4 *vs* 7 showed no statistical difference, $0.05 < p < 0.1$).

Discussion

The Pax8 transcription factor is required for mammalian morphogenesis of the thyroid gland, and it is essential for the thyrocite-specific promoter activation of the TPO and TG genes [9-11]. In humans, PAX8 mutation carriers have been reported to be hypothyroids with thyroid hypoplasia [2,15-27]. Most of the known mutations are monoallelic and localized in the paired box domain. They evidence a functional DNA-binding impairment, suggesting that hypothyroidism could be secondary to PAX8 haploinsufficiency.

In the present report we describe different members of the same family carrying the same PAX8 variant at the heterozygous state: the R133W substitution, replacing the last conserved arginine of the DNA-binding paired-box domain with a tryptophan residue, and characterized by a prediction of likely being a damaging substitution. The family members carrying the substitution evidence a remarkable

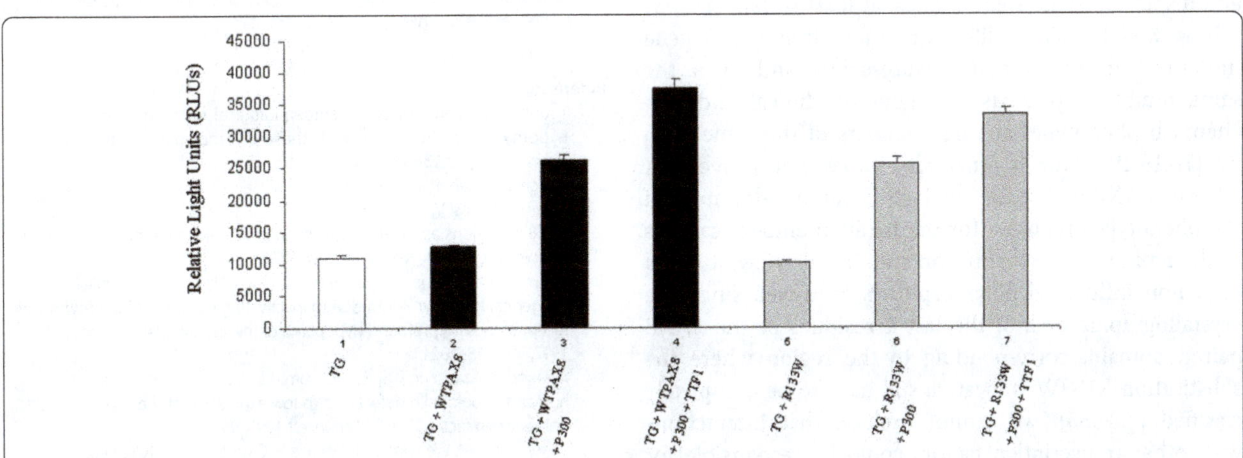

Figure 3 The intensity of luminescence production in HEK293 cells is reported in relative light units (RLUs). Firefly luciferase activities were normalized to the Renilla luciferase activity derived from cotransfected pRL-TK internal control vector (see text).

phenotypic variability, from congenital hypothyroidism associated with thyroid hypoplasia, to mild subclinical hypothyroidism with thyroid hypoplasia and nodules.

In order to verify the actual role of the R133W variant in the development of the thyroid phenotype, we carried out *in vitro* functional studies in the TG promoter, known to be a genetic target of the Pax8 transcription factor. On the TG promoter, the Pax8 protein interacts with several other transcription factors in the formation of complexes targeting several regulatory regions [20]. The general transcriptional coactivator p300 has been shown to be essential in mediating Pax8 activation on both the TG and the rat thyroperoxidase (TPO) promoters. It plays a crucial role in the functional synergism between Pax8 and NKX2.1 in thyroid specific gene expression [20,30]. In order to assess whether R133W mutation was able to efficiently recruit p300 and assemble the transcriptional coactivation complex [20], we employed HEK293 cells. These cells, indeed, are deficient in endogenous p300 because of expression of the adenovirus E1A protein [30,31], which sequestrates p300 into the cytosol.

Functional studies of R133W-PAX8 in the HEK293 cells show comparable activation of the TG promoter of both the mutated and the wild-type Pax8. Furthermore, R133W-Pax8, similarly to the wild-type, is able to recruit p300 to synergistically transactivate the TG promoter.

Evaluation of 282 alleles belonging to either healthy or hypothyroid subjects revealed that R133W-PAX8 does not seem to be a common polymorphism and therefore it is probably a rare variant.

It is well known that persistent stimulation by increased plasma TSH levels leads to thyroid proliferation and often nodule formation [32,33]. This clinical observation could account for the similar phenotype of subjects II-3 and III-1, evidencing thyroid nodules, and for the substantial difference in the propositus, patient III-2, who was treated from birth with substitutive therapy, and displayed no thyroid nodules, at least so far.

It is well known in literature that often PAX8 gene mutations display variable expressivity, and even the same mutation gives rise to different clinical and biochemical phenotypes among members of the same family [16,18,19]. Our *in vitro* data does not prove that R133W-PAX8 is directly involved in the development of the phenotypes reported for the family members carriers of the aminoacidic substitution and, in this view, it could be a non influential polymorphism. However, since the crystallographic data of the last 4 residues of the PAX8 paired domain, corresponding to the region where the substitution R133W is located, still have to be completely clarified [7,34,35], we cannot exclude that interactions with other transcription factors could be responsible for the variable phenotypic expressivity evidenced in the reported family.

Conclusions

Although *in vitro* data do not prove that R133W-PAX8 is directly involved in the development of the different thyroid phenotypes reported for the heterozygous carriers of the same family, it is reasonable to conceive that the substitution described could have an impact *in vivo*, the condition where all the interactions with different protein complexes actually take place. For transcription factors such as Pax8, indeed, genetic, epigenetic and environmental factors are likely involved, and only a thorough understanding of all the possible actors entangled can deeply clarify the actual contribution of variant such as the R133W-PAX8.

Competing interests

The authors declare that they have no competing interests.

Authors' contributions

All the authors had full access to all of the data in the study and take responsibility for the integrity of the data and the accuracy of the data analysis. Moreover, all authors read and approved the final manuscript. MV conceived of the study, carried out the genetic analysis, contributed to the preparation and critical review of the manuscript. MC carried out the genetic and molecular analysis, contributed to the critical review of the manuscript. EF carried out the functional studies of the PAX8 gene variant. FT carried out the genetic and molecular analysis, contributed to the critical review of the manuscript. GV carried out the DNA extraction from control subjects. RG contributed to the recruitment of participants. PC helped to draft the manuscript. GDM carried out the molecular analysis. PA carried out the molecular analysis. AD carried out the molecular analysis. MT participated in the design of the study and in the coordination of genetic analysis and contributed to the critical review of the manuscript. AB participated in the design of the study and contributed to the critical review of the manuscript. FA conceived the study and participated in its coordination.

Acknowledgements

We are deeply grateful to proband's family members who kindly provided all the needed information.

Author details

[1]Department of Life and Reproduction Sciences, University of Verona, Piazzale Scuro 10, 37126 Verona, Italy. [2]Azienda Ospedaliera Universitaria Integrata di Verona, Verona, Italy. [3]Department of Endocrinology, Centro di Eccellenza AmbiSEN, University of Pisa, Pisa, Italy.

References

1. Toublanc JE: **Comparison of epidemiological data on congenital hypothyroidism in Europe with those of other parts in the world.** *Horm Res* 1992, **138:**230–235.
2. Macchia PE, Lapi P, Krude H, Pirro MT, Missero C, Chiovato L, Souabni A, Baserga M, Tassi V, Pinchera A, Fenzi G, Grüters A, Busslinger M, Di Lauro R: **PAX8 mutations associated with congenital hypothyroidism caused by thyroid dysgenesis.** *Nat Genet* 1998, **19:**83–86.
3. Abramowicz MJ, Duprez L, Parma J, Vassart G, Heinrichs C: **Familial congenital hypothyroidism due to inactivating mutation of the thyrotropin receptor causing profound hypoplasia of the thyroid gland.** *J Clin Invest* 1997, **99:**3018–3024.
4. Acebròn A, Aza-Blanc P, Rossi DL, Lamas L, Santisteban P: **Congenital human thyroglobulin defect due to low expression of the thyroid-specific transcription factor TTF-1.** *J Clin Invest* 1995, **96:**781–785.
5. Clifton-Bligh RJ, Wentworth JM, Heinz P, Crisp MS, John R, Lazarus JH, Ludgate M, Chatterjee WK: **Mutation of the gene encoding human TTF-2 associated with thyroid agenesis, cleft palate and choanal atresia.** *Nat Genet* 1998, **19:**399–401.

6. Nettore IC, Cacace V, De Fusco C, Colao A, Macchia PE: **The molecular causes of thyroid dysgeneis: a sistematic review.** *J Endocrinol Invest* 2013, **36:**654–664.
7. Xu W, Rould MA, Jun S, Desplan C, Pabo CO: **Crystal structure of a paired domain-DNA complex at 2.5 Å resolution reveals structural basis for Pax developmental mutations.** *Cell* 1995, **80:**639–650.
8. Jun S, Desplan C: **Cooperative interactions between paired domain and homeodomain.** *Development* 1996, **122:**2639–2650.
9. Van Vliet G: **Development of the thyroid gland: lessons from congenitally hypothyroid mice and men.** *Clin Gen* 2003, **63:**445–455.
10. Damante G, Tell G, Di Lauro R: **A unique combination of transcription factors controls differentiation of thyroid cells.** *Prog Nucleic Acid Res Mol Biol* 2001, **66:**307–356.
11. Plachov D, Chowdhury K, Walther C, Simon D, Guenet JL, Gruss P: **Pax8, a murine paired box gene expressed in the developing excretory system and thyroid gland.** *Development* 1990, **110:**643–651.
12. PascadiMagliano M, Di Lauro R, Zannini MS: **Pax8 has a key role in thyroid cell differentiation.** *Proc Natl Acad Sci U S A* 2000, **97:**13144–13149.
13. Di Palma T, Nitsch R, Mascia A, Nitsch L, Di Lauro R, Zannini M: **The paired domain-containing factor Pax8 and the homeodomain-containing factor TTF-1 directly interact and synergistically activate transcription.** *J Biol Chem* 2003, **278:**3395–3402.
14. Kozmik Z, Kurzbauer R, Dorfler P, Busslinger M: **Alternative splicing of Pax-8 gene transcripts is developmentally regulated and generates isoforms with different transactivation properties.** *Mol Cell Biol* 1993, **13:**6024–6035.
15. Vilain C, Rydlewski C, Duprez L, Heinrichs C, Abramowicz M, Malvaux P, Renneboog B, Parma J, Costagliola S, Vassart G: **Autosomal dominant transmission of congenital thyroid hypoplasia due to loss-of-function mutation of PAX8.** *J Clin Endocrinol Metab* 2001, **86:**234–238.
16. Congdon T, Nguyen LQ, Nogueira CR, Habiby RL, Medeiros-Neto G, Kopp P: **A novel mutation (Q40P) in PAX8 associated with congenital hypothyroidism and thyroid hypoplasia: evidence for phenotypic variability in mother and child.** *J Clin Endocrinol Metab* 2001, **86:**3962–3967.
17. Komatsu M, Takahashi T, Takahashi I, Nakamura M, Takahashi I, Takada G: **Thyroid dysgenesis caused by PAX8 mutation: the hypermutability with CpG dinucleotides at codon 31.** *J Pediatr* 2001, **139:**597–599.
18. Meeus L, Gilbert B, Rydlewski C, Parma J, Roussie AL, Abramowicz M, Vilain C, Christophe D, Costagliola S, Vassart G: **Characterization of a novel loss of function mutation of PAX8 in a familial case of congenital hypothyroidism with in-place, normal-sized thyroid.** *J Clin Endocrinol Metab* 2004, **89:**4285–4291.
19. De Sanctis L, Corrias A, Romagnolo D, Di Palma T, Biava A, Borgarello G, Gianino P, Silvestro L, Zannini M, Dianzani I: **Familial PAX8 small deletion (c.989–992delACCC) associated with extreme phenotype variability.** *J Clin Endocrinol Metab* 2004, **89:**5669–5674.
20. Grasberger H, Ringkananont U, LeFrancois P, Abramowicz M, Vassart G, Refetoff S: **Thyroid transcription factor 1 rescues PAX8/p300 synergism impaired by a natural PAX8 paired domain mutation with dominant negative activity.** *Mol Endocrinol* 2005, **19:**1779–1791.
21. Lanzerath K, Bettendorf M, Haag C, Kneppo C, Schulze E, Grulich-Henn J: **Screening for Pax8 Mutations in Patients with Congenital Hypothyroidism in South-West Germany.** *Horm Res* 2006, **66:**96–100.
22. Tonacchera M, Banco ME, Montanelli L, Di Cosmo C, Agretti P, De Marco G, Ferrarini E, Ordookhani A, Perri A, Chiovato L, Santini F, Vitti P, Pinchera A: **Genetic analysis of the PAX8 gene in children with congenital hypothyroidism and dysgenetic or eutopic thyroid glands: identification of a novel sequence variant.** *Clin Endocrinol (Oxf)* 2007, **67:**34–40.
23. Di Palma T, Zampella E, Filippone MG, Macchia PE, Risstalpers C, de Vroede M, Zannini M: **Characterization of a Novel Loss of Function Mutation of Pax8 Associated with Congenital Hypothyroidism.** *Clin Endocrinol (Oxf)* 2010, **73:**808–814.
24. Al Taji E, Biebermann H, Lìmanovà Z, Hnìkovà O, Zikmund J, Dame C, Grüters A, Lebl J, Krude H: **Screening for mutations in transcription factors in a Czech cohort of 170 patients with congenital and early-onset hypothyroidism: identification of a novel PAX8 mutation in dominantly inherited early-onset non-autoimmune hypothyroidism.** *Eur J Endocrinol* 2007, **156:**521–529.
25. Jo W, Ishizu K, Fujieda K, Tajima T: **Congenital Hypothyroidism Caused by a PAX8 Gene Mutation Manifested as Sodium/Iodide Symporter Gene Defect.** *J Thyroid Res.* 2010:619013. doi:10.4061/2010/619013.
26. Hermanns P, Grasberger H, Refetoff S, Pohlenz J: **Mutations in the NKX2.5 gene and the PAX8 promoter in a girl with thyroid dysgenesis.** *J Clin Endocrinol Metab* 2011, **96:**E977–E981.
27. Carvalho A, Hermanns P, Rodrigues AL, Sousa I, Anselmo J, Bikker H, Cabral R, Pereira-Duarte C, Mota-Vieira L, Pohlenz J: **A new PAX8 mutation causing congenital hypothyroidism in three generations of a family is associated with abnormalities in the urogenital tract.** *Thyroid* 2013, **23:**1074–1078.
28. Camilot M, Teofoli F, Vincenzi M, Federici F, Perlini S, Tatò L: **Implementation of a Congenital Hypothyroidism Newborn Screening Procedure with Mutation Detection on Genomic DNA Extracted from Blood Spots: The Experience of the Italian Northeastern Reference Center.** *Genet Test* 2007, **11:**387–390.
29. Adzhubei IA, Schmidt S, Peshkin L, Ramensky VE, Gerasimova A, Bork P, Kondrashov AS, Sunyaev SR: **A method and server for predicting damaging missense mutations.** *Nat Methods* 2010, **7:**248–249.
30. De Leo R, Miccadei S, Zammarchi E, Civitareale D: **Role for p300 in Pax 8 induction of thyroperoxidase gene expression.** *J Biol Chem* 2000, **275:**34100–34105.
31. Zannini M, Francis-Lang H, Plachov D, Di Lauro R: **Pax-8, a paired domain-containing protein, binds to a sequence overlapping the recognition site of a homeodomain and activates transcription from two thyroid-specific promoters.** *Mol Cell Biol* 1992, **12:**4230–4241.
32. Niedziela M: **Pathogenesis, diagnosis and management of thyroid nodules in children.** *Endocr Relat Cancer* 2006, **13:**427–453.
33. Gerschpacher M, Göbl C, Anderwald C, Gessl A, Krebs M: **Thyrotropin Serum Concentrations in Patients with Papillary Thyroid Microcancers.** *Thyroid* 2010, **20:**389–392.
34. Xu HE, Rould MA, Xu W, Epstein JA, Maas RL, Pabo CO: **Crystal structure of the human Pax6 paired domain-DNA complex reveals specific roles for the linker region and carboxy-terminal subdomain in DNA binding.** *Genes Dev* 1999, **13:**1263–1275.
35. Codutti L, van Ingen H, Vascotto C, Fogolari F, Corazza A, Tell G, Quadrifoglio F, Viglino P, Boelens R, Esposito GJ: **The solution structure of DNA-free Pax-8 paired box domain accounts for redox regulation of transcriptional activity in the pax protein family.** *J Biol Chem* 2008, **283:**33321–33328.

3

Familial multinodular goiter syndrome with papillary thyroid carcinomas: mutational analysis of the associated genes in 5 cases from 1 Chinese family

Shunyao Liao[1*], Wenzhong Song[2*], Yunqiang Liu[3], Shaoping Deng[1,4], Yaming Liang[1], Zhenlin Tang[2], Jiyuan Huang[2], Dandan Dong[5] and Gang Xu[5]

Abstract

Background: Familial papillary thyroid cancer (fPTC) is recognized as a distinct entity only recently and no fPTC predisposing genes have been identified. Several potential regions and susceptibility loci for sporadic PTC have been reported. We aimed to evaluate the role of the reported susceptibility loci and potential risk genomic region in a Chinese familial multinodular goiter (fMNG) with PTC family.

Methods: We sequenced the related risk genomic regions and analyzed the known PTC susceptibility loci in the Chinese family members who consented to join the study. These loci included (1) the point mutations of the *BRAF* and *RET*; (2) the possible susceptibility loci to sporadic PTC; and (3) the suggested potential fMNG syndrome with PTC risk region.

Results: The members showed no mutations in the common susceptible *BRAF* and *RET* genomic region, although contained several different heterozygous alleles in the *RET* introns. All the members were homozygous for PTC risk alleles of rs966423 (C) at chromosome 2q35, rs2910164 (C) at chromosome 5q24 and rs2439302 (G) at chromosome 8p12; while carried no risk allele of rs4733616 (T) at chromosome 8q24, rs965513 (A) or rs1867277 (A) at chromosome 9q22 which were associated with radiation-related PTC. The frequency of the risk allele of rs944289 (T) but not that of rs116909374 (T) at chromosome 14q13 was increased in the MNG or PTC family members.

Conclusions: Our work provided additional evidence to the genetic predisposition to a Chinese familial form of MNG with PTC. The family members carried quite a few risk alleles found in sporadic PTC; particularly, homozygous rs944289 (T) at chromosome 14q13 which was previously shown to be linked to a form of fMNG with PTC. Moreover, the genetic determinants of radiation-related PTC were not presented in this family.

Keywords: Familial papillary thyroid carcinomas, Multinodular goiter syndrome, Mutational analysis, Genetic association, Risk alleles

* Correspondence: shunyaol@yahoo.com; wz360@hotmail.com
[1]Diabetes & Endocrinology Center, Sichuan Academy of Medical Science, Sichuan Provincial People's Hospital, Chengdu 610072, China
[2]Department of Thyroid Disease & Nuclear Medicine, Sichuan Academy of Medical Science, Sichuan Provincial People's Hospital, Chengdu 610072, China
Full list of author information is available at the end of the article

Background

PTC is the most prevalent malignancy of the thyroid gland. There has been an increasing incidence of PTC worldwide for the past few decades. The etiology of PTC is related to environmental, hormonal and genetic factors. About 5-15% of PTC patients show a familial occurrence, and fPTC is recognized as a distinct entity only in recent years [1,2]. Families with accumulation of PTCs show an inherited trait of the disease and patients with fPTC often have early age at disease onset and increased severity in successive generations, also, fPTC patients frequently present more aggressive tumors with increased incidence of multifocality, local invasion, lymph node metastases than the sporadic PTC [2,3]. Generally, fPTC is diagnosed when three or more family members have PTC and in the absence of other known associated syndromes [1,2]. PTC has a significant gender bias with much more women affected than men; it is especially suggestive for the familial predisposition when men or children were diagnosed with PTC [1,4]. While, because families share the same environment and a common genetic background, it is difficult to distinguish between environmental and genetic contributing factors, and also because the majority of fPTC pedigrees are small in size and may present with a variety of additional benign thyroid nodules, the genetic predisposition to fPTC is unknown and the molecular alterations at the origin of the pathology are only now beginning to emerge [1,5,6].

Sporadic PTC is known to be associated with point mutation of the *BRAF* genes and chromosomal rearrangements of *RET/PTC*. The *BRAF* encodes a serine/threonine-protein kinase which plays a role in regulating the MAP kinase/ERKs signaling pathway and affects cell division, differentiation and secretion; point mutations in *BRAF* are found in up to 45% PTC cases [7]. The *RET* protooncogene is one of the receptor tyrosine kinases, cell-surface molecules that transduce signals for cell growth and differentiation; rearrangements of the *RET* are found in about 35% of sporadic PTC [7]. Although somatic mutations of the genes like *BRAF* and *RET* exclusively play a causative role in sporadic thyroid cancer development, germline mutations of single nucleotide polymorphisms (SNPs) in these genes were also reported to act as modifiers in the cancer process [8,9], it needs to mention here that in a Chinese population, SNPs of *BRAF* were shown to be associated with PTC [10], and thus it is intriguing to verify these mutations in fPTC families.

Recent studies based on population stratification have made progresses to identify several single nucleotide polymorphisms (SNPs) associated with PTC risk. For examples, (1) It was discovered that rs966423 at 2q35, locating into the intron region of the disrupted in renal carcinoma 3 gene (*DIRC3*), was significantly associate with European nonmedullary thyroid cancer (NMTC) by the genome-wide studies [11]. *DIRC3* predicted a non coding RNA transcript with unknown function, the first 2 exons of *DIRC3* replaced exon 1 of *HSPBAP1* and formed a DIRC3-HSPBAP1 fusion transcript, which are associated with chromatin remodeling and stress response; (2) It was reported that the heterozygosity G/C of SNP rs2910164 at 5q24 within the precursor of *microRNA-146a* predisposed to PTC by altering expression of miR146a target genes in the Toll-like receptor and cytokine signaling pathway [12,13]; (3) The genome-wide study also identified that chromosomal 8q24 was associated with the risk of various cancers, particularly, rs4733616 at 8q24 was founded to be possibly associated with PTC risk in 26 European families [14-16]; (4) The rs2439302, located in the intron of *HRG-beta1c* at 8p12,was reported to be associated with *neuregulin 1* (*NRG1*) and confer risk of thyroid cancer [11]. HRG-beta1c is one of the NRG1 isoforms and interacts with tyrosine kinase to increase its phosphorylation on tyrosine residues, playing critical roles in the growth and development of multiple organ system; (5) It was repeatedly observed that the rs965513 at 9q22.33 were the strong association signal for NMTC in European people [16-19] and it was proposed that the rs965513 might linked to the nearest thyroid transcription factor of forkhead family (*FOXE1*) gene, which likely plays a crucial role in thyroid morphogenesis; furthermore, some research indicated that rs1867277 within the *FOXE1* 5′ UTR is also a causal variant in thyroid cancer susceptibility [16,20]; (6) Finally, both rs944289 and rs116909374 on 14q13.3 were observed to be strongly associated with NMTC in European people [11,16-19,21]. Nonetheless, all these genetic associations found by the genome-wide association studies have not been investigated in a family based study.

In addition, a few potential regions for harboring an fPTC gene have been reported: chromosomal region 1q21 linked to fPTC with papillary renal neoplasia [22], 2q21 linked to familial NMTC type 1 syndrome [23], and the telomere abnormalities and chromosome fragility might display in fPTC family [24]; Specifically, familial NMTC and its relationship with familial MNG are recognized as distinct clinical entities, and the molecular pathophysiology of MNG and PTC is different, indeed MNG1 is located at 14q [25]; however, one study in a kindred with MNG and PTC suggested that 14q32 linked to a form of inherited MNG syndrome with a significant risk of progression to PTC [26].

In the present report we studied 2 PTCs and 3 MNGs obtained from members of one Chinese family. This family was ascertained through initial identification of the proband, a 35-year-old men (III2, Figure 1). The probands's mother, 5 maternal aunts and 1 younger first cousin were diagnosed with MNG or PTC by different hospitals in China. The mode of inheritance in the family appeared to

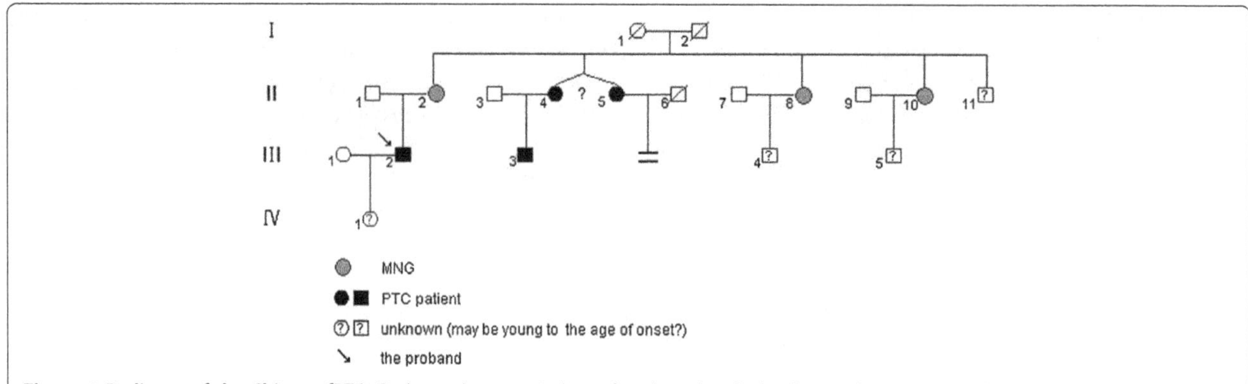

Figure 1 Pedigree of the Chinese fPTC. Circles and squares indicate female and male family members, respectively. The proband is indicated by an arrow.

be autosomal dominant. For the purpose to improve our understanding of the PTC predisposition, based on the recent progresses in genetic studies about PTC, we analyzed in this Chinese family (1) the point mutations of the *BRAF* and *RET*; (2) the possible susceptibility loci to sporadic PTC; and (3) the suggested potential fMNG syndrome with PTC risk region.

Methods

Patients

The fMNG with PTC pedigree is reported in Figure 1. The clinical and pathological findings are summarized in Table 1.

The study protocol was approved by the Review Board of Clinical Research of the Sichuan Provincial hospital, and by the Research & Ethics Committee of Sichuan Medical Research Institution. The blood samples were collected from the proband (III2), proband's parents (II1 & 2) and maternal aunts (II5, 8, & 10) with their written informed consent.

A 35-year-old man (Figure 1 III2) came to our observation: the man complained both his lymph nodes containing palpable lump for more than 10 days, initial ultrasound examinations revealed an 1.9 × 1.4 cm solid mass with irregular & indefinite border, sand calcification and blood flow in his right neck, and also 2 small nodule goiters in his left neck; The thyroid function tests showed the man was euthyroid; both the fine needle aspiration cytological and thyroidectomy specimen pathologic examinations disclosed that the architecture and nuclear features of the neoplasm in his both necks were typical for PTC (Figure 2A) and immunohistochemical staining confirmed the diagnosis (Figure 2B, C, D); After the total thyroidectomy and radioactive iodine treatment, the patient is now doing well. Interestingly, in terms of fMNG with PTC, the patient's mother is diagnosed with MNG in bilateral thyroid and underwent a total thyroidectomy in Chongqing, China (Figure 1 II2). Both of the patient's maternal twin aunts and a younger male cousin were diagnosed with MNG and PTC by different hospitals in Beijing and Chongqing, China, respectively; the other two maternal aunts were diagnosed with MNG by different hospitals in Chengdu and Dazhou, China, respectively (Figure 1 II8&10).

DNA extraction

The whole blood was collected from the medial cubital vein into heparin anticoagulant tubes. The total DNA was purified using the spin protocol of QIAamp DNA Blood Mini Kit according to the manufacturer's directions (Qiagen, Hilden, Germany). The purified DNA was resuspended in TE buffer and stored at 4 °C. Gel electrophoresis and spectrophotometric determination were used to DNA quantification and quality analysis. The OD260/OD280 ratio of DNA samples were between 1.8-2.0 and concentration was more than 100 ng/ml.

Table 1 Clinical and pathological study of the collected samples

Members	Sex	Age at diagnosis	Histology	sizes for PTCs and MNGs	Surgical treatment
II1	male	64	normal		
II2	female	62	bilateral MNG	MNG (1.2 cm), suspicious lesion	completion thyroidectomy
III2	male	35	bilateral MNG with PTC	PTC in MNG, PTC (1.6 cm)	completion thyroidectomy
II5	female	56	bilateral MNG with PTC	PTC in MNG, PTC (1.5 cm)	completion thyroidectomy
II8	female	45	bilateral MNG	MNG (0.3 cm)	
II10	female	41	MNG in right thyroid	MNG (0.6 cm)	

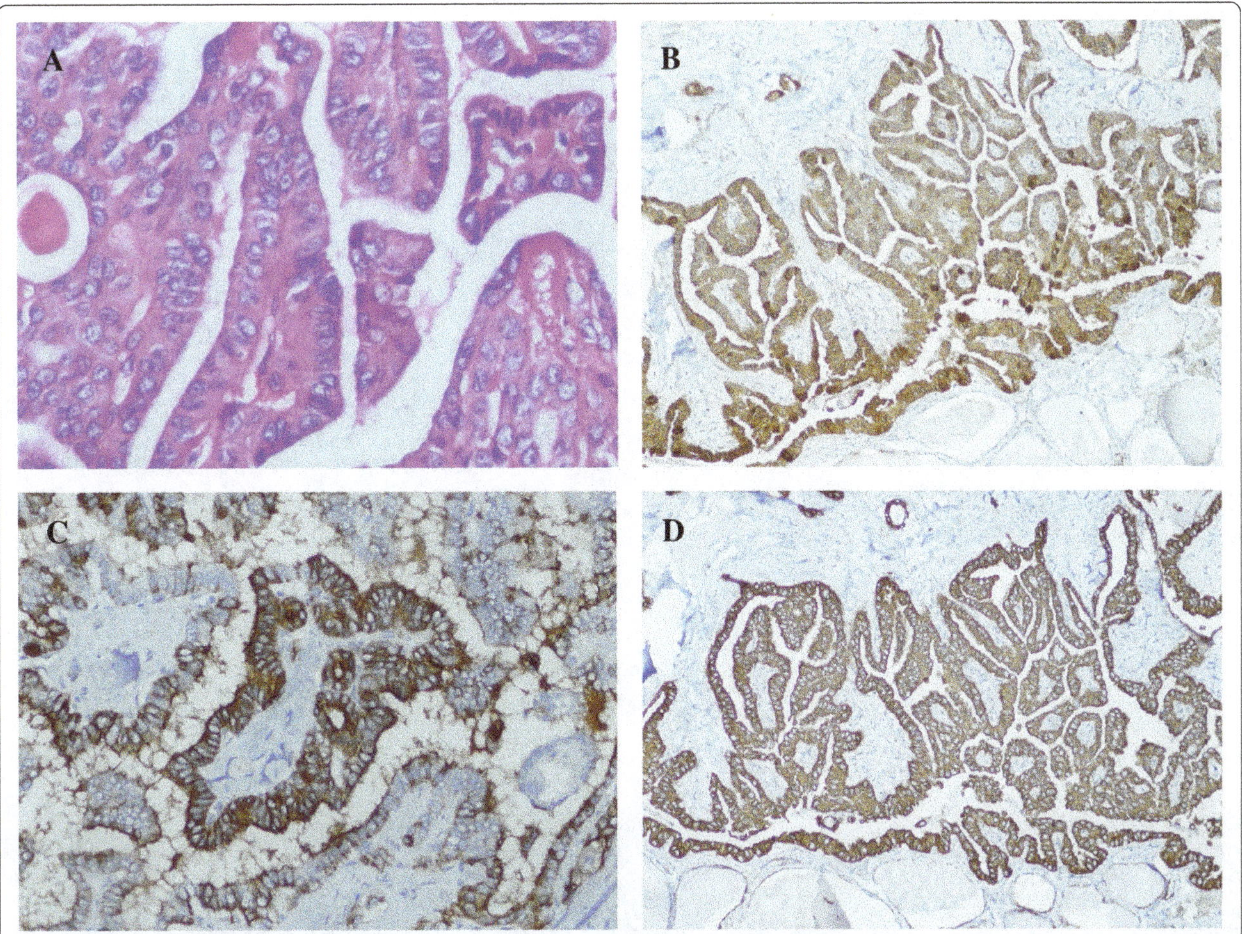

Figure 2 The histological features of the proband's papillary carcinoma. A: The cytological feature: crowded oval nuclei, nuclear grooves, clearing, elongation and overlapping (HE × 400). **B**: Galectin-3 showed predominantly cytoplasmic staining with occasional nuclear staining (×200). **C**: HBME1 showed positive diffuse membrane (×200). **D**: Cytokeratin 19 showed strong, predominantly cytoplasmic staining (×200).

Genetic mutational analysis

The potential regions and susceptibility loci investigated in the study were listed in Table 2. Sequencing was performed on PCR-amplified products using primers (Table 2) according to the published sequences or self-designed with Primer Premier 6.1 (PREMIER Biosoft, Palo Alto CA). The PCR amplifications were performed using ABI GeneAmp PCR System 9700 (Applied Biosystems, Foster City, CA). The PCR reaction system included 2U *Pfu* DNA polymerase (Thermo Fisher Scientific Inc, USA), 50pmol of each sense and antisense primers, 1 × reaction buffer (20 mM Tris–HCl pH8.8, 10 mM KCl, 10 mM $(NH4)_2SO_4$, 1% (v/v) Triton X-100), 250 μM dNTP, 2.0 mM $MgCl_2$ and 200 ng genomic DNA in a total volume of 50 μl. The PCR cycling parameters were followed the recommendations for *Pfu* DNA polymerase according to the manufacturer. Precautions were taken to prevent PCR contamination, and indeed, in each experiment DNA template negative samples were run in parallel. The PCR products were resolved by electrophoresis in a 2% agarose gel stained with ethidium bromide and purifed using the QIAquick PCR purification kit (Qiagen). Purified PCR products were sequenced directly in both orientations using standard procedures with an ABI PRISM 3100 Genetic Analyzer (ABI, CA). The sequences were confirmed with two independent PCRs from two independent DNA samples.

Results

The identification for the fMNG with PTC

The histological features of the proband' papillary carcinoma were shown in Figure 2. The members of the Chinese family were diagnosed with MNG and PTC by different hospitals in China; the affected individuals showed typical MNG or MNG with PTC, bilateral and multicentric nodes. In this Chinese family, there were 2 first-degree blood relatives were diagnosed with bilateral MNG and PTC, 5 second-degree blood relatives including a pair of twin sisters were diagnosed with MNG or PTC; Also among these family members, 2 men (III2

Table 2 Sequences of the primers

Clinical channel	Primers	Localization & product
BRAF at Chr7q34: 140,433,812-140,624,564(190,752 bp)		
exon15: 176,372-176,490 (119 bp) K601E: 176,431(A → G) rs121913364: 140,453,134 V600E: 176,429 (T → A) rs113488022: 140,453,136	5'-TGCTTGCTCTGATAGGAAAATG-3' 5'-CCACAAAATGGATCCAGACA-3'	Chr7:140,453,250-140,453,078 (173 bp) intron: 176,315-176,371 exon15:176,372-176,487 (116 bp)
RET at Chr10q11.2: 43,572,517-43,625,799		
exon5: 34,308-34,503 (196 bp) R313Q: 34,378(G → A) rs77702891: 43,601,894 R330Q: 34,429(G → A) rs80236571: 43,601,945	5'-CTTTCCTCACAACCCCCTCC-3' 5'-AGAGCGAGCACCTCATTTCC-3'	Chr10: 43,601,341-43,602, 077 (737 bp) intron: 33, 825–34,307&34,504-34,561 exon5: 34,308-34,503 (196 bp) STS: 33,825-34,398
exon8: 40,031-40,156 (126 bp) G533C: 40,105(G → T) rs75873440: 43,607,621	5'-CCTGTGCAGTCAGCAAGAGA-3' 5'-CCTGTTCCCATGCCCTGATT-3'	Chr10: 43,607,577-43,608,444 (868 bp) exon8: 40,061-40,155 (96 bp) intron: 40,156-40,784&40,896-40,928 exon9: 40,785-40,895 (111 bp)
exon10: 41,488-41,607(120 bp) C609R: 41,553(T → C) rs77558292: 43,609,069 C609Y: 41,554(G → A) rs77939446: 43,609,070 C611W: 41,561 (C → G) rs80069458: 43,609,077 C618R/G: 41,580(T → C/G) rs76262710: 43,609,096 C618S: 41,581(G → C) rs79781594: 43,609,097 C620R: 41,586(T → C) rs77316810: 43,609,102 C620F/S/Y: 41,587(G → A/C/T) rs77503355: 43,609,103 C620W: 41,588(C → G) rs79890926: 43,609,104 cds-indel: 41,562_41,588del27 rs121913313: 43,609,078_43,609,104del27	5'-GGAAACCTGGATCCCACAGG-3' 5'-GGGAGGGAAGTTTCATGGGG-3'	Chr10: 43,608,459-43,609,249 (791 bp) intron: 40,943-41,487&41,608-41,557 exon10: 41,488-41,607 (120 bp) STS: 41558-41733
exon12: 44,516-44,663 (148 bp)	5'-GTGGGCCCAATGTGTGGATA –3' 5'-CTCTTCAGGGTCCCATGCTG-3'	Chr10: 43,611,512-43,612,272 (761 bp) intron: 43,996-44,515&44,664-44,756 exon10: 44,516-44,663 (148 bp)
exon13: 46, 305–46,412 (108 bp) S765P: 46,313(T → C) rs75075748: 43,613,829 E768E: 46,324(G → A/C) rs78014899: 43,613,840 V778I: 46,352(G → A) rs75686697: 43,613,868 L790F: 46,390(G → C) rs75030001: 43,613,906 Y791F: 46,392(A → T) rs77724903: 43,613,908	5'-CGGGGAATTTCTGTGGACGA-3' 5'-ATGGCAGTGTCACACCAGAG-3'	Chr10: 43,613,496-43,614,200 (705 bp) intron: 45,980-46,304&46,413-46,684 exon13: 46, 305–46,412 (108 bp) misc_difference: 46,327
exon14: 47, 463–47,677 (215 bp) V804M: 47,480(G → A/T) rs79658334: 43,614, 996	5'-GAGGCAGAGAGCAAGTGGTT-3' 5'-AATAGCACGAGTCGTCAGGC-3'	Chr10: 43,614,767-43,615,517 (751 bp) intron: 47,251-47, 462&47,678-48,001 exon14: 47, 463–47,677 (215 bp)
exon15: 48,013-48,135 (123 bp) S891A: 48,076(T → G) rs75234356: 43,615,592 cds-indel: 48,051_48,053delAGCinsTTT rs121913306 43,615,567_43,615,567delins R897Q: 48,095(G → A) rs76087194: 43,615,611 cds-indel: 48,097_48,108del12 rs121913309: 43,615,613_43,615,624del12	5'-TCTCACAGGGGATGCAGTATCTG-3' 5'-GAGGCTGAGCGGAGTTCTAATTG-3'	Chr10: 43,615,159-43,615,837 (679 bp) exon14: 47,643-47,677 (35 bp) intron: 47,678-48,012&48,136-48,321 exon15: 48,013-48,135 (123 bp)
exon16: 49, 878–49,948 (71 bp) M918T: 49,900(T → C) rs74799832: 43,617,416 R912P: 49,882(G → C/T) rs78347871: 43,617,398	5'-GCTCCAGCCCCTTCAAAGAT-3'5'-CTTTGAGCAGTTTGGGGCAC-3'	Chr10: 43,617,229-43,617,941 (713 bp) intron: 49,713-49, 877&49, 949–50,425 exon16: 49,878-49,948 (71 bp) STS: 49,832-50,007
exon17: 51, 603–51,740 (138 bp)R972G: 51,715(A → G) rs76534745: 43,619,231	5'-CTCTGATGGGAGTGGCTTGG-3'5'-CCACTCAGGCACCCCTTAAC-3'	Chr10: 43,618,871-43,619,601 (713 bp) intron: 51,355-51, 602&51,741-52,085 exon17: 51, 603–51,740 (138 bp)
2q35		
DIRC3 (noncoding RNA):218,148,746-218,621,316 (472571 bp)rs966423:218,310,340	5'-CGGCCTCGACCAACACTTAT-3' 5'-ACTGGGCGTCTCAACTACAATCTG –3'	Chr2: 218,310,115-218,310,537(423 bp) located in the intron region of DIRC3,
5q24		
Pre-miR-146a: 159,912,359-159,912,457(99 bp) rs2910164: 159,912,418	5'-ATTTTACAGGGCTGGGACAG-3' 5'-TCTTCCAAGCTCTTCAGCAG-3'	Chr5: 159,912,297-159,912,523(227 bp)
8q24		
rs4733616: 128,662,095	5'-CACCGGGGATTGGAAGAGATAAG-3' 5'- TGAAGCCACAGGGGAGAAAAGT –3'	Chr8:128,661,750-128,662,159(410 bp)
8p12		
NRG1 transcript variant *HRG-beta1c*: 31,496,820-32,622,558(1,125,738 bp) rs2439302: 32,432,369	5'-AATGCAAGAATGGCCTAACACAAT-3' 5'-AACCTGGGGSSSSSTCTGAAGC-3'	Chr8: 32,432,326-32,432,660(334 bp) located in intron of NRG1

Table 2 Sequences of the primers *(Continued)*

9q22.33		
rs965513:100,556,109	5'-CCGGCTTGAGTTCAGGTATGTAGT-3' 5'-CCAGGCTCAGGTTATGTCTTTGTT-3'	Chr9: 100,555,758-100,556,177(420 bp)
9q22		
FoxE1: 100,615,537-100,618,997(3,460 bp)rs1867277: 100,615,914	5'-AGACCAGCTGCAGCCACCCCAACC-3' 5'-GTCTCGCCGCGCTCTTCCTTCACG-3'	Chr9: 100,615,806-100,616,270(465 bp)located in the STS of FoxE1
14q13.3		
rs944289: 36,649,246	5'-CCAGTGGCCCCGCAGGTT-3'5'-GAAAAGCACGTCTCCCCACAGTCC-3'	Chr14: 36,648,944-36,649,435(492 bp)
rs116909374: 36,738,361	5'-TGTAATGGCAGCTCTTGACCTT-3' 5'-ACCTTTGATTGCCCTTAGTTTGA-3'	Chr14: 36,738,229-36,738,674(446 bp)

and III3), 35 and 25 years old respectively, were diagnosed with MNG and PTC (Figure 1); As the family members resided in different cities and denied radiation exposure, no other neoplasia syndromes or somatic genetic alterations in the tumor DNA was observed, according to diagnostic criteria of familial MNG with PTC [6], we considered the Chinese family presented hereditary predisposition to PTC.

The comparison of the susceptibility loci

In the current study, we investigated the exon 15 of *BRAF*, since several SNPs in the genomic region were reported to contribute to PTC in a Chinese population [8] and the transversions in exon 15 are the common morphotype-specific mutation in adult sporadic PTC. The results were shown in Table 3: the examined *BRAF* sequences involved these susceptibility loci carried no risk alleles and were the same as common TT at $BRAF^{T1799A}$ and AA at $BRAF^{A1801G}$. No any other genetic mutation was found in the family members.

We also investigated all the known *RET* susceptibility loci to family thyroid diseases in this Chinese family. Either, no known *RET* susceptibility loci was mutational in the family members. However, it needs to mention that in the genomic regions which we sequenced, the *RET* introns contained certain differences among the family members, such as introns between exon 4 and 5 (rs35800403 & rs2742243), between 11 and 12 (rs2256550), between 14 and 15 (rs11238441 & rs2472737) (Table 3), and also, there was a new C to T heterozygous allele in the upstream of rs111306965 in the genome of memberII8 andII10 by repeatedly sequencing. Additionally, rs1800863 in exon 15 contained variants of synonymous code substitution in the genome of several family members (II2, II5 & II10).

With respect to the other susceptibility loci identified, as shown in Table 3, all the members from the Chinese family had equal sequences in the (1) *DIRC3* susceptibility locus at 2q35, (2) *Pre-miR-146a* susceptibility locus at 5q24, (3) *NRG1* transcript variant *HRG-beta1c* susceptibility locus at 8p12, (4) susceptibility loci of 8q24, and (5) susceptibility loci of 9q22. Noticeably, all the family members including the proband's father without thyroid disease were homozygous for the risk alleles of (1) rs966423 (CC) in *DIRC3*, (2) rs2910164 (CC) in *Pre-miR-146a* and (3) rs2439302 (GG) in *HRG-beta1c*; While all these members from the Chinese family contained no risk allele of (4) rs4733616 at 8q24, (5) rs965513 and rs1867277 at 9q22.

For the susceptibility loci of 14q13.3, as 14q was reported to be specifically linked with MNG1 and a form of MNG with PTC [25,26], it is worth to mention that the risk T allele of rs944289 was presented in the sequences of the most family members affected with thyroid disease (II2 & II8, MNG; II5 & III2, MNG with PTC; Table 1). The sequence result in Table 3 showed that both MNG with PTC family members II5 and III2 were heterozygous (CT) and the 2 MNG family members II2 and II10 were homozygous (TT) at rs944289 locus (Table 3). While for another susceptibility locus of rs116909674 at 14q13.3 which we checked, none of the studied Chinese family members carried the risk alleles.

Discussion

The Chinese family presented hereditary predisposition to PTC, but currently the genetic incline to fPTC is unknown. With the aim of understanding the involvement of genetic factors underlying fPTC, we analyzed the reported possible PTC susceptibility genetic regions by sequence in the Chinese family members who consented to join the study. First, it is worthy to mention that no risk allele of rs965513 (A) or rs1867277 (A) at 9q22 was observed among the Chinese family members. These susceptibility loci of *FOXE1* at 9q22 were related to radiation-induced PTC [19], hence it may be reasonable that the *FOXE1* risk alleles were not presented in the familial form of MNG with PTC, as the members denied radiation exposure and resided in quite different environment. Either, the Chinese family members carried no risk allele of rs4733616 (T) at 8q24 which has been shown to be associated with sporadic PTC in Europeans [14-16], but the pathogenic role of the allele is currently unknown.

Table 3 Sequences of susceptibility loci in the family members

Chromosome	*BRAF* at Chr7q34		*RET* at Chr10q11.2: 43,572,517-43,625,799								
	rs121913364	rs113488022	rs35800403	rs2742243	rs77702891	rs80236571	rs75873440	rs77558292	rs77939446	rs80069458	
Locus	140,453,134 exon15	140,453,136 exon15	43,601,415 intron	43,601,749 intron	43,601,894 exon5	43,601,945 exon5	43,607,621 exon8&9	43,609,069 exon10	43,609,070 exon10	43,609,077 exon10	
Allele	A:germline G: germline somatic A → G missense	A:germline; somatic C:somatic T:germline T → A missense	G/C	T/C	A:germline G:germline G → A missense	A:germline G:germline G → A missense	G:germline T:germline G → T missense	T:germline C:germline T → C missense	G:germline A: germline G → A missense	C:germline G:germline C → G missense	
II1 normal	TT	AA	GC	TC	GG	GG	GG	TT	GG	CC	
II2 MNG	TT	AA	GG	TT	GG	GG	GG	TT	GG	CC	
III2 PTC	TT	AA	GC	TC	GG	GG	GG	TT	GG	CC	
II5 PTC	TT	AA	GG	TT	GG	GG	GG	TT	GG	CC	
II8 MNG	TT	AA	GC	TC	GG	GG	GG	TT	GG	CC	
II10 MNG	TT	AA	GG	TT	GG	GG	GG	TT	GG	CC	
Chromosome	*RET* at Chr10q11.2: 43,572,517-43,625,799										
	rs76262710	rs79781594	rs77316810	rs77503355	rs79890926	rs121913313	rs2256550	rs75075748	rs78014899	rs75686697	rs75030001
Locus	43,609,096 exon10	43,609,097 exon10	43,609,102 exon10	43,609,103 exon10	43,609,104 exon10	43,609,104 exon10	43,611,865 exon12	43,613,829 exon13	43,613,840 exon13	43,613,868 exon13	43,613,906 exon13
Allele	C:germline G: germline T: germline T → C&T → G missense	C:germline G: germline G → C missense	C:germline T:germline T → C missense	A:germline C:germline G:germline T:germline G → A& G → C& G → T missense	C:germline G:germline C → G missense	not availiable cds-indel	T/C intron	C:germline T:germline T → C missense	A:unkown C: somatic G: germline G → A& G → C cds-synon	A:germline G:germline G → A missense	C:unkown G:germline G → C missense
II1 normal	TT	GG	TT	GG	CC	no del	TC	TT	GG	GG	GG
II2 MNG	TT	GG	TT	GG	CC	no del	TT	TT	GG	GG	GG
III2 PTC	TT	GG	TT	GG	CC	no del	TC	TT	GG	GG	GG
II5 PTC	TT	GG	TT	GG	CC	no del	TT	TT	GG	GG	GG
II8 MNG	TT	GG	TT	GG	CC	no del	TC	TT	GG	GG	GG
II10 MNG	TT	GG	TT	GG	CC	no del	TT	TT	GG	GG	GG
Chromosome	*RET* at Chr10q11.2: 43,572,517-43,625,799										
	rs77724903	rs79658334	rs11238441	new	rs2472737	rs121913306	rs75234356	rs76087194	rs121913309	rs1800863	rs78347871
Locus	43,613,908 exon13	43,614,996 exon14	43,615,382 intron	43,615,404 intron	43,615,505 intron	43,615,567 exon15	43,615,592 exon15	43,615,611 exon15	43,615,613 exon15	43,615,633 exon15	43,617,398 exon16
Allele	A:germline T: germline A → T missense	A:unkown G: germline T: germline G → A &G → T missense	C/T	C/T	G/A	AGC: germline TTT:somatic cds-indel	G:germline T:germline T → G missense	A:germline G:germline G → A missense	not availiable cds-indel	not availiable C/ G cds-synon	C:germline G:germline G → C missense

Table 3 Sequences of susceptibility loci in the family members *(Continued)*

II1 normal	AA	GG	CC	CC	GA	AGC	TT	GG	no del	CC	GG
II2 MNG	AA	GG	CT	CC	GG	AGC	TT	GG	no del	CG	GG
III2 PTC	AA	GG	CC	CC	GA	AGC	TT	GG	no del	CC	GG
II5 PTC	AA	GG	CT	CC	GG	AGC	TT	GG	no del	CG	GG
II8 MNG	AA	GG	CC	CT	GA	AGC	TT	GG	no del	CC	GG
II10 MNG	AA	GG	CT	CT	GG	AGC	TT	GG	no del	CG	GG

The SNP alleles are shown as the reference/variant, referring to NCBI Build 36.3; the common to mutant is showed by "→"; the risk allele is indicated with an asterisk and outlined if presented in the family members, and the different sequences among the family members are shadowed.

Our results verified that, for the predisposition to familial form of PTC and radiation-related PTC, their mechanism of PTC susceptibility did not completely overlap each other, since the genetic determinants associated with radiation-related PTC were not presented in the Chinese family members with PTC and MNG.

It is also noticeable that all the family members were homozygous for the risk alleles of rs966423 (CC) at 2q35, rs2910164 (CC) at 5q24 and rs2439302 (GG) at 8p12. All these susceptibility loci have been reported to associate with sporadic PTC [11,13], but currently the pathogenic functions of these alleles are not known well. We think all these risk alleles might contribute jointly to the development of MNG and PTC in the Chinese family members; while considering the risk alleles also presented in the proband's father with normal thyroid, it is possible that different pathogenic mechanisms exist to activate the tumor transformation in the family members with thyroid disease.

Interestingly, we observed that the frequency of T risk allele of rs944289 at 14q13.3 locus was increased in these MNG and PTC Chinese family members (C: T = 0.4:0.6 vs 0.571:0.429 in normal people). Several studies suggested the possible genetic predisposition of 14q to familial PTC [25] while no association between the radiation-related PTC and 14q13.3 [19]. Also, family nontoxic MNG locus maps to chromosome 14q [24]. Further research suggested that rs944289 was located in a CEBP-alpha/CEBP-beta binding element in the 5-prime UTR of a thyroid-specific lincRNA gene, papillary thyroid carcinoma susceptibility candidate 3 (*PTCSC3*), *PTCSC3* had the characteristics of a tumor suppressor, the rs944289 T risk allele reduced *PTCSC3* promoter activation and thereby predisposes to PTC [21]. Nevertheless, the tumor suppression mechanism of *PTCSC3* is currently unknown. In addition, the thyroid transcription factor of NK2 homeobox 1, *NKX2-1*, is also located in the 14q13.3; *NKX2-1* regulates the expression of thyroid-specific genes involved in morphogenesis. But how rs944289 was associated with *NKX2-1* remains to be investigated. Also, we investigated PTC susceptibility locus of rs116909374 (T) locating between *PTCSC3* and *NKX2-1* at the same 14q, the family members carried no risk allele at all. Hence, our current work implied the possible role of rs944289 in familial MNG with PTC. Whereas, it is surprise that heterozygosity as CT rather than homozygosity as TT presented in the fPTC family members; the same phenomenon was once suggested as a possible special form of genetic epistasis in the rs2910164 allele of *pre-miR-146a* gene [12], which may also contributed to this Chinese fMNG with PTC as shown by the study. Briefly, our results in the Chinese family agreed that rs944289 but not rs116909374 at 14q13.3 locus might be associated with genetic predisposition to familial form of MNG with PTC; it will be intriguing to further analyze the pathogenic link between rs944289 and the disease.

As we failed to detect somatic genetic alterations in the tumor DNA, such as the *BRAF* and *RET* proto-oncogene in the Chinese family members, in the current study, we investigated the genomic region containing the *BRAF* susceptible variants in sporadic PTC, and also all the known *RET* susceptibility loci to thyroid diseases (Tables 2 and 3). Our sequencing results confirmed that the *BRAF* and *RET* mutations were not germline mutations or susceptibility genetic events in this Chinese family. However, we noticed that in the sequenced *RET* genetic region, several different heterozygous alleles were presented among the Chinese family members, and most alleles were in the intron region. Recently, the chromosomal fragile sites breakage was proposed to cause PTC by forming chromosome rearrangement [26]. The chromosomal fragile sites are regions of the genome with a high susceptibility to forming DNA breaks and are often associated with cancer. Exposure to a variety of external factors such as chemotherapeutic, dietary and environmental compounds can induce and accelerate the fragile site breakage. Several intron regions of *RET* were identified as DNA breakage region. Hence, we are wondering if it is possible that the polymorphisms of introns could link to the structural difference in the *RET* region and could impact the related chromosome architecture and thyroid gene expression, albeit there was no *RET* mutation in the cancerous thyroid. Interestingly, there were 2 related facts to be considered: (1) it was shown that transfecting thyroid cells with *RET* produced morphological changes in nuclei that mimicked those seen in PTC [27]; (2) it is curious that the *RET* gene is not expressed in the thyroid follicular cells from which PTC develops, but rearrangements of the *RET* are found in PTC cases [28]. Hence, we think it will be intriguing to investigate the association between the genomic structural of *RET* region and the regulation mechanism of *RET*.

Our work may provide additional evidence to the genetic predisposition to familial form of MNG with PTC. Due to unavailability of samples and the complex of pathogenesis, the current studied Chinese family was small and limited. Nonetheless, for complex diseases like PTC, there may be many genes influencing risk as well as the effects of environment, also, it is much more difficult to collect pedigrees with multiple affected relatives and there is no guarantee of the same (or any) gene (SNP) segregating in these family. To provide insights into the genetic risk factors for familiar PTC, more researches are needed.

Conclusions

Based on our current investigation in the Chinese fMNG with PTC, the risk allele homozygote of rs966423 (CC) at 2q35, rs2910164 (CC) at 5q24 and rs2439302 (GG) at

8p12 could contribute to the fMNG with PTC, while the other identified risk alleles for sporadic PTC or radiation-related PTC might not be involved. Also, corresponding to the previous studies on the association between chromosome 14q and fMNG with PTC, our work approved that rs944289 but not rs116909374 at 14q13 locus might be associated with genetic predisposition to a Chinese family MNG with PTC. Though several different heterozygous alleles in the *RET* introns presented, the common *BRAF* and *RET* mutations were not susceptibility genetic events in this Chinese family.

Competing interests
The authors have non-financial competing interests.

Authors' contributions
SY L, YQ L and WZ S designed the molecular genetic studies, participated in the sequence alignment and drafted the manuscript. DD D and G X carried out the immunohistochemical assay. SP D and YM L have been involved in revising the manuscript critically. ZL T, JY H participated in data acquisition and helped to draft the manuscript. All authors read and approved the final manuscript.

Acknowledgments
We thank the members of the Chinese fMNG with PTC family for their essential contribution to scientific research. We thank Dr. Hongji Yang and the colleagues in Department of General Surgery, Sichuan Academy of Medical Science, Sichuan Provincial People's Hospital, for their support and collaboration.

Funding
This study was supported by the research grants (to Wenzhong Song and to Shunyao Liao) from Sichuan Provincial Health Department, China (100450,120074).

Author details
[1]Diabetes & Endocrinology Center, Sichuan Academy of Medical Science, Sichuan Provincial People's Hospital, Chengdu 610072, China. [2]Department of Thyroid Disease & Nuclear Medicine, Sichuan Academy of Medical Science, Sichuan Provincial People's Hospital, Chengdu 610072, China. [3]Department of Medical Genetics and Division of Morbid Genomics, State Key Laboratory of Biotherapy, West China Hospital, Sichuan University, Chengdu 610041, China. [4]Department of Surgery, Harvard Medical School, Massachusetts General Hospital, Boston, MA, USA. [5]Department of Pathology, Sichuan Academy of Medical Science, Sichuan Provincial People's Hospital, Chengdu 610072, China.

References

1. Nosé V: **Familial thyroid cancer: a review.** *Mod Pathol* 2011, **24**(Suppl 2):S19–S33.
2. Khan A, Smellie J, Nutting C, Harrington K, Newbold K: **Familial nonmedullary thyroid cancer: a review of the genetics.** *Thyroid* 2010, **20**(7):795–801. Review.
3. Bonora E, Tallini G, Romeo G: **Genetic predisposition to familial nonmedullary thyroid cancer: an update of molecular findings and state-of-the-Art studies.** *J Oncol* 2010, **2010**. 385206.
4. Hemminki K, Eng C, Chen B: **Familial risks for nonmedullary thyroid cancer.** *J Clin Endocrinol Metab* 2005, **90**(10):5747–5753.
5. Morrison PJ, Atkinson AB: **Genetic aspects of familial thyroid cancer.** *Oncologist* 2009, **14**(6):571–577.
6. Musholt TJ, Musholt PB, Petrich T, Oetting G, Knapp WH, Klempnauer J: **Familial papillary thyroid carcinoma: genetics, criteria for diagnosis, clinical features, and surgical treatment.** *World J Surg* 2000, **24**(11):1409–1417.
7. Nikiforov YE, Nikiforova MN: **Molecular genetics and diagnosis of thyroid cancer.** *Nat Rev Endocrinol* 2011, **7**(10):569–580.
8. Shifrin AL, Ogilvie JB, Stang MT, Fay AM, Kuo YH, Matulewicz T, Xenachis CZ, Vernick JJ: **Single nucleotide polymorphisms act as modifiers and correlate with the development of medullary and simultaneous medullary/papillary thyroid carcinomas in 2 large, non-related families with the RET V804M proto-oncogene mutation.** *Surgery* 2010, **148**(6):1274–1280.
9. Shifrin AL, Fay A, Kuo YH, Ogilvie J: **Response to "Single nucleotide polymorphisms and development of hereditary medullary thyroid cancer in V804M RET families: disease modification or linkage disequilibrium? ".** *Surgery* 2012, **151**(6):902–903.
10. Zhang Q, Song F, Zheng H, Zhu X, Song F, Yao X, Zhang L, Chen K: **Association between single-nucleotide polymorphisms of BRAF and papillary thyroid carcinoma in a Chinese population.** *Thyroid* 2013, **23**(1):38–44.
11. Gudmundsson J, Sulem P, Gudbjartsson DF, Jonasson JG, Masson G, He H, Jonasdottir A, *et al*: **Discovery of common variants associated with low TSH levels and thyroid cancer risk.** *Nat Genet* 2012, **44**(3):319–322.
12. Jazdzewski K, Murray EL, Franssila K, Jarzab B, Schoenberg DR, de la Chapelle A: **Common SNP in pre-miR-146a decreases mature miR expression and predisposes to papillary thyroid carcinoma.** *Proc Natl Acad Sci USA* 2008, **105**(20):7269–7274.
13. Jazdzewski K, Liyanarachchi S, Swierniak M, Pachucki J, Ringel MD, Jarzab B, de la Chapelle A: **Polymorphic mature microRNAs from passenger strand of pre-miR-146a contribute to thyroid cancer.** *Proc Natl Acad Sci USA* 2009, **106**(5):1502–1505.
14. Neta G, Yu CL, Brenner A, Gu F, Hutchinson A, Pfeiffer R, Sturgis EM, Xu L, Linet MS, Alexander BH, Chanock S, Sigurdson AJ: **Common genetic variants in the 8q24 region and risk of papillary thyroid cancer.** *Laryngoscope* 2012, **122**(5):1040–1042.
15. He H, Nagy R, Liyanarachchi S, Jiao H, Li W, Suster S, Kere J, de la Chapelle A: **A susceptibility locus for papillary thyroid carcinoma on chromosome 8q24.** *Cancer Res* 2009, **69**(2):625–631.
16. Jones AM, Howarth KM, Martin L, Gorman M, Mihai R, Moss L, Auton A, Lemon C, Mehanna H, Mohan H, Clarke SE, Wadsley J, Macias E, Coatesworth A, Beasley M, Roques T, Martin C, Ryan P, Gerrard G, Power D, Bremmer C, Consortium TCUKIN, Tomlinson I, Carvajal-Carmona LG: **Thyroid cancer susceptibility polymorphisms: confirmation of loci on chromosomes 9q22 and 14q13, validation of a recessive 8q24 locus and failure to replicate a locus on 5q24.** *J Med Genet* 2012, **49**(3):158–163.
17. Gudmundsson J, Sulem P, Gudbjartsson DF, Jonasson JG, Sigurdsson A, Bergthorsson JT, *et al*: **Common variants on 9q22.33 and 14q13.3 predispose to thyroid cancer in European populations.** *Nat Genet* 2009, **41**(4):460–464.
18. Matsuse M, Takahashi M, Mitsutake N, Nishihara E, Hirokawa M, Kawaguchi T, Rogounovitch T, Saenko V, Bychkov A, Suzuki K, Matsuo K, Tajima K, Miyauchi A, Yamada R, Matsuda F, Yamashita S: **The FOXE1 and NKX2-1 loci are associated with susceptibility to papillary thyroid carcinoma in the Japanese population.** *J Med Genet* 2011, **48**(9):645–648.
19. Takahashi M, Saenko VA, Rogounovitch TI, Kawaguchi T, Drozd VM, Takigawa-Imamura H, Akulevich NM, Ratanajaraya C, Mitsutake N, Takamura N, Danilova LI, Lushchik ML, Demidchik YE, Heath S, Yamada R, Lathrop M, Matsuda F, Yamashita S: **The FOXE1 locus is a major genetic determinant for radiation-related thyroid carcinoma in Chernobyl.** *Hum Mol Genet* 2010, **19**(12):2516–2523.
20. Landa I, Ruiz-Llorente S, Montero-Conde C, Inglada-Pérez L, Schiavi F, Leskelä S, *et al*: **The variant rs1867277 in FOXE1 gene confers thyroid cancer susceptibility through the recruitment of USF1/USF2 transcription factors.** *PLoS Genet* 2009, **5**(9):e1000637.
21. Jendrzejewski J, He H, Radomska HS, Li W, Tomsic J, Liyanarachchi S, Davuluri RV, Nagy R, de la Chapelle A: **The polymorphism rs944289 predisposes to papillary thyroid carcinoma through a large intergenic noncoding RNA gene of tumor suppressor type.** *Proc Natl Acad Sci USA* 2012, **109**(22):8646–8651.
22. Malchoff CD, Sarfarazi M, Tendler B, Forouhar F, Whalen G, Joshi V, Arnold A, Malchoff DM: **Papillary thyroid carcinoma associated with papillary renal neoplasia: genetic linkage analysis of a distinct heritable tumor syndrome.** *J Clin Endocrinol Metab* 2000, **85**(5):1758–1764.
23. McKay JD, Lesueur F, Jonard L, Pastore A, Williamson J, Hoffman L, *et al*: **Localization of a susceptibility gene for familial nonmedullary thyroid carcinoma to chromosome 2q21.** *Am J Hum Genet* 2001, **69**(2):440–446.
24. Cantara S, Pisu M, Frau DV, Caria P, Dettori T, Capezzone M, Capuano S, Vanni R, Pacini F: **Telomere abnormalities and chromosome fragility in patients affected by familial papillary thyroid cancer.** *J Clin Endocrinol Metab* 2012, **97**(7):E1327–E1331.

25. Bignell GR, Canzian F, Shayeghi M, Stark M, Shugart YY, Biggs P, *et al*: **Familial nontoxic multinodular thyroid goiter locus maps to chromosome 14q but does not account for familial nonmedullary thyroid cancer.** *Am J Hum Genet* 1997, **61**(5):1123–1130.
26. Bakhsh A, Kirov G, Gregory JW, Williams ED, Ludgate M: **A new form of familial multi-nodular goiter with progression to differentiated thyroid cancer.** *Endocr Relat Cancer* 2006, **13**(2):475–483.
27. Fischer AH, Bond J, Taysavang P, Battles OE, Wynford-Thomas D: **Papillary thyroid carcinoma oncogene (RET/PTC) alters the nuclear envelope and chromatin structure.** *Am J Pathol* 1998, **153**(5):1443–1450.
28. Kitamura Y, Minobe K, Nakata T, Shimizu K, Tanaka S, Fujimori M, Yokoyama S, Ito K, Onda M, Emi M: **Ret/PTC3 is the most frequent form of gene rearrangement in papillary thyroid carcinomas in Japan.** *J Hum Genet* 1999, **44**(2):96–102.

4

A case of thyroid metastasis from pancreatic cancer

Alessandro P Delitala[1*], Gianpaolo Vidili[2], Alessandra Manca[2], Upinder Dial[3], Giuseppe Delitala[2] and Giuseppe Fanciulli[2]

Abstract

Background: Thyroid metastases are clinically rare, and usually occur in patients with a history of prior malignancy and when there are metastases elsewhere. Metastases of pancreatic carcinoma to the thyroid are extremely rare, with only three cases reported in the literature.

Case presentation: We report a patient who had a pancreatic carcinoma with metastasis to the thyroid as initial clinical presentation of the disease. A 63-year-old man with a history of weight loss and fatigue presented with cervical lymphadenopathies and a large nodule in the right lobe of the thyroid. A fine needle aspiration of the nodule gave inconclusive cytological results for the origin of the neoplastic cells. An ultrasound-guided core biopsy revealed the presence of a poorly differentiated adenocarcinoma infiltrating the thyroid with atrophic thyroid follicles. Immunohistochemical staining of the lesion was strongly positive for Cytokeratin 19 suggesting a pancreatic origin of the metastasis. A contrast CT scan demonstrated an enlargement of the pancreatic body, dilatation of the pancreatic duct, diffuse retroperitoneal, paraaortic and cervical lymphadenopathy and secondary lesions in the liver.

Conclusion: Metastases to the thyroid from pancreatic carcinoma are extremely rare. A core biopsy of the lesion excluded a thyroid carcinoma and permitted the diagnosis of the primary neoplasm.

Keywords: Contrast enhanced ultrasonography, Core-biopsy, Pancreatic adenocarcinoma, Thyroid metastasis

Background

The thyroid gland is a known but unusual site for metastatic tumours from various primary sites. Although clinically apparent metastases from nonthyroid malignancies (NTMs) to the thyroid gland are uncommon, metastases to the thyroid have been reported in 1.4-3.0% of all patients who had surgery for thyroid malignancy [1,2]. Moreover, a wide range of prevalence, from 1.9% to 24%, has been reported from autopsy series [3,4]. The most common NTMs that metastasize to the thyroid are kidney, colorectal, lung and breast carcinomas.

Metastasis of pancreas carcinoma to the thyroid is extremely rare and only three cases have been previously reported. We present a case of thyroid metastasis from a pancreatic carcinoma in which the metastasis was the initial clinical presentation.

* Correspondence: aledelitala@tiscali.it
[1]Department of Biomedical Science, University of Sassari, Sassari, Viale San Pietro 8, 07100 Sassari, Italy
Full list of author information is available at the end of the article

Case presentation

We present the case of a Caucasian 63-year-old man who had an 8 –week history of 10 kilogram weight loss, profound fatigue and cervical lymphadenopathy.

As an outpatient he underwent a neck ultrasonography (US) in another center which identified a big hypoechoic lesion in the right lobe with ill-defined margins. Cytological analysis of the lesion was defined as malignancy (Figure 1A) according to the Bethesda System for reporting thyroid cytopathology [5] and the patient was referred for possible thyroidectomy. Thyroid function tests showed the following results: thyrotropin level 5.5 μU/ml (normal 0.46-4.68), free triiodothyronine 3.12 pg/ml (normal 2.75-5.26), and free thyroxine 1.07 ng/dl, (normal 0.77-2.19). Antibodies against thyroperoxidase and against thyroglobulin were negative, and serum calcitonin was normal (8 pg/ml, normal < 18).

Subsequently, he referred to our ward to perform further analysis. Neck US was repeated using a high frequency linear probe (15 L8W, 7.5-14 MHz, Acuson Sequoia 512, Siemens, Mountain View, California, USA).

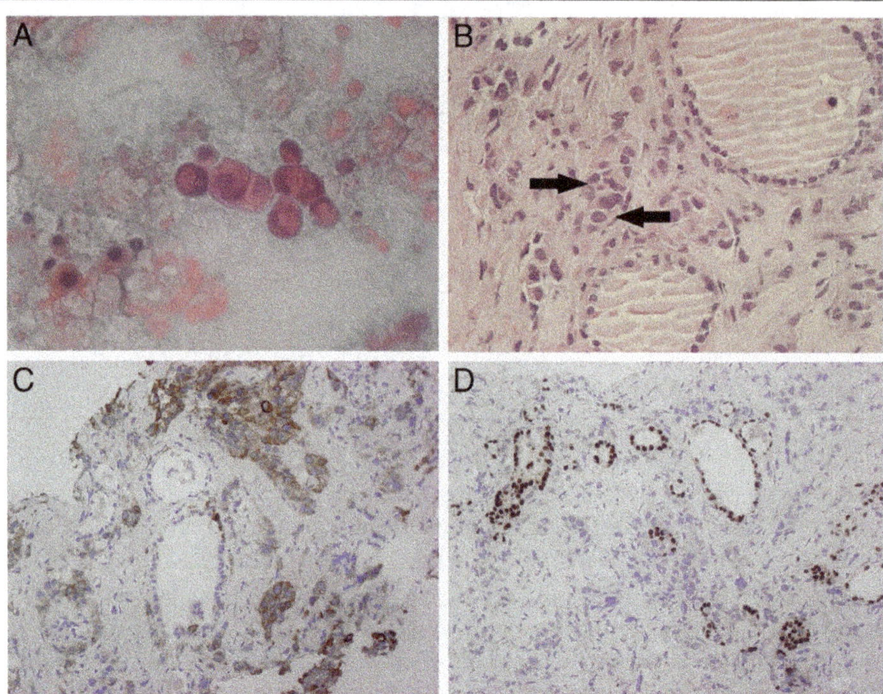

Figure 1 Cytological and histological aspects of the nodule. (A) Thyroid fine needle aspiration (Papanicolaou, magnitude 600 X). A high power field showing a cluster of neoplastic cells in a necrotic background. **(B)** Thyroid core biopsy (hematoxilin and eosin, magnitude 400 X): thyroid tissue infiltrated by poorly differentiated adenocarcinoma (arrows). **(C)** Thyroid core biopsy (CK19, magnitude 200 X): Strong cytoplasmic positivity in neoplastic cells. **(D)** Thyroid core biopsy (TTF-1, magnitude 200 X): nuclear positivity in follicular cells.

A thyroid hypoechoic mass of 30 mm in the maximum longitudinal size was detected in the right lobe of the gland, associated with round and enlarged lymph nodes in laterocervical part of the neck, especially on the right side. After conventional US, a contrast enhancement US (CPS, Siemens, Mountain View, California; Sonovue, Bracco, Italy) focused to the thyroid gland and lymph node was performed (Figure 2). Nodule and lymph node showed a similar pattern. In the central part, they exhibited a hypovascular aspect in all phases of contrast US (typical for malignant lesions), except for the presence of small vessels. The enhancement was located only in the peripheral part of both nodule and lymph node.

An US-guided core biopsy (Selectcore Inrad, 20 gauge, 10 cm in length) of the nodule was performed.

On microscopic examination, histological sections revealed a pseudoglandular proliferation of atypical epithelial cells embedded in a fibrous stroma with atrophic thyroid follicles (Figure 1B). Furthermore, on immunohistochemical findings, thyrocytes showed immunoreactivity for thyroid transcription factor-1 (TTF-1) in spite of negativity in the neoplastic cells (Figure 1D). All these features were consistent with the diagnosis of metastatic pancreatic adenocarcinoma. Therefore, we measured tumor markers which revealed elevated carcinoembryonic antigen (15.98 ng/mL, normal <5), cancer antigen 19–9 (8731.52 U/ml, normal <37), and slightly elevated cancer antigen 125 (240.10 U/ml, normal <35). Additional laboratory blood tests were consistent with biliary obstruction and liver damage.

A contrast CT scan demonstrated an enlargement of the pancreatic body with a 22 mm hypodense lesion with ill-defined margins, dilatation of the pancreatic duct, diffuse retroperitoneal, paraaortic and cervical lymphadenopathy and secondary lesions in the liver (1–4.2 cm) (Figure 3). A needle biopsy of the largest hepatic lesion revealed hepatic tissue infiltrated by poorly differentiated adenocarcinoma which was similar to the neoplastic tissue found in the right lobe of the thyroid.

The patient referred to the oncology unit for palliative treatment, and died two months later.

Discussion

The thyroid gland is believed to be a rare site of metastatic disease. It has been hypothesized that the fast arterial flow through the thyroid and the high oxygen saturation and iodine content within the thyroid might inhibit the growth of metastatic malignant cells [3]. NTMs seem to occur more frequently in glands that were also abnormal. These abnormalities included goiter, thyroiditis, benign and malignant primary neoplasm. In particular, malignant metastases were most commonly found concomitantly with goiters and follicular thyroid adenomas [6]. These data support the hypothesis that the abnormal blood supply

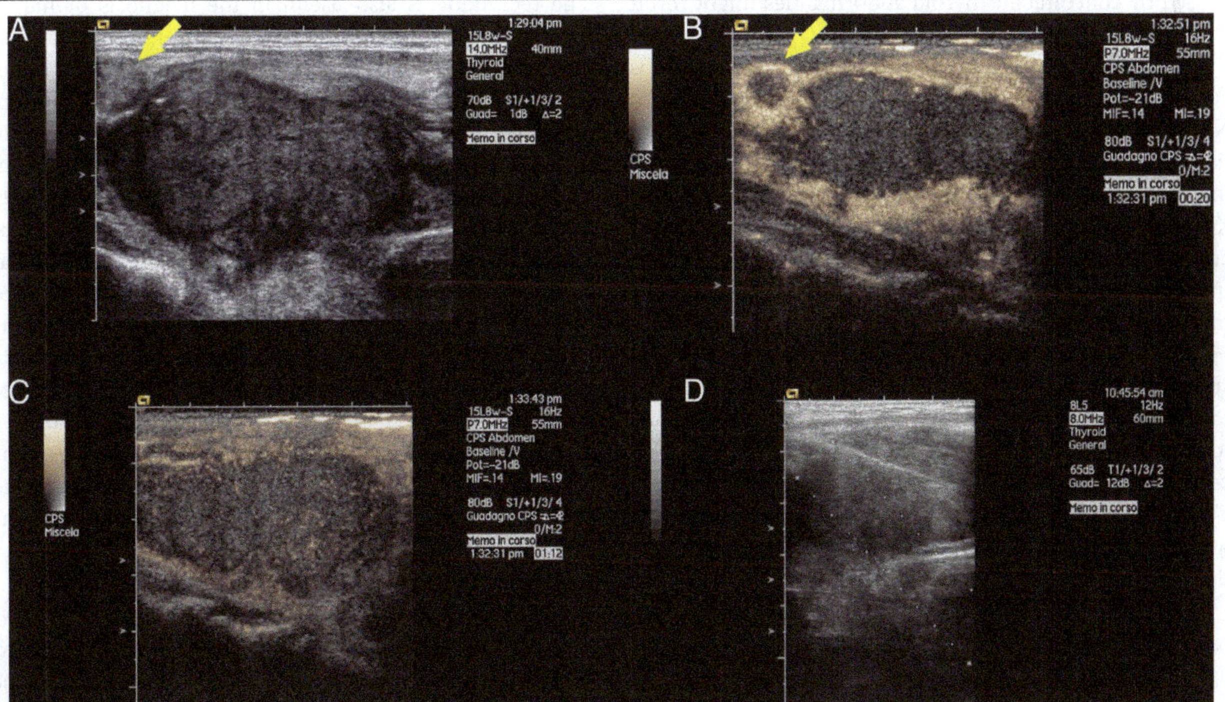

Figure 2 Thyroid ultrasound with contrast enhancement and biopsy. Longitudinal view of the right lobe of the thyroid gland performed with linear probe (7.5-14 Mhz) in conventional ultrasound **(panel A, D)** and after contrast enhancement ultrasound **(panel B,C)**. Panel A shows a hypoechoic lesion of the right lobe of the thyroid gland. The yellow arrow indicates a metastatic lymph node located close to the upper pole of the right lobe. Panel B shows the hypovascular aspect of the nodule and lymph node after contrast injection. The enhancement is located only in the peripheral part both of nodule and lymph node as well. Panel C shows the enhancement in the venous phase which is still located only in the peripheral part of the nodule, except for the presence of small tiny vessels located also in the central part. Panel D show the path of the needle inserted inside of the nodule.

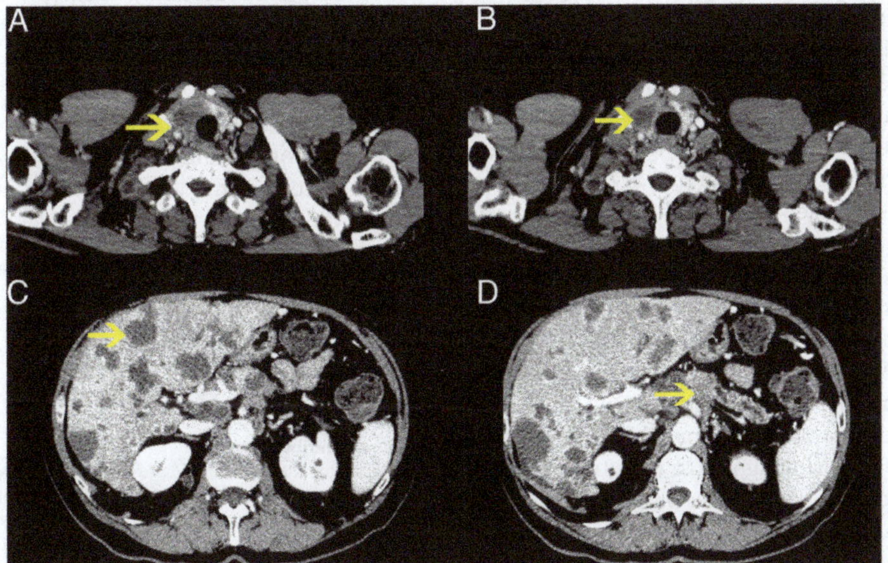

Figure 3 CT scan of the body. In panel **A** and **B** the yellow arrows indicate the big mass of the right lobe of the thyroid gland. In panel **C** the yellow arrow indicates one of the multiple secondary liver lesions. In panel **D** the yellow arrow indicates the pancreatic cancer located in the body with dilatation of the pancreatic duct.

caused by concomitant thyroid abnormalities might result in decreased oxygen and iodine content.

The reported prevalence of metastasis to the thyroid is variable, since the prevalence of thyroid metastasis from NTMs ranges from 1.9% to 24% in autopsy studies in patients with a known history of neoplasm. This wide range may be mainly explained by different population studied (few cases in most of the studies) and by the predominance of the type of primary cancer included in the series (patients with renal cancer had an increased prevalence of metastasis to thyroid gland).

However, a very recent review of the literature clearly suggests that clinically significant metastases of NTMs to the thyroid are not rare. In particular, the most common NTMs that metastasize to the gland are renal cell, colorectal, lung, breast carcinoma and sarcoma [2,6]. Thus, metastasis to the thyroid should be considered when a thyroid lesion is detected in the follow-up of patients with a history of cancer.

According a MEDLINE search, there are only three reported cases of thyroid metastasis from pancreatic malignant tumour.

The first was reported by Eriksson et al. [7] in a 54 year-old men with disseminated pancreatic carcinoma. Interestingly, this patient had a transient thyrotoxicosis due to a destructive thyroiditis caused by the massive invasion of the organ by tumour cells. Percutaneous biopsy of the gland excluded the presence of thyroiditis and demonstrated the presence of carcinoma. Autopsy showed an adenocarcinoma of the pancreatic tail with widespread metastasis. In particular, in the areas involved by the tumour, invasion and disruption of thyroid follicles by tumour cells were frequent.

The second patient was reported by Hsiao et al. [8] in a 45-year-old male with a previously diagnosed intraductal papillary-mucinous carcinoma of the pancreas. Adenocarcinoma metastatic to the thyroid was proven pathologically only after thyroidectomy, as cytodiagnosis of the thyroid aspirate did not proven the primary site of the lesion. The patient died one week after the surgery.

The third case has been reported by Kelly et al. [9] in a 38-year-old man with obstructive jaundice and epigastric pain who underwent a pancreatic-duodenectomy and, eight weeks later, a total thyroidectomy. The histology of the thyroid was similar to that of the pancreatic specimen.

Metastatic lesions in the thyroid gland could range from overt hypothyroidism with myxedema (3) to hyperthyroidism/thyrotoxicosis (7), although most of patients did not show any thyroid dysfunction. The prognosis essentially refers to the primary site of the cancer, and the overall survival time is not significantly different in cancer patients with or without thyroid metastasis [10].

Fine needle aspiration (FNA) is the most common and useful investigation in the diagnosis of thyroid pathology. The technique is also useful in the diagnosis of malignant metastasis to the thyroid. However, FNA may not yield a definitive diagnosis in all cases, particularly when the metastatic cells are poorly differentiated. Therefore histology and immunochemistry is usually necessary in order to differentiate primary thyroid carcinomas from metastatic neoplasm. Percutaneous core biopsy has been shown to be superior to the FNA in patients with prior non diagnostic FNA of thyroid nodules [11]. In our patient microscopic examination of the specimen obtained by core biopsy revealed the presence of a poorly differentiated carcinoma with a strong cytoplasmatic positivity for Cytokeratin 19 [12], and negative staining for thyroglobulin and TTF-1 [13], thus favouring the diagnosis of metastatic tumour over a primary thyroid cancer. The association of this immunohistochemical finding and clinical and biochemical data clearly indicated that the thyroid lesion was a metastatic pancreatic carcinoma.

Conclusions

Our case represents the fourth case reported in the literature of pancreatic adenocarcinoma metastatic to the thyroid, and the first in whom the thyroid metastasis was the initial clinical presentation of the pancreatic disease. The core biopsy of the thyroid lesion, providing more tissue (with retained cellular architecture) compared to the FNA, allowed the identification of the primary neoplasm. Moreover, we describe for the first time the behavior of the ultrasound contrast agent in a thyroid lesion, secondary to a metastatic pancreatic adenocarcinoma.

Metastases of NTM to thyroid gland are uncommon and their identification could be challenging. We suggest that the use of ultrasound-guided core biopsy could help the physician in the diagnosis.

Consent

Written informed consent was obtained from the patient for publication of this Case report and accompanying images. A copy of the written consent is available for review by the Editor of this journal.

Abbreviations

NTMs: Nonthyroid malignancies; US: Ultrasonography; TTF-1: Thyroid transcription factor-1; FNA: Fine needle aspiration.

Competing interest

The authors declare that they have no competing interests.

Authors' contributions

APD: wrote the manuscript, GPV: performed contrast enhanced ultrasonography and core-biopsy, AM: performed immunohistochemical staining of the lesion, DU: data collection, GD: reviewed and edited manuscript, GF: reviewed and edited manuscript. All authors read and approved the final manuscript.

Author details

[1]Department of Biomedical Science, University of Sassari, Sassari, Viale San Pietro 8, 07100 Sassari, Italy. [2]Department of Clinical and Experimental

Medicine, University of Sassari, Azienda Ospedaliera Universitaria, Sassari, Italy. [3]Department of Pathology, University of Sassari, Azienda Ospedaliera Universitaria, Sassari, Italy.

References

1. Nakhjavani MK, Gharib H, Goellner JR, van Heerden JA: **Metastasis to the thyroid gland. A report of 43 cases.** *Cancer* 1997, **79**:574–578.
2. Wood K, Vini L, Harmer C: **Metastasis to the thyroid gland: the Royal Marsden experience.** *Eur J Surg Oncol* 2004, **30**:583–588.
3. Willis RA: **Metastatic tumours in the thyroid gland.** *Am J Pathol* 1931, **7**:187–208.
4. Mortensen JD, Woolner LB, Bennet WA: **Secondary malignant tumours of the thyroid gland.** *Cancer* 1956, **9**:306–309.
5. Cibas ES, Alisz NCI: **Thyroid State of the Science Conference. The Bethesda system for reporting thyroid cytopathology.** *Am J Clin Pathol* 2009, **2009**(132):658–665.
6. Chung AY, Tran TB, Brumund KT, Weisman RA, Bouvet M: **Metastases to the thyroid: a review of the literature from the last Decade.** *Thyroid* 2012, **22**:258–268.
7. Eriksson M, Aimani SK, Mallette LE: **Hyperthyroidism from metastasis of pancreatic adenocarcinoma.** *JAMA* 1977, **238**:1276–1278.
8. Hsiao PJ, Tsai KB, Lai FJ, Yeh KT, Shin SJ, Tsai JH: **Thyroid metastasis from intraductal papillary-mucinous carcinoma of the pancreas. A case report.** *Acta Cytol* 2000, **44**:1066–1072.
9. Kelly ME, Kinsella J, d'Adhemar C, Swan N, Ridgway PF: **A rare case of thyroid metastasis from pancreatic adenocarcinoma.** *J Pancreas* 2011, **12**:37–39.
10. Mirallié E, Rigaud J, Mathonnet M, Gibelin H, Regenet N, Hamy A, Bretagnol F, de Calan L, Le Néel JC, Kraimps JL: **Management and prognosis of metastases to the thyroid gland.** *J Am Coll Surg* 2005, **200**:203–207.
11. Samir AE, Vij A, Seale MK, Desai G, Halpern E, Faquin WC, Parangi S, Hahn PF, Daniels GH: **Ultrasound-guided percutaneous thyroid nodule core biopsy: clinical utility in patients with prior nondiagnostic fine-needle aspirate.** *Thyroid* 2012, **22**:461–467.
12. Alexander J, Krishnamurthy S, Kovacs D, Dayal Y: **Cytocheratin profile of extrahepatic pancreatobiliary epithelia and their carcinomas.** *Appl Immunohistochem* 1997, **5**:216–222.
13. Holzinger A, Dingle S, Bejarano PA, Miller MA, Weaver TE, DiLauro R, Whitsett JA: **Monoclonal antibody to thyroid transcription factor-1: production, characterization, and usefulness in tumor diagnosis.** *Hybridoma* 1996, **15**:49–53.

5

Serum homocysteine levels are decreased in levothyroxine-treated women with autoimmune thyroiditis

Maciej Owecki[1*], Jolanta Dorszewska[2], Nadia Sawicka-Gutaj[1], Anna Oczkowska[2], Michał K Owecki[2], Michał Michalak[3], Jakub Fischbach[1], Wojciech Kozubski[2] and Marek Ruchała[1]

Abstract

Background: Hyperhomocysteinemia is a well-known cardiovascular risk factor and its elevation is established in overt hypothyroidism. Since some authors suggest that chronic autoimmune thyroiditis per se may be considered as a novel risk factor of atherosclerosis independent of thyroid function, the analysis of classical cardiovascular risk factors might be helpful in evaluation the causative relationship. Data concerning the impact of thyroid autoimmunity in euthyroid state on homocysteine (Hcy) level is lacking. The aim of this study was to evaluate Hcy level in context of anti-thyroperoxidase antibodies (TPOAbs) in euthyroidism.

Methods: It is a case–control study. 31 euthyroid women treated with levothyroxine (L-T4) due to Hashimoto thyroiditis (HT) and 26 females in euthyroidism without L-T4 replacement therapy were enrolled in the study. All women with HT had positive TPOAbs. Forty healthy females negative for TPOAbs comparable for age and body mass index (BMI) participated in the study as controls. Exclusion criteria were a history of any acute or chronic disease, use of any medications (including oral contraceptives and vitamin supplements), smoking, alcoholism.

Results: TPOAbs titers were higher in both groups of HT patients versus the healthy controls. Hcy levels were found to be significantly lower in treated HT patients (Me 11 μmol; IQR 4.2 μmol) as compared with healthy controls (Me 13.35 μmol; IQR 6.34 μmol; $p = 0.0179$). In contrast, no significant difference was found between non treated HT and control group in Hcy level. The study groups and the controls did not differ in age and BMI. Furthermore, levels of TSH, FT4, TC, LDL, HDL and TAG did not differ between the study group and the control group.

Conclusion: The main finding of the study is a decrease in Hcy level in treated HT as compared with healthy controls. Based on our observations one can also assume that correct L-T4 replacement was associated here with a decrease of Hcy. Furthermore, it seems that non treated HT in euthyroidism is not associated with Hcy increase, in contrast to overt hypothyroidism. This may be just another argument against the concepts about the role of "euthyroid HT" in the development of atherosclerosis.

Keywords: Homocysteine, Thyroid, Autoimmunity, Hashimoto disease

* Correspondence: mowecki@ump.edu.pl
[1]Department of Endocrinology, Metabolism and Internal Medicine, Poznan University of Medical Sciences, Przybyszewskiego St. 49, 60-355 Poznań, Poland
Full list of author information is available at the end of the article

Background

Homocysteine (Hcy) is a sulfur-containing amino acid naturally found in human blood and its metabolism is based on two divergent pathways: transsulfuration and remethylation [1]. Hcy has been investigated as a risk factor for cardiovascular disease since 1969, when McCully observed that two patients with homocystinuria were affected with extensive atherosclerosis and arterial thrombosis [2]. Since the association between elevated level of Hcy and increased risk of coronary heart disease was established [3,4], the issue whether there is a causal relation still remains unclear [5,6].

To date, hypothyroidism is considered as an independent risk factor for atherosclerosis. However, the atherogenic lipid profile does not fully explain the increased cardiovascular morbidity in hypothyroid individuals. For that reason, the possible association between hypothyroid state and Hcy concentration was suggested. Interestingly, increased Hcy level in overt hypothyroidsm was found in many studies [7-9]. Additionally, normalization of Hcy level was achieved after euthyroidism restoration [10]. In sharp contrast with the above mentioned results, decreased Hcy concentration was found in hyperthyroidism [11].

The possible mechanism responsible for increased Hcy level in hypothyroidism also remains a matter of recent debate. Firstly, the observed hyperhomocysteinemia may reflect impaired renal Hcy clearance. Hypothyroidism probably reduces glomerular filtration rate leading to increased creatinine and Hcy levels [12-14]. Secondly, impaired liver metabolism of Hcy linked with hypothyroidism may contribute to hyperhomocysteinemia. Decreased activity of both enzymes, methionine synthase and methylenetetrahydrofolate reductase was established in thyroidectomized rats and may also explain the elevated level of Hcy in hypothyroidism [15-17].

In contrast to overt thyroid disorders, data concerning Hcy concentration among patients with subclinical hypothyroidism (SH) is contradictory. Some studies showed that, despite atherogenic lipid profile in SH, Hcy level is not increased [18,19]. On the other hand, Hcy concentration was reported to be higher as compared with euthyroid controls [20].

In view of those controversies, and considering the fact that numerous thyroid disorders are caused by autoimmune disturbances, we hypothesized that it might be the autoimmunity against thyroid gland that initially affects Hcy production, even in pre-clinical phases of thyroid disorders. Therefore, the aim of this study was to evaluate Hcy level in context of anti-thyroperoxidase antibodies (TPOAbs) rather than thyroid function. To achieve this goal, Hcy concentration was determined in otherwise healthy and euthyroid women with, and without chronic autoimmune thyroiditis. The criterion of euthyroidism let us exclude the possible influence of thyroid dysfunction *per se* on Hcy concentrations.

Methods

Thirty one euthyroid women treated with levothyroxine (L-T4) due to Hashimoto thyroiditis (HT) at the outpatient clinic of the Department of Endocrinology, Metabolism and Internal Medicine and twenty six females with chronic autoimmune thyroiditis in euthyroidism without L-T4 replacement therapy were enrolled in the study (Table 1). All women with HT had positive TPOAbs. Forty healthy females negative for TPOAbs comparable for age and body mass index (BMI) participated in the study as controls (Table 1).

All subjects and controls were euthyroid, either spontaneously, or under L-T4 medication. None of the patients and the controls had a history of any acute or chronic disease, including diabetes mellitus, hypertension, angina

Table 1 Characteristics of the study groups and the controls

	Non treated Hashimoto (n = 26)	Treated Hashimoto (n = 31)	Controls (n = 40)	p
Age (yr)	43 (17)	38 (18)	35.5 (15)	ns
BMI (kg/m^2)	22.8 (3.6)	22.6 (4)	21.8 (5.40)	ns
TSH (mU/L)	1.64 (2.08)	2.07 (3.14)	1.54 (1.5)	ns
FT4 (pmol/L)	14.7 (2.27)^{a}	17.13 (5.11)^{b}	15.52 (2.23)^{a,b}	p = 0.0019
TPOAbs (IU/mL)	242 (290)^{b}	300 (391)^{b}	9 (5.5)^{a}	p < 0.0001
Hcy (μmol)	11 (4.2)^{a,b}	10.8 (6.9)^{a}	13.35 (6.34)^{b}	p = 0.0179
[Mean ± SD]	[10.33 ± 3.36]^{a,b}	[9.84 ± 4.24]^{a}	[12.97 ± 6.71]^{b}	
TC (mg/dl)	207 (64)	205 (60)	196 (51)	ns
LDL (mg/dl)	118.5 (50.6)	121 (45.6)	110.9 (37.4)	ns
HDL (mg/dl)	57 (30)	67 (16)	65 (15.5)	ns
TAG (mg/dl)	75 (38)	83 (47)	82 (46)	ns

Results are expressed as medians, followed by interquartile ranges given in brackets.
a,b – values followed by the same letters do not differ significantly at p < 0.05.

pectoris, evidence of any kidney or liver disorder. Exclusion criteria were also use of any medications (including oral contraceptives and vitamin supplements), smoking, alcoholism.

All subjects underwent physical examination with recording of height, weight, heart rate, systolic and diastolic blood pressure. Blood samples were obtained after an overnight fast. In patients with HT blood samples were drawn before the ingestion of usual morning L-T4 medication. Serum levels of thyrotropin hormone (TSH), free thyroxine (FT4), TPOAbs, Hcy, total cholesterol (TC), low-density lipoprotein (LDL), high-density lipoprotein (HDL), triacylglycerol (TAG) were evaluated.

TSH and FT4 were measured using the electrochemiluminescence technique in Cobas E 601 (norm ranges: TSH 0.27–4.2 mU/l; FT4 11.5–21.0 pmol/l). TPOAbs were measured by radioimmunoassay (norm range: <34 IU/ml).

Serum Hcy levels were assessed by high-performance liquid chromatography (HPLC). The analyzed plasma thiol compounds (Hcy, Fluka Germany) were diluted with water at 2:1 ratio and reduced using 1% TCEP (Tris-(2-carboxyethyl)-phosphin-hydrochloride; Applichem, Germany) at 1:9 ratio. Subsequently, the sample was deproteinized using 1 M $HClO_4$ (at 2:1 ratio) and applied to the HPLC/EC system.

To determine thiol concentration the samples were fed to the HPLC system (P580A; Dionex, Germany) coupled to an electrochemical detector (CoulArray 5600; ESA, USA). The analysis was performed in Termo Hypersil BDS C18 column (250 mm × 4.6 mm × 5 μm) (Germany) in isocratic conditions, using the mobile phase of 0.15 M phosphate buffer, pH 2.9, supplemented with 12.5-17% acetonitrile. The system was controlled, and the data were collected and processed using Chromeleon software (Dionex, Germany).

The study was approved by the Poznan University of Medical Sciences Ethical Commitee, and informed consent was signed by every subject.

Comparison of analyzed parameters between three groups (HT patients versus healthy controls) was performed by Kruskal-Wallis test with Dunn's post-hoc tests because data did not follow normal distribution. Normality was analyzed by Shapiro-Wilk's test. Results were presented as medians and interquartile ranges (IQR). Spearman's correlation coefficient was used to measure the strength of relationship of analyzed parameters. All tests were performed two-tailed and were considered as significant at $p < 0.05$. Statistical analyses were performed with Statistica 10 (StatSoft Inc., Poland) and MedCalc version 10.3.2 (MedCalc Software, Mariakerke, Belgium) .

Results

Descriptive characteristics for the study groups and the control group are shown in Table 1.

The study groups and the controls did not differ in age and BMI.

TSH levels of treated and non treated HT patients were similar to those of control subjects. FT4 concentrations of treated HT patients were significantly higher as compared with non treated HT and did not differ from controls (Figure 1). TPOAbs titers were higher in both groups of HT patients versus the healthy controls.

Hcy levels were found to be significantly lower in treated HT patients as compared with healthy controls (Figure 2). In contrast, no significant difference was found between non treated HT and control group in Hcy level.

In treated HT females Hcy level was negatively correlated with age ($p = 0.017289$; $r = -0.42$). In contrast, correlation between Hcy and age was not found in non treated HT and in controls. No significant associations were found between Hcy and BMI, waist circumference, TSH, FT4, TPOAbs in all of HT patients and in healthy females. Furthermore, levels of TC, LDL, HDL and TAG did not differ between the study groups and the control group.

Discussion

In this study, we investigated the influence of thyroid autoimmunity on Hcy concentrations. To achieve this goal, we used very strict criteria of enrollment, and we excluded the possible influence of hypothyroidism by including only patients who were euthyroid, obviously either spontaneously, or under medication. With this novel approach, we came to somewhat surprising conclusions that we discuss beneath.

We showed here that non treated HT and treated HT females had comparable TPOAbs, however treated HT group had higher level of FT4. Moreover, FT4 in treated HT and healthy controls did not differ indicating sufficient replacement therapy. The main finding of the study is a decrease in Hcy level in treated HT as compared with healthy controls.

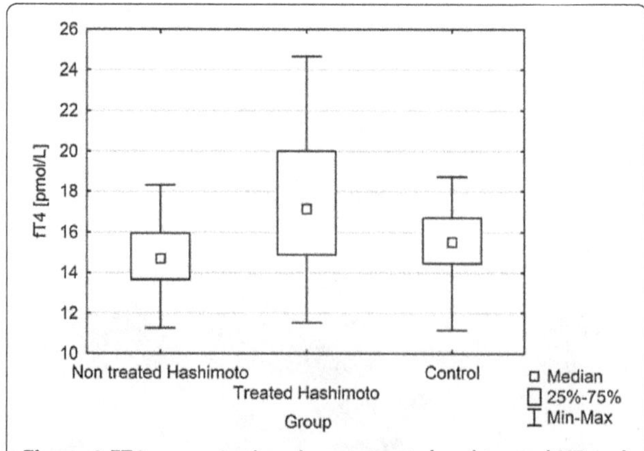

Figure 1 FT4 concentrations in non treated and treated HT and in controls.

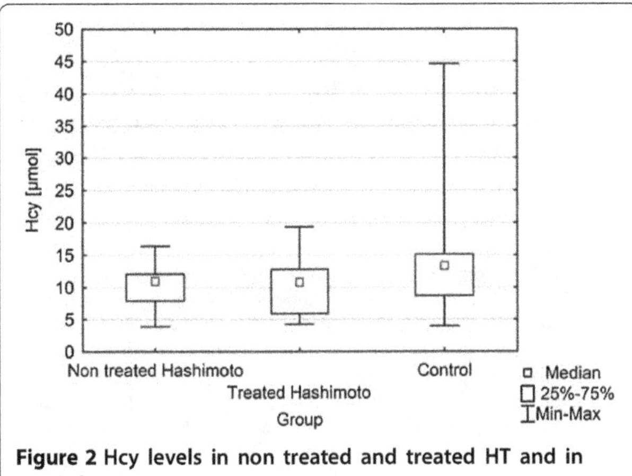

Figure 2 Hcy levels in non treated and treated HT and in controls.

Obviously, our findings should be understood in a broader context of the association between thyroid autoimmunity and atherosclerosis. Indeed, some authors suggest that chronic autoimmune thyroiditis per se may be considered as a novel risk factor of atherosclerosis independent of thyroid function [21-24]. Currently, however, the causative relationship between thyroid autoimmunity and increased risk of atherosclerosis has not yet been established. A few studies which were addressing this question investigated the effect of thyroid autoimmunity on lipid profile, abdominal obesity, fasting glucose and homeostasis model assessment (HOMA) insulin resistance, as well as carotid intima-media thickness (CIMT) [25-27]. However, in contrast to our study group, the study populations were not uniform, therefore the conclusions of these investigations are not comparable. Tamer et al. found that euthyroid HT ($n = 84$) patients had higher LDL level as compared with controls ($n = 150$) ($p = 0.0042$) [25]. Moreover, TPOAbs level was negatively correlated with HDL ($p = 0.031$; $r = -0.137$) and positively with TAG ($p = 0.013$; $r = 0.158$) and waist circumference ($p = 0.048$; $r = 0.128$). Ciccone et al. established that overweight or obese women with HT have increased IMT as compared with controls [27]. They suggested that the autoimmunity in HT patients is an independent factor that might accelerate atherosclerosis. However, they also found that HT patients had higher TSH levels and lower FT3.

It must be emphasized here that the effect of both hypothyroidism and hyperthyroidism on Hcy concentration has been investigated in many studies before. However, data concerning the impact of thyroid autoimmunity in euthyroid state on Hcy level is lacking.

To our knowledge, there was only one report of Hcy in context of thyroid autoimmunity in euthyroid premenopausal females with Hashimoto thyroiditis recently reported by Topaloglu et al. [26]. In this research, the study population was divided into two subgroups: first with TSH ≤ 2.5 IU/L and second with TSH > 2.5 IU/L. The controls were age-matched. CIMT was the only one evaluated parameter that was significantly higher in the study group regardless of TSH. CIMT was positively correlated with antithyroglobulin antibodies ($p = 0.014$; $r = 0.328$). In contrast to our results, Hcy level did not differ between the study and the control groups. However, in our study the control group had comparable BMI with the study group, therefore the body weight did not have any effect on the Hcy comparison. In contrast, Topaloglu et al. had a control group with BMI much lower than the study group ($p < 0.001$). Therefore, the potential influence of this co-variable on the Hcy analysis should be taken into consideration. New insight into the discussed problem was given in recently published research concerning Hcy level in patients with atrophic glossitis or burning mouth syndrome and autoimmune thyroiditis [28]. Wang et al. found increased Hcy level in these patients independently of thyroid function. Majority of the studied group positive for antithyroid antibodies (anti-thyroglobulin antibodies or antithyroid microsomal antibodies) was euthyroid. However, despite normal thyroid function in 85.8% of investigated individuals abnormal high blood Hcy level was established. Authors suggested that this finding was linked with vitamin B12 deficiency confirmed among this group.

Our study has some strengths and limitations. The main limitation of the present study is the number of patients who underwent the evaluation. However, it should be underlined, that all subjects were euthyroid females without any comorbidities and they did not take any medication. The only one difference between treated HT females and controls were TPOAbs. In our opinion, the homogeneity of subjects examined was the strength of this work that could balance its limitations.

Serum FT4 concentration is considered as an independent determinant of Hcy level [29]. As was mentioned above, Hcy level is generally decreased in hyperthyroid patients in contrast to hypothyroid subjects, who have higher Hcy concentration. Moreover, restoration of thyroid function leads to normalization of Hcy concentration. In general, our study and control groups were euthyroid, but this state was achieved by L-T4 replacement therapy in a group of treated HT women. This group had lower Hcy levels than normal controls, despite similar FT4 levels. A possible explanation of this finding is the fact that, in spite of similar hormone concentrations, these patients differed in that had different sources of thyroxine: it was endogenous in one group, and exogenous in the other. In our opinion, there is a causative relationship between L-T4 replacement therapy and decreased Hcy levels. Patients who are on L-T4 therapy have daily changes of FT4 serum concentration that result from pharmacokinetic properties of this medication. The maximum FT4 concentration occurs approximately two hours after the drug ingestion [30]. Moreover, there is a transient increase of FT4 serum level after ingestion of L-T4 for 5 hours [31]. Since FT4 directly influences Hcy concentration, during this time Hcy metabolism is similar to hyperthyroid state and it may lead to decreased Hcy levels in treated HT patients in contrast to healthy controls, in whom FT4 output is adjusted to real needs and the rate of physiological elimination .

Conclusions

The main finding of the study is a decrease in Hcy level in treated HT as compared with healthy controls. Our study adds further evidence to the debate on possible association between chronic autoimmune thyroiditis and atherosclerosis. It seems that non treated HT in euthyroidism is not associated with Hcy increase, in contrast to overt hypothyroidism. This may be just another argument against the concepts about the role of "euthyroid HT" in the development of atherosclerosis, which is of quite importance considering the high prevalence of high TPOAbs titers in Europe. Furthermore, that Hcy was lower in the treated group may point to the beneficial role of L-T4 treatment in general. Correct L-T4 replacement was associated here with a decrease of Hcy. In conclusion, L-T4 treatment may further add to medical approach aimed at atherosclerosis risk reduction with regard to Hcy decrease in L-T4-treated women with chronic autoimmune thyroiditis. This last concept, however, as drawn only from a cross-sectional setting, requires further investigation in observational studies.

Competing interests

The authors declare that there are no conflicts of interests.

Authors' contributions

MO conceived of the study, and participated in its design and coordination and recruitment of patients, drafted the manuscript; JD participated in design of the study, carried out the high-performance liquid chromatography and helped to draft the manuscript; NSG collected and analyzed the data, prepared the manuscript, performed the statistical analysis and the literature review; AO carried out the immunoassays and high-performance liquid chromatography; MKO participated in design of the study and coordination; MM performed the statistical analysis, helped to draft the manuscript; JF participated in design of the study and recruitment of patients; WK corrected the manuscript, approved the final version of the manuscript; MR corrected the manuscript, approved the final version of the manuscript. All authors read and approved the final manuscript.

Funding

The total cost of measurements (immunoassays and high-performance liquid chromatography techniques) were funded by Poznan University of Medical Sciences Internal Funding. The funder had no role in study design, data collection and analysis, decision to publish, or preparation of manuscript. The authors have not been paid to carry out the study and write the manuscript.

Author details

[1]Department of Endocrinology, Metabolism and Internal Medicine, Poznan University of Medical Sciences, Przybyszewskiego St. 49, 60-355 Poznań, Poland. [2]Department of Neurology, Poznan University of Medical Sciences, Przybyszewskiego St. 49, 60-355 Poznań, Poland. [3]Department of Informatics and Statistics, Poznan University of Medical Sciences, Dąbrowskiego St. 79, 60-529 Poznań, Poland.

References

1. Selhub J: **Homocysteine metabolism.** *Annu Rev Nutr* 1999, **19**:217–246.
2. McCully KS: **Vascular pathology of homocysteinemia: implications for the pathogenesis of arteriosclerosis.** *Am J Pathol* 1969, **56**:111–128.
3. Homocysteine Studies Collaboration: **Homocysteine and risk of ischemic heart disease and stroke: a meta-analysis.** *JAMA* 2002, **288**:2015–2022.
4. Klerk M, Verhoef P, Clarke R, Blom HJ, Kok FJ, Schouten EG: **MTHFR Studies Collaboration Group MTHFR 677C→T polymorphism and risk of coronary heart disease: a meta-analysis.** *JAMA* 2002, **288**:2023–2032.
5. Thampi P, Stewart BW, Joseph L, Melnyk SB, Hennings LJ, Nagarajan S: **Dietary homocysteine promotes atherosclerosis in apoE-deficient mice by inducing scavenger receptors expression.** *Atherosclerosis* 2008, **197**:620–629.
6. Clarke R, Halsey J, Bennett D, Lewington S: **Homocysteine and vascular disease: review of published results of the homocysteine-lowering trials.** *J Inherit Metab Dis* 2011, **34**:83–91.
7. Nedrebø BG, Ericsson UB, Nygård O, Refsum H, Ueland PM, Aakvaag A, Aanderud S, Lien EA: **Plasma total homocysteine levels in hyperthyroid and hypothyroid patients.** *Metabolism* 1998, **47**:89–93.
8. Morris MS, Bostom AG, Jacques PF, Selhub J, Rosenberg IH: **Hyperhomocysteinemia and hypercholesterolemia associated with hypothyroidism in the third US National Health and Nutrition Examination Survey.** *Atherosclerosis* 2001, **155**:195–200.
9. Gunduz M, Gunduz E, Kircelli F, Okur N, Ozkaya M: **Role of surrogate markers of atherosclerosis in clinical and subclinical thyroidism.** *Int J Endocrinol* 2012. doi:10.1155/2012/109797.
10. Lien EA, Nedrebø BG, Varhaugh JE, Nygard O, Aakvaag A, Ueland PM: **Plasma total homocysteine levels during short-term iatrogenic hypothyroidism.** *J Clin Endocrinol Metab* 2000, **85**:1049–1053.
11. Nedrebø BG, Nygård O, Ueland PM, Lien EA: **Plasma total homocysteine in hyper- and hypothyroid patients before and during 12 months of treatment.** *Clin Chem* 2001, **47**:1738–1741.
12. Diekman MJ, van der Put NM, Blom HJ, Tijssen JG, Wiersinga WM: **Determinants of changes in plasma homocysteine in hyperthyroidism and hypothyroidism.** *Clin Endocrinol (Oxf)* 2001, **54**:197–204.
13. Lien EA, Nedrebø BG, Varhaug JE, Nygård O, Aakvaag A, Ueland PM: **Plasma tHcy levels during short-term iatrogenic hypothyroidism.** *J Clin Endocrinol Metab* 2000, **85**:1049–1053.
14. Nedrebø BG, Nygård O, Ueland PM, Lien EA: **Plasma tHcy in hyper- and hypothyroid patients before and during 12 months of treatment.** *Clin Chem* 2001, **47**:1738–1741.
15. Chan MM, Stokstad EL: **Metabolic responses of folic acid and related compounds to thyroxine in rats.** *Biochimica Biophysica Acta* 1980, **632**:244–253.
16. Nair CP, Viswanathan G, Noronha JM: **Folate-mediated incorporation of ring-2-carbon of histidine into nucleic acids: influence of thyroid hormone.** *Metabolism* 1994, **43**:1575–1578.
17. Ayav A, Alberto JM, Barbe F, Brunaud L, Gerard P, Merten M, Gueant JL: **Defective remethylation of homocysteine is related to decreased synthesis of coenzymes B2 in thyroidectomized rats.** *Amino Acids* 2005, **28**:37–43.
18. Luboshitzky R, Aviv A, Herer P, Lavie L: **Risk factors for cardiovascular disease in women with subclinical hypothyroidism.** *Thyroid* 2002, **12**:421–425.
19. Atabek ME, Pirgon O, Erkul I: **Plasma homocysteine concentration in adolescents with subclinical hypothyroidism.** *J Pediatr Endocrinol Metab* 2003, **16**:1245–1248.
20. Sengul E, Cetinarslan B, Tarkun I, Canturk Z, Turemen E: **Homocysteine concentrations in subclinical hypothyroidism.** *Endocr Res* 2004, **30**:351–359.
21. Bastenie PA, Vanhaelst L, Golstein J, Smets P: **Asymptomatic autoimmune thyroiditis and coronary heart disease.Cross-sectional and prospective studies.** *Lancet* 1977, **2**:155–158.

22. Hak AE, Pols HA, Visser TJ, Drexhage HA, Hofman A, Witteman JC: **Subclinical hypothyroidism is an independent risk factor for atherosclerosis and myocardial infarction in elderly women: the Rotterdam study.** *Ann Intern Med* 2000, **132:**270–278.
23. Nyirenda MJ, Clark DN, Finlayson AR, Read J, Elders A, Bain M, Fox KA, Toft AD: **Thyroid disease and increased cardiovascular risk.** *Thyroid* 2005, **15:**718–724.
24. Zoller B, Li X, Sundquist J, Sundquist K: **Risk of subsequent ischemic and hemorrhagic stroke in patients hospitalized for immune-mediated diseases: a nationwide follow-up study from Sweden.** *BMC Neurol* 2012, **12:**41.
25. Tamer G, Mert M, Tamer I, Mesci B, Kilic D, Arik S: **Effects of thyroid autoimmunity on abdominal obesity and hyperlipideamia.** *Endokrynol Pol* 2011, **62:**421–428.
26. Topaloglu O, Gokay F, Kucukler K, Burnik FS, Mete T, Yavuz HC, Berker D, Guler S: **Is autoimmune thyroiditis a risk factor for early atherosclerosis in premenopausal women even if in euthyroid status?** *Endocrine* 2013, **44:**145–151.
27. Ciccone MM, De Pergola G, Porcelli MT, Scicchitano P, Caldarola P, Lacoviello M, Pietro G, Giorgino F, Favale S: **Increased carotid IMT in overweight and obese women affected by Hashimoto's thyroiditis: an adiposity and autoimmune linkage?** *BMC Cardiovasc Disord* 2010, **10:**22.
28. Wang YP, Lin HP, Chen HM, Kuo YS, Lang MJ, Sun A: **Hemoglobin, iron, and vitamin B12 deficiencies and high blood homocysteine levels in patients with anti-thyroid autoantibodies.** *J Formos Med Assoc* 2012. doi:10.1016/j.jfma.2012.04.003.
29. Orzechowska-Pawilojc A, Sworczak K, Lewczuk A, Babinska A: **Homocysteine, folate and cobalamin levels in hypothyroid women before and after treatment.** *Endocr J* 2007, **54:**471–476.
30. Colucci P, Seng Yue C, Ducharme M, Benvenga S: **A review of the pharmacokinetics of levothyroxine for the treatment of hypothyroidism.** *Eur Endocrinol* 2013, **9:**40–47.
31. Ain KB, Pucino F, Shiver TM, Banks SM: **Thyroid hormone levels affected by time of blood sampling in thyroxine-treated patients.** *Thyroid* 1993, **3:**81–85.

6

Increased vertebral morphometric fracture in patients with postsurgical hypoparathyroidism despite normal bone mineral density

Maira L Mendonça[1], Francisco A Pereira[1], Marcello H Nogueira-Barbosa[1], Lucas M Monsignore[1], Sara R Teixeira[1], Plauto CA Watanabe[2], Lea MZ Maciel[1] and Francisco JA de Paula[1,3*]

Abstract

Background: The mechanism behind parathyroid hormone (PTH) activation of bone remodeling is intimately dependent on the time of exposure of bone cells to hormone levels. Sustained high PTH levels trigger catabolism, while transitory elevations induce anabolism. The effects of hypoparathyroidism (PhPT) on bone are unknown. The objective was to study the impact of PhPT on bone mineral density (BMD), on the frequency of subclinical vertebral fracture and on mandible morphometry.

Methods: The study comprised thirty-three postmenopausal women, 17 controls (CG) and 16 with PhPT (PhPTG) matched for age, weight and height. Bone mineral density (BMD) of lumbar spine, total hip and 1/3 radius, radiographic evaluation of vertebral morphometry, panoramic radiography of the mandible, and biochemical evaluation of mineral metabolism and bone remodeling were evaluated in both groups.

Results: There were no significant differences in lumbar spine or total hip BMD between groups. There was marked heterogeneity of lumbar spine BMD in PhPTG (high = 4, normal = 9, osteopenia = 1, and osteoporosis = 2 patients). BMD was decreased in the 1/3 radius in PhPTG $P < 0.005$). The PhPTG group exhibited an increased frequency of morphometric vertebral fractures and decreased mandible cortical thickness.

Conclusion: The study suggests that vertebral fragility occurs in PhPT despite normal or even high BMD. The current results encourage further studies to evaluate the use of panoramic radiography in the identification of osteometabolic disorders, such as PhPT and the development of a more physiological treatment for PhPT.

Keywords: Postsurgical hypoparathyroidism, Osteoporosis, Morphometric fracture, Parathyroid hormone, Panoramic radiography

Background

During this decade a remarkable advance has occurred in the knowledge about the molecular and cellular action of PTH on bone [1,2], whereas little progress has been made regarding the physiological role of PTH secretion in bone mass development and homeostasis [3]. There are few lines of evidence suggesting that individuals with normal bone mass have greater PTH release in response to physiological stimuli (hyperphosphatemic diet or modest hypocalcemia) than osteoporotic patients [4,5]. In contrast, several studies have demonstrated increased bone mass in patients with chronic postsurgical hypoparathyroidism, (PhPT) [6,7]. However, to date no study has addressed fracture susceptibility in patients with PhPT [6,8].

Although the risk of fracture increases significantly with decreasing BMD, large observational studies have demonstrated that osteoporotic fractures can occur across a wide spectrum of BMDs [9,10]. Most likely, these events are related not only to bone mass quantity but also to bone quality, a component not captured by DXA measurements [10,11]. Great efforts are being currently devoted to the determination of clinical conditions associated with a high

* Correspondence: fjpaula@fmrp.usp.br
[1]Department of Internal Medicine, School of Medicine of Ribeirão Preto, University of São Paulo, São Paulo, Brazil
[3]Department of Internal Medicine, School of Medicine of Ribeirão Preto, University of São Paulo, Av. Bandeirantes 3900, Ribeirão Preto, SP 14049-900, Brazil

fracture risk despite an apparent protection by normal or increased BMD. Algorithms that combine BMD with identifiable independent risk factors to estimate a 10-year absolute fracture risk are now being used to provide a more holistic evaluation of absolute fracture risk over a 10-year period [12]. Attempts to further refine the algorithms have been made by taking into account novel variables such as type 2 diabetes mellitus, cardiovascular disease, asthma and use of tricyclic antidepressants in addition to the traditional variables of fracture risk assessment (FRAX) [13]. In addition, the use of other specific bone sites which are largely assessed by radiological exams can potentially be used for the early recognition of osteoporosis [14]. Approximately 1 in 3 of all radiological examinations is made by dentists [15]. Dental panoramic radiographs provide images of the jaws and there is evidence that jaw BMD and radiomorphometric indices developed for this site can be potentially used for the preventive diagnosis of osteoporotic patients [16,17] and of fracture susceptibility [18]. The OSTEODENT study suggested that an automatic measurement of mandible cortical bone thickness on panoramic radiographs is a valid test for the diagnosis of osteoporosis in women aged 45 to 70 years [18]. Bone mass of the mandible have never been evaluated in patients with chronic PhPT.

The present study was designed to evaluate BMD (lumbar spine, total hip, femoral neck, 1/3 radius and total body), vertebral subclinical fracture and cortical thickness in the inferior region of the mandible in a homogenous group of patients with chronic PhPT. All patients were women previously submitted to thyroidectomy due to atoxic benign multinodular goiter. Additionally, we assessed serum levels of insulin-like growth factor (IGF-I), receptor activator of nuclear factor-κB ligand (RANK-L), osteoprotegerin (OPG), 25-hydroxyvitamin D (25-OH-D), and bone remodeling markers [serum osteocalcina (OC) and urinary deoxypyridinoline (DPD)].

Subjects and methods

Subjects

The study was conducted on 33 postmenopausal women whose clinical characteristics are shown in Table 1. The study group included 16 patients with PhPT (PhPTG) followed up at the Outpatient Clinic of Osteometabolic Disorders of the University Medical Center, School of Medicine of Ribeirão Preto, University of São Paulo (FMRP-USP). The diagnosis of permanent PhPT was established by the concomitant presence of low circulatory levels of calcium and PTH after thyroidectomy, as well as by the requirement of continued calcium and vitamin D treatment to maintain serum calcium levels within the normal range.

The control group (CG) consisted of 17 adult women, matched to the PhPTG for age, weight, height and body mass index (BMI) (Table 1). The general exclusion criteria established for both groups were a personal or family history of osteometabolic disorders, alcohol abuse, smoking, hepatic or renal disease, or using medications known to interfere with mineral metabolism (anabolic steroids, glucocorticoids, anticonvulsants, diuretics or medication for the treatment of osteoporosis). Additionally, no woman, in both group had premature ovarian failure. The study was approved by the Ethics Committee of the School of Medicine of Ribeirão Preto, University of

Table 1 Clinical characteristics and biochemical evaluation of control subjects (CG) and of patients with postsurgical hypoparathyroidism (PhPTG)

	CG (n = 17)	PhPTG (n = 16)	Estimated difference [C.I.(95%)]	p-value
Age (year)	58.0 ± 6.1	62.3 ± 8.9	−4.31(−9.69;1.06)	P = 0.2
Weight(kg)	71.8 ± 13.7	72.6 ± 10.9	−0,82(−9.63;7.98)	P = 0.9
Height (m)	1.58 ± 6.4	1.54 ± 7.9	4.18(−0.95;9.31)	P = 0.8
BMI (kg/m^2)	28.5 ± 5.5	30.3 ± 4.2	−1.84(−5.33;1.65)	P = 0.4
Duration of PhPT	-	15.3 ± 12.4		
Total calcium (mmol/L)	2.43 ± 0.13*	2.05 ± 0.21	1.45(0.95;1.96)	P <0.0001
Ca X Pi	3.11 ± 0.63	3.21 ± 0.59	−1.15(−6.51;4.21)	P = 0.50
Albumin (g/L)	44.1 ± 2.4*	42.3 ± 1.8	0.18(0.02;0.33)	P < 0.05
Phosphorus (mmol/L)	1.29 ± 0.22*	1.57 ± 0.32	−0.86(−1.46;-0.27)	P < 0.05
Alkaline phosphatase (U/L)	235.4 ± 65.8	198.1 ± 37.14	37.29(−1;75.58)	P = 0.09
Creatinine (µmol/L)	57.96 ± 7.63*	69.39 ± 21.35	−0.30(−0.15;-0.005)	P < 0.05
PTH (ng/L)	42.0 ± 18.7*	5.9 ± 4.6	36.05(26.23;45.88)	P < 0.0001
25-hydroxyvitamin D (nmol/L)	82.0 ± 35.02	100.8 ± 31.47	−18.9(−42.6;4.85)	P = 0.11
IGF-I (µg/L)	68.76 ± 43.55	51.94 ± 19.15	16.83(−7.33;40.98)	P = 0.53

São Paulo (9523/2008). All subjects gave written informed consent.

The PhPT group had been on treatment for 15.3 ± 12.4 years, with daily intake of elemental calcium, calcitriol and L-thyroxin of 1713 ± 419 mg, 0.33 ± 0.18 µg and 99.3 ± 42.1 µg, respectively. The treatment target was to maintain serum total calcium in the lower limit of normal reference values and to keep serum levels of phosphorus and TSH in the normal range. We excluded from this group all individuals with a history of hyperthyroidism and those with a diagnosis of thyroid cancer, as well as individuals with a diagnosis of pseudohypoparathyroidism and autoimmune hypoparathyroidism.

Methods

Blood and urine collections and radiographic documentation were performed on two days. On the first day, blood and second void urine were samples collected in the morning between 7:00 and 9:00 after a 10–12 hour fast and kept in an ice-chilled container until centrifugation. Serum aliquots were stored at –70°C until assessment, with all determinations being carried out in the same assay. Subsequently, the volunteers were taken to the Image Center of the University Hospital, FMRP-USP, for DXA (dual energy X-ray absorptiometry) scan in total body, lumbar spine, proximal femur and forearm and standard thoracic and lumbar spine X-rays. On the second day, the individuals went to the Radiology Service of the Dental School of Ribeirão Preto, USP, to perform digital panoramic radiography.

Serum levels of calcium, phosphorus, alkaline phosphatase and creatinine were determined with an automatic biochemical analyzer (KoneLab 6.0, Winer, Argentina) on the day of blood collection. Serum IGF-I was measured by enzyme immunoassay [intra-assay coefficient of variation (CV) = 9.5%; Immunodiagnostic Systems, Fountain Hills, AZ]. Also, serum OC (CV = 5.6%; Quidel, San Diego, CA, USA), 25-OH-D (CV = 7.2%; Immunodiagnostic System, Fountain Hills, AZ), OPG (CV = 5.6%; Quidel, San Diego, CA, USA) and RANKL (CV = 6.8%; Biomedica, Austria) and urinary DPD (CV = 6.7%; Quidel, San Diego, CA, USA), were measured by enzyme immunoassay. Serum PTH was measured by chemiluminescence (CV = 4.7%; SIEMENS, Los Angeles, CA, USA).

Bone mineral density

BMD was measured by DXA at the femoral neck, total hip, lumbar spine (L1-L4) and distal radius by a trained radiologic technician (Hologic 4500 W densitometer, Hologic Inc., Bedford, MA, USA). *In vivo* precision was 1.2% for L1-L4, 2.3% for femoral neck, 2.7% for total hip and 1.7% for 1/3 radius, respectively. BMD values were expressed as g/cm^2 and T-Score.

Vertebral morphometry

Lateral thoracic and lumbar spine radiographs were taken for each patient and images were digitized using a Vidar DiagnosticPro scanner with a spatial resolution of 84 m and the gray scale represented by 8 bits/pixel. Six points were marked with electronic calipers on each of the 13 vertebral bodies from T4 to L4 using K-PACS Workstation software, v 1.6.0. These points were positioned on the outer edge of the upper and lower endplates. Using the six points, the anterior, middle and posterior heights were determined for each vertebral body in millimeters. Image analysis was carried out by consensus between 2 radiologists, both performed by blind assessment. A senior musculoskeletal radiologist reviewed all images in which any of the measured vertebral height ratios in a single film was <0.75 and also solved difficult cases when any doubt was present regarding the positioning of the calipers or to check if the encountered deformity was related to pathologies other than insufficiency fractures. The last analysis was also performed by blind assessment.

The criteria of vertebral deformity were: 1) more than a 20% reduction between two of the above measures and/or a 20% reduction in the relation between any one of the above measurements and the measurement of the corresponding region of the vertebral body immediately superior or inferior to each vertebral body analyzed, or 2) a reduction ≥ 4 mm in the absolute vertebral height value in relation to the other heights in the same vertebral body and in relation to the similar height in the immediate neighboring vertebral bodies.

Panoramic radiograph

All panoramic radiographs were obtained with an RX Veraviewepocs Digital Panoramic instrument (J. Morita Co). Digital images were examined with RADIOIMP software (Radiomemory, Brazil). In this panoramic images, the thickness of the inferior cortical region of the mandible bone were measured on both sides and in two regions (mental and goniac). The digital panoramic radiograph was inserted into the software and calibrated using magnification (30%) and resolution (300 d.p.i.) factors [19]. The projected areas of interest are used for the determination of the Mental Index and Goniac Index, as previously described [20,21].

Statistical analysis

All statistical analyses were performed using SAS 9.0 software (SAS/STAT® User's guide version 9.0, Cary, NC, USA: SAS Institute Inc., 2002). The Student t–test was applied using the PROC *T* TEST of the SAS 9.0 software to compare the results of the two groups. To determine the association of the variables of interest (BMD with hypoparathyroidism duration, IGF-I and 25-OH-D, simple linear regression models were adjusted, yielding the regression coefficients and R-square, through the REG procedure of the SAS 9.0 software. Considering the method described by Hsieh et al. [22] for determining the sample size required for the estimation of a correlation coefficient and for linear regression models, a sample of size 16 is sufficient for estimating a correlation coefficient equal to 0.65 with a level of significance of 0.05 and a power of 0.20. Thus, it was established that the sample size in each group should be at least 16. Data are expressed as mean ± SD.

Results

Table 1 shows that both groups were appropriately matched for age (range: CG = 49–70 vs PhPTG = 45–77 years), weight (range: CG = 46-94.6 vs PhPTG = 54.8–98.5 Kg) height (range: CG = 1.47–1.74 vs PhPTG = 1.47–1.69 m), BMI (range: CG = 16.9–36.1 vs PhPTG = 23.3–38.0 kg/m^2). The duration of postsurgical hypoparathyroidism ranged from 2 to 44 years (mean = 15.3 ± 12.4 years). Both groups presented normal serum creatinine levels (CG = 57.96 ± 7.63 μmol/L vs PhPTG = 69.39 ± 21.35 μmol/L). All volunteers had creatinine clearance above 60 ml/min. The serum levels of TSH were normal in PhPT group (PhPTG = 2.6 ± 1.0 mIU/L).

Serum levels of total calcium (CG = 2.43 ± 0.13 vs PhPTG = 2.05 ± 0.21 mmol/L; $P < 0.0001$), total calcium corrected by albumin (CG = 2.39 ± 0.21 vs PhPTG = 2.01 ± 0.26 mmol/L, $P < 0.005$), as well as PTH (CG = 4.45 ± 1.99 vs PhPTG = 0.63 ± 0.49 pmol/L, $P < 0.0001$) were significantly lower in PhPTG. The control group showed significantly lower serum phosphorus levels than PhPTG (CG = 1.29 ± 0.22 vs PhPTG = 1.57 ± 0.32 mmol/L, $P <$ 0.01). The groups showed nonsignificant differences in circulatory levels of 25-OH-D and IGF-I (Table 1).

Circulatory levels of the biochemical marker of bone formation, OC, were significantly lower in PhPTG (6.75 ± 2.36 μg/L) than in CG (9.64 ± 2.54 μg/L), $P < 0.01$, whereas there was no significant difference in urinary excretion of DPD (CG = 7.44 ± 3.0 vs PhTHG = 11.15 ± 13.16 nmol/mmol creatinine; p = 0.77). Both groups presented similar serum levels of RANKL (CG = 0.26 ± 0.21 vs PhPTG = 0.29 ± 0.27 pg/dl; p = 0.57) and OPG (CG = 0.094 ± 0.012 vs PhPTG = 0.1 ± 0.025 pmol/L; p = 0.44).

Total body BMD was slightly higher in PhPTG (0.923 ± 0.13 g/cm^2) than in CG (0.904 ± 0.10 g/cm^2). The mean values of lumbar spine BMD did not differ significantly between groups (CG = 0.970 ± 0.15 g/cm^2 vs PhPTG = 1.093 ± 0.26 g/cm^2). However, there was wide heterogeneity of T-score distribution within PhPTG, with 4 patients presenting a high T-score (> + 2.0 SD), 9 patients presenting a normal T-score (between +2 and −1.0 SD), 1 patient presenting a T-score compatible with osteopenia, and 2 patients presenting L1-L4 BMD compatible with osteoporosis (T-score < −2.5 SD) (Figure 1). Lumbar spine BMD was also evaluated after exclusion of the dominant vertebral body when there was a difference higher than 1 SD between two contiguous vertebral bodies. The results obtained in this second evaluation did not differ significantly from those obtained in the first evaluation (CG = 0.970 ± 0.153 vs PhPTG = 1.088 ± 0.250 g/cm^2). Both groups showed similar BMD values in femoral neck (CG = 0.826 ± 0.111 vs PhPPG = 0.865 ± 0.159 g/cm^2) and total hip (CG = 0.961 ± 0.145 vs PhPTG = 0.953 ± 0.162 g/cm^2) (Figure 1). However, BMD values for the 1/3 radius were significantly lower in PhPTG compared to control group (CG = 0.630 ± 0.07 vs PhPTG = 0.570 ± 0.09, $P < 0.05$) (Figure 1).

Table 2 shows that 10 of the 16 PhPTG patients (63%) had morphometric vertebral fractures, as opposed to only 2 CG individuals. The table also shows that morphometric vertebral fractures were not restricted to individuals with a low bone mass. Actually, 3 of the 4 patients with a BMD T-score above + 2SD had subclinical fractures in the thoracic and/or lumbar spine.

There was a significant correlation between the duration of postsurgical hypoparathyroidism and lumbar spine BMD (Figure 2). However, there was no correlation between the duration of postsurgical hypoparathyroidism and vertebral fracture. There was no correlation between BMD and serum IGF-I levels or between BMD and serum 25-OH-D levels.

There was no significant difference between groups regarding inferior cortical thickness in the region of the mandible angle (goniac). Inferior cortical thickness in the mental mandible was significantly decreased in PhPTG (Table 2). There was no significant correlation between lumbar spine BMD and cortical thickness in the mental region of the mandible. However, this last index was significantly and positively correlated with 1/3 distal forearm BMD (Figure 2).

Discussion

Skeletal fracture has not been considered a potential problem in postsurgical hypoparathyroidism, especially after clinical investigation, based on surrogate parameters, have shown that BMD is preserved or even enhanced in PhPT [7,23]. The present study demonstrated that patients with PhPT have marked heterogeneity in lumbar spine BMD, usually exhibiting high or normal bone mass, while densitometric osteoporosis is uncommon. Paradoxically, we have observed a high frequency of morphometric fracture of lumbar and thoracic vertebrae in patients with PhPT, which is not restricted to those with low bone mass. A previous nonvertebral fracture was present in one patient of the PhPT group, while no individual of the control group sustained clinical fracture. In addition, our results show that panoramic radiography of the mandible is a useful tool for the recognition of bone disorders in PhPT. These results are of great significance in the clinical

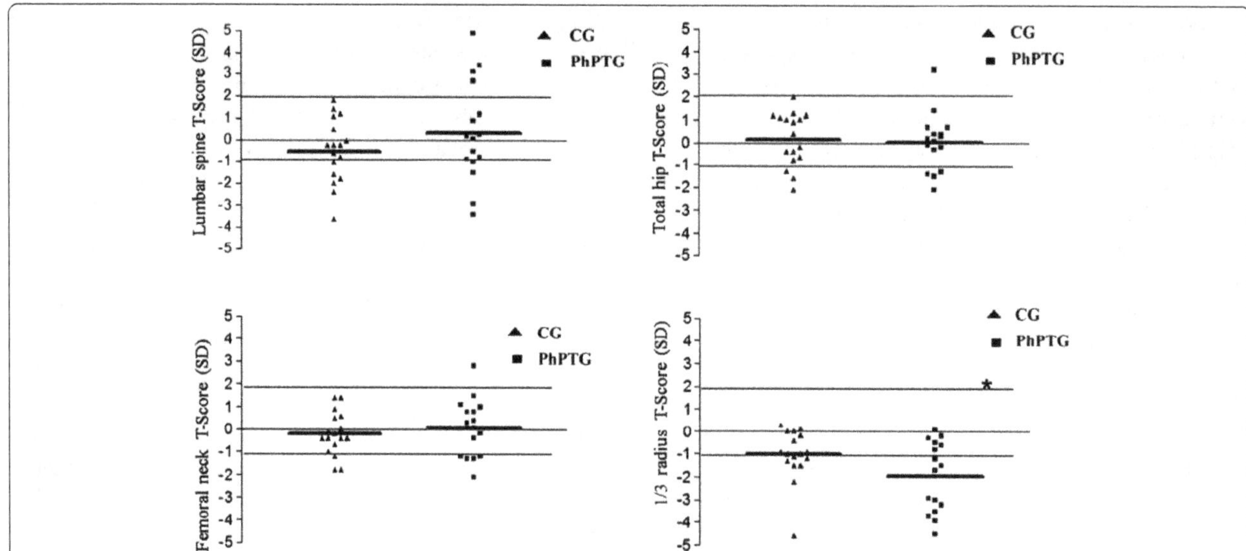

Figure 1 Distribution of bone mineral density values of lumbar spine (A), femoral neck (B), total hip (C) and 1/3 d forearm (D) of the control group (CG) and of the postsurgical hypoparathyroidism group (PhPTG).

setting since these data correspond to the first evidence of increased risk of fractures in postsurgical hypoparathyroidism. Therefore, these preliminary results encourage further investigation of the etiopathogenesis and prevalence of this condition and a more appropriate approach to the management of this particular group of patients.

There are studies showing a differential impact of PhPT on diverse bone sites, the increase in BMD being higher in the lumbar spine than in the proximal femur [23], whereas forearm BMD was not positively affected [24]. For Instance, Duan et al. evaluated 10 postmenopausal women harboring postsurgical hypoparathyroidism. The duration

Table 2 Number of vertebral fractures, bone mineral density (T-score) and mental index in the control group (CG) and postsurgical hypoparathyroidism group (PhPTG)

CG	Vertebral fracture	T-score (L1-L4)	MI *	PhTPG	Vertebral fracture	T-score (L1-L4)	MI
1	0	−2	3.02	**1**	0	2.7	3.36
2	0	1.2	3.59	**2**	0	0.3	2.80
3	0	0.0	3.60	**3**	0	−0.8	1.82
4	0	−1.8	3.32	**4**	3 (T6, T7, T11)	0.2	3.35
5	4 (T5, T6, T7, T11)	1.8	3.9	**5**	6 (T6, T8, T9, T10, T11, T12)	3.1	3.09
6	0	−1.6	3.48	**6**	3 (T6, T8, T11)	−3.4	2.32
7	2 (T5, T6)	−0.6	3.37	**7**	0	−0.9	2.20
8	0	−3.6	1.66	**8**	3 (L1, L3, L4)	−0.5	3.50
9	0	−0.2	4.44	**9**	1 (T5)	1.2	3.30
10	0	−1	4.04	**10**	0	−1.5	2.26
11	0	−2.4	3.25	**11**	8 (T7, T8, T10, T11, L1, L2, L3, L4)	3.4	4.22
12	0	−0.2	2.74	**12**	1 (T11)	4.9	3.35
13	0	0.5	3.54	**13**	1 (L4)	−1	2.02
14	0	1.1	3.30	**14**	0	0.1	3.44
15	0	−0.8	4.21	**15**	2 (T7, T8)	−2.9	2.05
16	0	1.4	2.81	**16**	1 (T11)	0.9	1.38
17	0	−0.2	4.39	-	-	-	-
Mean ± SD	-	−0.49 ± 1.47	3.45 ± 0.68	-	-	0.36 ± 2.28	2.79 ± 0.78

*Indicates a significant difference between groups, $P < 0.05$.

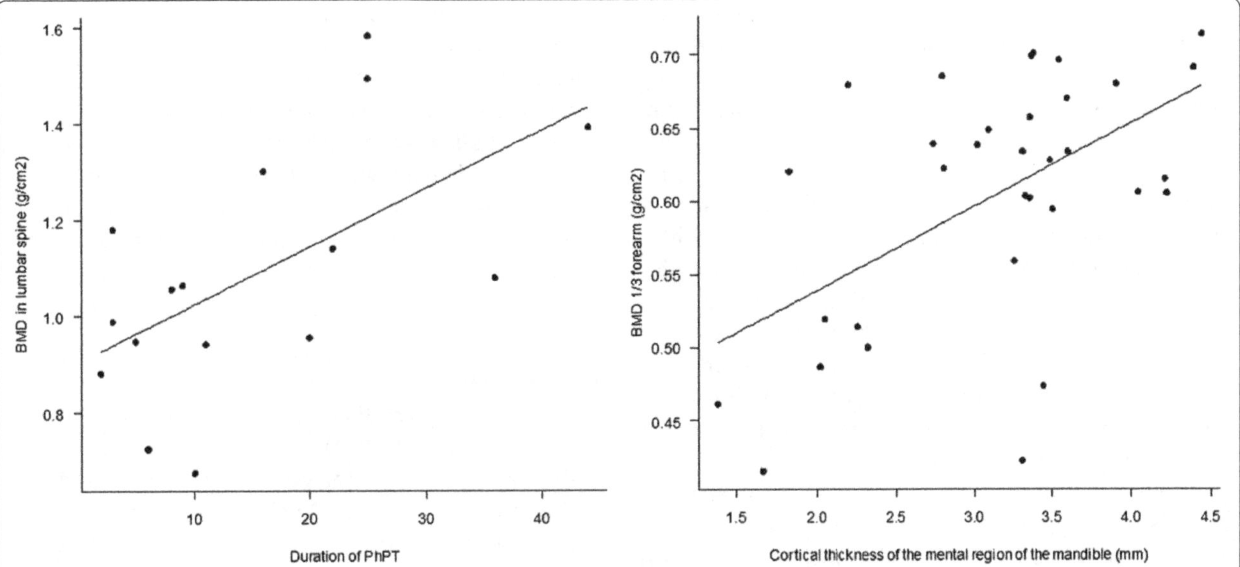

Figure 2 (Right) Correlation between bone mineral density in lumbar spine and duration of postsurgical hypoparathyroidism ($p = 0.03$ adjusted by TSH; $R2 = 0.35$) and (Left) correlation between bone mineral density and cortical thickness of the mental region of the mandible ($p < 0.01$; $R2 = 0.30$).

of PhPT in this group varied from 0.5 to 51 yr. These authors observed that BMD in patients with hypoparathyroidism was higher when compared with the age predicted mean at the lumbar spine and proximal femur, but not at the distal radius [25]. The present study replicates this spectrum on a different level, with BMD being only slightly increased in the lumbar spine due to wide heterogeneity among patients and being modestly decreased in the proximal femur of PhPT patients, whereas bone mass was decreased in the distal forearm. The divergences between studies are probably due to differences in the profile of the patients examined. Different from other studies, we adopted more rigid criteria for the selection of volunteers. Patients with previous diagnosis of thyroid cancer and hyperthyroidism were excluded, ultimately avoiding the inclusion of individuals affected by other disorders associated with bone loss and fracture. Another difference is that previous studies included pre- and postmenopausal women, whereas only postmenopausal women participated in the present study. Akin to other studies, our patients showed a great variability in the duration of PhPT [25]. This aspect can, at least in part, account for the large variation of BMD values in patients with PhPT. The relevance of this point is reinforced by the strong positive correlation between PhPT duration and BMD.

It should be mentioned that BMD assessment by DXA in PhPT was comparable to that described in primary hyperparathyroidism. It is well known that cortical bone is preferentially affected by primary hyperparathyroidism, and the same pattern was observed in PhPT. It should be pointed out that the control group also had distal forearm BMD within the osteopenia range, a fact possibly related to population characteristics, since the same profile was observed in normal individuals in previous studies performed in our laboratory [25]. However, PhPT patients showed significantly lower distal forearm BMD compared to control individuals. Furthermore, the panoramic radiography of the mandible was especially useful to capture the reduction in cortical thickness in another bone site.

Despite the BMD of the lumbar spine, 63% of patients with PhPT showed at least one morphometric fracture in the dorsal/lumbar spine, and morphometric fractures were also detected in patients showing high bone mass. No study has previously evaluated fracture susceptibility in PhPT. The results indicate deterioration of bone quality, the other component that assures bone strength. A previous study [6] detected by Fourier transform infrared imaging of transiliac biopsies that the collagen cross-link ratio was significantly higher in hypoparathyroid subjects compared to normal individuals. Based on these and other results the authors suggested that bone has low turnover rate and acquires a mature or hypermature profile in PhPTH [6]. Although, we have assessed only osteocalcin and DPD as biochemical bone markers of bone remodeling, our results support previous data obtained by bone histomorphometry. Decreased osteocalcin reflects reduced osteoblast activity in hypoparathyroidism. A reduced rate of bone remodeling which was reversed by intermittent administration of subcutaneous PTH has also been demonstrated by histomorphometric analysis in PhPT patients [7]. In support of these data we observed that osteocalcin levels were significantly lower in PhPT patients than in normal individuals. On a long-term basis, the impairment of bone renewal is implicated in inefficient repair of microdamage and ultimately in fracture susceptibility.

Other factors must be taken into account regarding impairment of bone strength in PhPT patients, especially in those with high BMD. Thickening of trabecular bone could compromise bone strength by reducing resilience [26,27]. In normal bone, the elastic properties of trabecular bone allow the skeleton to absorb energy by deforming reversibly when loaded [28]. Although the greater mineral content in the hypoparathyroid bone might produce greater material stiffness, it may do so at the expense of the ability of the bone to deform and thus to absorb and dissipate energy. Without elastic deformation, it is possible that hypoparathyroid bone could be vulnerable to structural failure. Because the effectiveness of bone in stopping cracks is directly proportional to the stiffness ratio across its internal interfaces, a homogeneous material will be less effective in slowing or stopping cracks initiated in the bone matrix, permitting cracks to grow more quickly to critical size and ultimately increase fracture risk [29,30].

Previous studies have shown that growth hormone deficiency impairs PTH circadian rhythm [31] and PTH action [32,33]. In order to detect hormonal alterations in the growth hormone (GH)/IGF-I axis, in the present study we assessed serum IGF-I levels and the results showed that PhPT patients have a lightly lower circulatory IGF-I level than control individuals. However, we did not measure GH secretion or GH/IGF-I sensitivity in PhPT patients. Additionally, vitamin D sufficiency was evaluated and all patients showed normal serum 25(OH)D levels conferring a convenient substrate supply for paracrine/autocrine synthesis of $1,25(OH)_2D$. Endocrine levels of $1,25(OH)_2D$ are largely dependent of PTH secretion, but all patients were taking physiological doses of calcitriol. Although, no woman of the control group was receiving calcium and vitamin D supplementation, they exhibited normal serum levels of 25-OHD. In agreement with these results, we did not observe a high frequency of hypovitaminosis D in this region of the state of São Paulo, Brazil, in previous studies [34,35]. As vitamin D deficiency is associated with worse bone outcome, it is likely that our groups were in advantageous conditions compared to other populations with a higher incidence of vitamin D deficiency [36].

Previous studies have shown increased serum levels of RANKL and maintained OPG levels in primary hyperparathyroidism [37]. Also, it was observed that intermittent administration of PTH to glucocorticoid-treated patients increases serum levels of RANKL and decreases serum levels of OPG [38]. In the present study no difference was detected in RANKL and OPG serum level of PhPT patients in comparison to control subjects. To our knowledge, no previous study addressed serum RANKL levels in postsurgical hypoparathyroidism. Although low PTH levels might be expected to provoke decreased RANKL levels, it should be considered that $1,25(OH)_2D$ stimulates RANKL synthesis.

The present study has some limitation; the number of patients studied was insufficient to definitively associate postsurgical hypoparathyroidism with increased fracture risk. However, these are important preliminary data for a more comprehensive study to examine the dissociation between bone fragility and bone mineral density in patients harboring postsurgical hypoparathyroidism.

Conclusions

Our results suggest that PhPT has a great impact on bone structure which is not necessarily detected by BMD density. Subclinical vertebral fracture was identified in more than 60% of PhPT patients, including those exhibiting high BMD. Panoramic radiography of the mandible should be thoroughly scrutinized to determine its place in the diagnosis or screening of osteoporosis. This site was useful to reveal cortical changes in PhPT. Panoramic radiography has the additional advantage of relying on a dentist for the screening of osteoporotic patients. The study encourages further investigation to determine the role of PTH as hormone replacement therapy in postsurgical hypoparathyroidism.

Abbreviations

BMD: Bone mineral density; BMI: Body mass index; CG: Control group; CV: Coefficient of variation; DPD: Urinary deoxypyridinoline; DXA: Dual energy X-ray absorptiometry; FMRP-USP: School of Medicine of Ribeirão Preto, University of São Paulo; IGF-I: Insulin-like growth factor; OPG: Osteoprotegerin; OC: Osteocalcin; PTH: Parathyroid hormone; PhPT: Hypoparathyroidism; PhPTG: Hypoparathyroidism group; RANK-L: Receptor activator of nuclear factor-κB ligand; 25-OH-D: 25-hydroxyvitamin D.

Competing interests

The authors declare no conflict of interests.

Authors' contributions

MLM participated in patient selection/sample collections, laboratory measurements and data analysis. FAP participated in sample collections, laboratory and bone mass measurerements. MHN-B participated in the study design and in the supervision of vertebral morphometry evaluation. LMM performed radiographic exams and the first blind evaluation of vertebral morphometry. SRT performed radiographic exams and the second blind evaluation of vertebral morphometry. PCAW performed radiographic exams of mandible and the correspondent evaluations. LMZM participated in patient selection, study design and laboratory evaluations. FJAdP participated in study design and laboratory measurements, supervised data collection and analysis and wrote the manuscript. All authors revised the manuscript. All authors read and approved the final manuscript.

Acknowledgments

M.L.M. received financial support from Coordenação de Aperfeiçoamento de Pessoal de Nível Superior (CAPES) and FJAP receive financial support from CNPq (306027/2011-9). This study received financial support from Fundação de Apoio ao Ensino Pesquisa e Assistência (FAEPA). We thank Sebastião Brandão Filho and Marta T. Nakao for technical assistance and Prof. Dr. Edson Z. Martinez for expert contribution on the statistical analysis.

Author details
[1]Department of Internal Medicine, School of Medicine of Ribeirão Preto, University of São Paulo, São Paulo, Brazil. [2]Department of Radiology, School of Dentistry of Ribeirão Preto, University of São Paulo, São Paulo, Brazil. [3]Department of Internal Medicine, School of Medicine of Ribeirão Preto, University of São Paulo, Av. Bandeirantes 3900, Ribeirão Preto, SP 14049-900, Brazil.

References

1. Jilka RL: **Molecular and cellular mechanisms of the anabolic effect of intermittent PTH.** *Bone* 2007, **40:**1434–1446.
2. Jilka RL, O'Brien CA, Bartell SM, Weinstein RS, Manolagas SC: **Continuous elevation of PTH increases the number of osteoblasts via both osteoclast-dependent and -independent mechanisms.** *J Bone Miner Res* 2010, **25:**2427–2437.
3. de Paula FJ, Rosen CJ: **Back to the future: revisiting parathyroid hormone and calcitonin control of bone remodeling.** *Horm Metab Res* 2010, **42:**299–306.
4. Pereira LC, Pereira FA, Sá MF, Foss MC, de Paula FJ: **Parathyroid hormone secretion in women in late menopause submitted to EDTA-induced hypocalcemia.** *Maturitas* 2008, **59:**91–94.
5. Silverberg SJ, Shane E, de la Cruz L, Segre GV, Clemens TL, Bilezikian JP: **Abnormalities in parathyroid hormone secretion and 1,25-diydroxyvitamin D3 formation in women with osteoporosis.** *N Engl J Med* 1989, **320:**277–281.
6. Rubin MR, Bilezikian JP: **Hypoparathyroidism: clinical features, skeletal microstructure and parathyroid hormone replacement.** *Arq Bras Endocrinol Metabol* 2010, **54:**220–226.
7. Rubin MR, Manavalan JS, Dempster DW, Shah J, Cremers S, Kousteni S, Zhou H, McMahon DJ, Kode A, Sliney J, Shane E, Silverberg SJ, Bilezikian JP: **Parathyroid hormone stimulates circulating osteogenic cells in hypoparathyroidism.** *J Clin Endocrinol Metab* 2011, **96:**176–186.
8. Laway BA, Goswami R, Singh N, Gupta N, Seith A: **Pattern of bone mineral density in patients with sporadic idiopathic hypoparathyroidism.** *Clin Endocrinol (Oxf)* 2006, **64:**405–409.
9. World Health Organization: *Assessment of fracture risk and its application to screening for postmenopausal osteoporosis.* Geneva: Switzerland; 1994.
10. Khosla S, Melton LJ 3rd: **Clinical practice. Osteopenia.** *N Engl J Med* 2007, **356:**2293–2300.
11. Kanis JA, Oden A, Johnell O, Johansson H, De Laet C, Brown J, Burckhardt P, Cooper C, Christiansen C, Cummings S, Eisman JA, Fujiwara S, Glüer C, Goltzman D, Hans D, Krieg MA, La Croix A, McCloskey E, Mellstrom D, Melton LJ 3rd, Pols H, Reeve J, Sanders K, Schott AM, Silman A, Torgerson D, van Staa T, Watts NB, Yoshimura N: **The use of clinical risk factors enhances the performance of BMD in the prediction of hip and osteoporotic fractures in men and women.** *Osteoporos Int* 2007, **18:**1033–1046.
12. Seeman E, Delmas PD: **Bone quality–the material and structural basis of bone strength and fragility.** *N Engl J Med* 2006, **354:**2250–2261.
13. Hippisley-Cox J, Coupland C: **Predicting risk of osteoporotic fracture in men and women in England and Wales: prospective derivation and validation of QFracture Scores.** *BMJ* 2009, **339:**b4229.
14. Vlasiadis KZ, Damilakis J, Velegrakis GA, Skouteris CA, Fragouli I, Goumenou A, Matalliotakis J, Koumantakis EE: **Relationship between BMD, dental panoramic radiographic findings and biochemical markers of bone turnover in diagnosis of osteoporosis.** *Maturitas* 2008, **59:**226–233.
15. Tanner R, Wall BF, Shrimpton PC, Hart D, Bungay DR: **Frequency of medical and dental x-ray examination in the UK.** 2000, NRPB-R320.
16. Devlin H, Allen P, Graham J, Jacobs R, Nicopoulou-Karayianni K, Lindh C, Marjanovic E, Adams J, Pavitt S, van der Stelt P, Horner K: **The role of the dental surgeon in detecting osteoporosis: the OSTEODENT study.** *Br Dent J* 2008, **204:**E16. discussion 560–561.
17. Watanabe PC, Farman A, Watanabe MG, Issa JP: **Radiographic signals detection of systemic disease. Orthopantomographic Radiography.** *Int J Morphol* 2008, **26:**915–926.
18. Horner K, Allen P, Graham J, Jacobs R, Boonen S, Pavitt S, Nackaerts O, Marjanovic E, Adams JE, Karayianni K, Lindh C, van der Stelt P, Devlin H: **The relationship between the OSTEODENT index and hip fracture risk assessment using FRAX.** *Oral Surg Oral Med Oral Pathol Oral Radiol Endod* 2010, **110:**243–249.
19. Bras J, van Ooij CP, Abraham-Inpijn K, Kusen GJ, Wilmink JM: **Interpretation of the mandibular angular cortex: a diagnostic tool in metabolic bone loss. Part I. Normal state and postmenopausal osteoporosis.** *Oral Surg* 1982, **53:**541–545.
20. Ledgerton D, Horner K, Devlin H, Worthington H: **Panoramic mandibular index as a radiomorphometric tool: an assessment of precision.** *Dentomaxillofac Radiol* 1997, **26:**95–100.
21. Taguchi A, Suei Y, Ohtsuka M, Otani K, Tanimoto K, Ohtaki M: **Usefulness of panoramic radiography in the diagnosis of postmenopausal osteoporosis in women. Width and morphology of inferior cortex of the mandible.** *Dentomaxillofac Radiol* 1996, **25:**263–267.
22. Hsieh FY, Bloch DA, Larsen MD: **A simple method of sample size calculation for linear and logistic regression.** *Stat Med* 1998, **17:**1623–1634.
23. Chan FK, Tiu SC, Choi KL, Choi CH, Kong AP, Shek CC: **Increased bone mineral density in patients with chronic hypoparathyroidism.** *J Clin Endocrinol Metab* 2003, **88:**3155–3159.
24. Rubin MR, Dempster DW, Zhou H, Shane E, Nickolas T, Sliney J Jr, Silverberg SJ, Bilezikian JP: **Dynamic and structural properties of the skeleton in hypoparathyroidism.** *J Bone Miner Res* 2008, **23:**2018–2024.
25. Duan Y, De Luca V, Seeman E: **Parathyroid hormone deficiency and excess: similar effects on trabecular bone but differing effects on cortical bone.** *J Clin Endocrinol Metab* 1999, **84:**718–722.
26. Currey J: **Structural heterogeneity in bone: good or bad?** *J Musculoskelet Neuronal Interact* 2005, **5:**317.
27. Rubin MR, Dempster DW, Kohler T, Stauber M, Zhou H, Shane E, Nickolas T, Stein E, Sliney J Jr, Silverberg SJ, Bilezikian JP, Müller R: **Three dimensional cancellous bone structure in hypoparathyroidism.** *Bone* 2010, **46:**190–195.
28. Lanyon LE, Baggott DG: **Mechanical function as an influence on the structure and form of bone.** *J Bone Joint Surg Br* 1976, **58-B:**436–443.
29. Turner CH: **Bone strength: current concepts.** *Ann N Y Acad Sci* 2006, **1068:**429–446.
30. Shane E, Burr D, Ebeling PR, Abrahamsen B, Adler RA, Brown TD, Cheung AM, Cosman F, Curtis JR, Dell R, Dempster D, Einhorn TA, Genant HK, Geusens P, Klaushofer K, Koval K, Lane JM, McKiernan F, McKinney R, Ng A, Nieves J, O'Keefe R, Papapoulos S, Sen HT, van der Meulen MC, Weinstein RS, Whyte M, American Society for Bone and Mineral Research: **Atypical subtrochanteric and diaphyseal femoral fractures: report of a task force of the American Society for Bone and Mineral Research.** *J Bone Miner Res* 2010, **25:**2267–2294.
31. Ahmad AM, Hopkins MT, Fraser WD, Ooi CG, Durham BH, Vora JP: **Parathyroid hormone secretory pattern, circulating activity, and effect on bone turnover in adult growth hormone deficiency.** *Bone* 2003, **32:**170–179.
32. Ahmad AM, Thomas J, Clewes A, Hopkins MT, Guzder R, Ibrahim H, Durham BH, Vora JP, Fraser WD: **Effects of growth hormone replacement on parathyroid hormone sensitivity and bone mineral metabolism.** *J Clin Endocrinol Metab* 2003, **88:**2860–2868.
33. White HD, Ahmad AM, Durham BH, Patwala A, Whittingham P, Fraser WD, Vora JP: **Growth hormone replacement is important for the restoration of parathyroid hormone sensitivity and improvement in bone metabolism in older adult growth hormone-deficient patients.** *J Clin Endocrinol Metab* 2005, **90:**3371–3380.
34. Ribeiro FB, Pereira Fde A, Muller E, Foss NT, de Paula FJ: **Evaluation of bone and mineral metabolism in patients recently diagnosed with leprosy.** *Am J Med Sci* 2007, **334:**322–326.
35. Pereira FA, de Castro JA, dos Santos JE, Foss MC, Paula FJ: **Impact of marked weight loss induced by bariatric surgery on bone mineral density and remodeling.** *Braz J Med Biol Res* 2007, **40:**509–517.
36. de Paula FJ, Rosen CJ: **Vitamin D safety and requirements.** *Arch Biochem Biophys* 2012, **523:**64–72.
37. Nakchbandi IA, Lang R, Kinder B, Insogna KL: **The role of the receptor activator of nuclear factor-kappaB ligand/osteoprotegerin cytokine system in primary hyperparathyroidism.** *J Clin Endocrinol Metab* 2008, **93:**967–973.
38. Buxton EC, Yao W, Lane NE: **Changes in serum receptor activator of nuclear factor-κB ligand, osteoprotegerin, and interleukin-6 levels in patients with glucocorticoid-induced osteoporosis treated with human parathyroid hormone (1–34).** *J Clin Endocrinol Metab* 2004, **89:**3332–3336.

7

The use of endobronchial ultrasound-guided transbronchial needle aspiration in the diagnosis of thyroid lesions

Roberto F Casal[1*], Mimi N Phan[1], Keerthana Keshava[2], Jose M Garcia[3], Horiana Grosu[2], D Ray Lazarus[1], Juan Iribarren[1] and Daniel G Rosen[4]

Abstract

Background: Non-palpable thyroid nodules can be difficult to access by conventional ultrasound-guided fine needle aspiration, particularly when they are intrathoracic. Many of these patients are subject to multiple follow up scans or invasive diagnostic procedures such as mediastinoscopy or surgical resection. We aim to describe the feasibility of endobronchial ultrasound-guided transbronchial needle aspiration (EBUS-TBNA) for diagnosis of thyroid lesions.

Methods: All EBUS-TBNA performed at our institutions from February 2010 to February 2013 were screened, and those in which a thyroid biopsy was performed were reviewed.

Results: We identified 12 cases of EBUS-TBNA thyroid biopsy. Nine patients had an indication for EBUS in addition to their thyroid lesions. The median age was 64 years (range 44 to 84 years), and 10 patients were male. Median lesion size was 22.5 mm (range, 10 to 43 mm). Five lesions were strictly intrathoracic. All cases were sampled with a 22G needle and rapid on-site cytologic examination. Adequate samples were obtained in all 12 cases. Malignancy was identified in 3 of the 12 patients (metastatic breast adenocarcinoma, large B-cell lymphoma, and metastatic lung adenocarcinoma). The remaining 9 samples were deemed to be benign nodules. Seven of these were confirmed by clinical follow-up (n = 3), biopsies (n = 3), or surgery (n = 1).
There were no EBUS-related complications.

Conclusions: EBUS-TBNA might be a safe and effective alternative for sampling thyroid lesions, particularly useful for those located below the thoracic inlet. Further prospective studies are required to compare its diagnostic yield and safety profile with standard techniques.

Keywords: EBUS-TBNA, Thyroid, Intrathoracic goiter

Background

Thyroid nodules occur in about 5-7% of the population, and of those, about 5% turn out to be malignant. Malignancy can be diagnosed through ultrasound-guided fine needle aspiration (US- FNA) with a low rate of complications and adequate samples for diagnosis in about 80% of cases, making it the procedure of choice [1-3]. Nevertheless, access to lesions that lie near the thoracic inlet or within the thoracic cavity can be difficult, risky, or even impossible with US- FNA. These cases typically lead to multiple follow up images or more invasive diagnostic modalities such as mediastinoscopy or surgical excision.

Endobronchial ultrasound-guided transbronchial needle aspiration (EBUS-TBNA) is now a well- established technique for sampling peribronchial and paratracheal lymph nodes and masses [4,5]. It plays a key role in mediastinal staging of lung cancer with comparable and even superior diagnostic yield than mediastinoscopy, and with an excellent safety profile [6-8]. Literature review reveals only a few case reports of EBUS-TBNA for

* Correspondence: casal@bcm.edu
[1]Section of Pulmonary and Critical Care Medicine, Baylor College of Medicine, Michael E. DeBakey VA Medical Center. 2002 Holcombe Blvd. Pulmonary Section 111i, Houston, TX 77030, USA

the diagnosis of intrathoracic thyroid lesions [9-11]. The aim of this study is to describe our experience of EBUS-TBNA for the sampling of thyroid lesions in terms of feasibility, diagnostic yield and safety profile.

Methods

After obtaining IRB approval, medical records from all EBUS-TBNA procedures performed on patients older than 18 years of age at the Michael E. DeBakey VA Medical Center (Houston, Texas) and at the New York Methodist Hospital (Brooklyn, New York) from February 2010 to February 2013 were reviewed. Due to the retrospective nature of the study, patient consent was waived by our local IRB (Institutional Review Board). We retrieved and analyzed those cases in which a thyroid biopsy was performed with EBUS-TBNA. Demographic and clinical data were obtained, including: baseline thyroid disease, size and location of thyroid lesion, indications for bronchoscopy, pre-procedure diagnoses, imaging reports prior to bronchoscopy and up to 12 months afterwards when available, description of techniques used in acquiring and processing the biopsy, documented complications of biopsy acquisition, pathology reports, and clinical reports up to 12 months after EBUS-TBNA. The result provided by EBUS-TBNA biopsy was compared to that of surgically removed thyroid specimens or US-FNA when available. Otherwise, the patient's clinical course and follow up images for up to 12 months were examined to determine if there was a correlation with the original diagnosis.

Results

We identified 12 cases of EBUS-TBNA thyroid biopsy. In 9 patients, the primary indication for EBUS-TBNA was sampling of mediastinal lymph nodes or masses, and biopsy of the thyroid was done in addition to this during the same procedure. In the remainder 3, biopsy of an intrathoracic thyroid lesion was the only indication for EBUS-TBNA. Eleven patients underwent the procedure via laryngeal mask airway under general anesthesia and one under moderate sedation via oropharynx. In all cases biopsies were performed using a real-time ultrasound biopsy bronchoscope (XBF-UC260F-OL8; Olympus Ltd.; Tokyo, Japan) in standard fashion. Only in one procedure the operator reported difficulty introducing the needle through the tracheal wall due to the acute angle necessary to reach the lesion. Samples were obtained with a dedicated 22-gauge needle (NA-201SX; Olympus Ltd.; Tokyo, Japan), with an average of 4 passes. On-site cytology examination was available in all procedures. Needle aspirates were smeared onto slides and air-dried or fixed in 95% alcohol, collecting the remaining aspirate for cell-block preparation. Slides were processed immediately using Romanowsky technique (Diff- Quik®) and/or Pap- staining. The characteristics of each patient are summarized in Table 1. The median age was 64 years (range 44 to 84 years), and 10 patients (83%) were male. Median lesion size in the short axis was 22.5 mm (range, 10 to 43 mm). Eleven lesions (92%) were on the left thyroid lobe and one on the right. Five lesions (42%) were strictly intrathoracic. Adequate samples were obtained in all 12 cases (see examples in Figure 1). Malignancy was identified in 3 (25%) patients: metastatic adenocarcinoma of the breast, large B-cell lymphoma, and metastatic adenocarcinoma of lung origin. There was thyroid tissue in the background of these biopsies confirming thyroid sampling. These were *de novo* diagnosis of malignancy for each patient. The remaining 9 samples were deemed to be benign lesions (follicular nodules = 8, multinodular goiter = 1,). Seven of these 9 benign diagnoses were confirmed by clinical-radiographic follow-up (n = 3), CT-guided or US-FNA (n = 3), or surgery (n = 1). Based on the clinical and radiographical (i.e. radionuclide scanning, follow-up ultrasound) behavior of these lesions, they were all presumed to be benign. The diagnosis of multinodular goiter was made with histopathology from surgical resection. There were no EBUS-related complications. Of note, one of the patients who underwent a subsequent US-FNA developed a large hematoma as a complication of the procedure.

Discussion

Ultrasound-guided FNA is the procedure of choice for sampling of thyroid nodules [12]. Nevertheless, for those lesions located below the thoracic inlet, the procedure becomes challenging and it imposes a higher risk since the needle trajectory is close to many vital structures. Our case series demonstrates that EBUS-TBNA is a feasible diagnostic approach for these lesions, being potentially safe and effective as well.

As previously mentioned, US-FNA provides diagnostically useful information in about 80% of thyroid nodules and has an average sensitivity of about 95% in patients with malignant thyroid nodules [13]. In our limited experience, EBUS-TBNA has provided cytologic samples comparable to those of US-FNA. Moreover, the EBUS scope also allowed us to characterize the gland and lesion in question providing ultrasonographic characteristics that can predict malignancy: solid mass, microcalcifications, increased vascularity, irregular borders [3]. Nevertheless, the authors could not over emphasize the fact that the decision to sample any thyroid lesion should always be made together with the managing endocrinologist. The diagnostic work up of the thyroid nodule has been extensively reviewed elsewhere in the literature and it is not within the scope of our manuscript [1,3,13,14].

Our malignancy rate was much higher (3/12, 25%) than that expected for thyroid nodules in the general

Table 1 Patient characteristics

Subject	Baseline thyroid disease	Indication for procedure	Size (mm)**	Strictly intrathoracic	Diagnosis
1	Multinodular goiter	Multiple lung masses, enlarged mediastinal LNs	19	No	Follicular nodule
2	None	Lung mass w/ enlarged hilar LNs	26	No	Large B-cell lymphoma
3	None	Lung mass	20	No	Follicular nodule
4*	None	Enlarged mediastinal LNs	20	Yes	Metastatic breast adenocarcinoma
5	None	Superior mediastinal mass	25	Yes	Follicular nodule
6	None	Lung mass	18	No	Follicular nodule
7	Subclinical hypothyroidism	Lung mass	33	Yes	Follicular nodule
8	Subclinical hyperthyroidism	Enlarged mediastinal LNs	32	Yes	Follicular nodule
9	None	Lung mass, enlarged mediastinal LNs	10	No	Metastatic lung adenocarcinoma
10	None	Lung mass w/ enlarged hilar LNs	33	No	Follicular nodule
11	None	Substernal thyroid mass	44	No	Follicular nodule
12*	None	Incidentally found anterior mediastinal mass	16	Yes	Multinodular goiter

*Patients number 4 and 12 were the only female in this study.
**Measured in the short axis.

population (5%). Moreover, all malignancies were metastatic to the thyroid, and none were primary thyroid neoplasms. We, indeed, found the most common non-thyroid malignancies that involve the thyroid: lymphoma, breast cancer, and lung cancer. This is likely because our population was referred for EBUS-TBNA of mediastinal lymph nodes or masses, hence with a much higher pre-test probability of having a malignancy outside the thyroid. The need to sample the thyroid, in addition to their lung or mediastinal lesions, was to rule out a second primary cancer. Four of our patients had an incidental finding of an 18-fluorodeoxyglucose avid thyroid nodule by positron emission tomography (PET) scan. Three of these four were confirmed to be malignant with EBUS-TBNA. A systematic review from Shie and coworkers found the prevalence of incidental focal abnormalities detected by PET in the thyroid gland to be roughly 1% (571 from 55160 patients) [15]. Of these

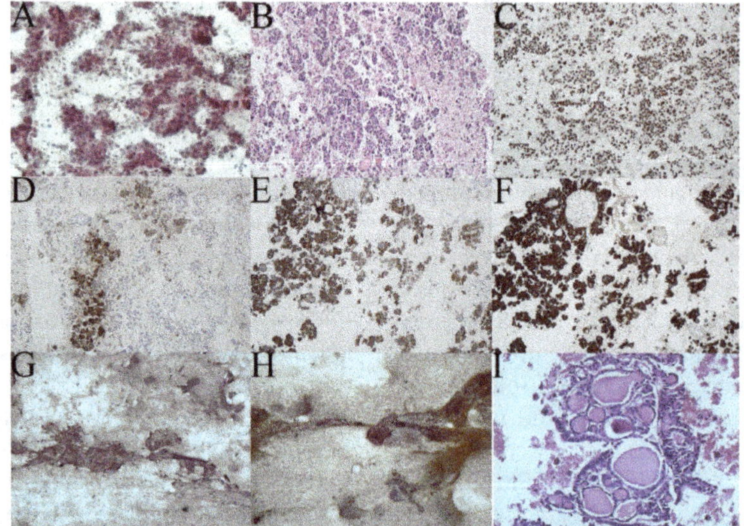

Figure 1 Representative microphotographs from EBUS-guided thyroid aspirations. Representative microphotographs from EBUS procedure: **(A)** papanicoulau stained smear and **(B)** cell block showing a poorly differentiated adenocarcinoma with papillary features. Immunohistochemistry showed these tumor cells with strong and diffuse positivity for TTF1 **(C)**, focal staining for carcinoembryonic antigen **(D)**, strong diffuse positivivty for CK7 **(E)**, and strong diffuse positivity for pancytokeratin. **(G)** and **(H)** show papanicoulau stained smear with clusters of benign follicular cells and colloid. **(I)** Cell block preparation showing thyroid follicles with colloid consistent with follicular nodule.

incidentally found thyroid nodules 33.2% were malignant in origin, which suggests that these findings need to be confirmed by cytology or histology.

Wakeley and Mulvany divided intrathoracic goiters into three types based on location and extent: "a", small substernal extension of a mainly cervical thyroid goiter; "b", partial intrathoracic goiter wherein the major portion of the goiter is situated within the thorax; and "c", complete intrathoracic goiter wherein the goiter lies entirely within the thoracic cavity [16,17]. Following this classification, in our small series, 5 patients were type "a", 2 patients were type "b", and 5 type "c".

Ultrasound guided-FNA complications are typically minor and self-limited such as local pain and small hematomas. More severe complications occur in less than 5% of cases: large hematoma, infection, needle track seeding of malignancy, recurrent laryngeal nerve palsy [2]. EBUS-TBNA has also been demonstrated to be an extremely safe procedure with an overall complication rate of less than 2% [8]. Data on patients undergoing EBUS-TBNA in the American College of Chest Physicians Quality Improvement Registry, Evaluation and Education (AQuIRE) database found that out of 1,317 patients at six hospitals, complications occurred in 19 patients only. There were no infectious complications, and pneumothorax, which occurred in 7 patients, was in fact associated with the addition of transbronchial lung biopsy [8]. Of note, there has been a recent report of an EBUS-TBNA biopsy of a cystic thyroid nodule which resulted in a thyroid abscess [18]. Unlike US-FNA, a completely aseptic technique, EBUS- TBNA implies passing the needle through the working channel of the bronchoscope that might be contaminated with oropharyngeal flora and/or tracheobronchial secretions. Physicians should be aware of this potential risk of infection, and cystic lesions in particular should be avoided.

Conclusions

To the best of our knowledge, this is the first series to describe the use of EBUS-TBNA for the sampling of thyroid lesions. In patients with intrathoracic thyroid lesions, EBUS-TBNA could potentially prevent complications associated with more invasive procedures, or reduce cost and anxiety associated with close follow-up and repeat imaging. We hope our results will prompt prospective comparisons between EBUS-TBNA, US-FNA and surgical approach to thoroughly assess its yield and safety profile. Until then, EBUS-TBNA should be reserved for intrathoracic thyroid lesions that are not amenable for US-FNA.

Abbreviations

EBUS-TBNA: Endobronchial ultrasound-guided transbronchial needle aspiration; US-FNA: Ultrasound-guided fine needle aspiration; PET: Positron emission tomography.

Competing interests

The authors declare that they have no competing interests.

Authors' contributions

MP, KK, HG, JG, DR, and RFC conceived the study. MP, KK, JI, and DRL collected the data. DR evaluated cytology samples. All authors participated in the design of the study and helped to draft the manuscript. All authors read and approved the final manuscript.

Author details

[1]Section of Pulmonary and Critical Care Medicine, Baylor College of Medicine, Michael E. DeBakey VA Medical Center. 2002 Holcombe Blvd. Pulmonary Section 111i, Houston, TX 77030, USA. [2]Division of Pulmonary and Critical Care Medicine, New York Methodist Hospital, Brooklyn, NY, USA. [3]Division of Endocrinology, Diabetes and Metabolism, Baylor College of Medicine, Houston, TX, USA. [4]Department of Pathology and Immunology, Baylor College of Medicine, Houston, TX, USA.

References

1. Hegedus L: **The thyroid nodule.** *N Engl J Med* 2004, **351**:1764–1771.
2. Polyzos SA, Anastasilakis AD: **Clinical complications following thyroid fine-needle biopsy: a systematic review.** *Clin Endocrinol (Oxf)* 2009, **71**:157–165.
3. Cooper DS, Doherty GM, Haugen BR, Kloos RT, Lee SL, Mandel SJ, Mazzaferri EL, McIver B, Pacini F, Schlumberger M, Sherman SI, Steward DL, Tuttle RM: **Revised American Thyroid Association management guidelines for patients with thyroid nodules and differentiated thyroid cancer.** *Thyroid* 2009, **19**:1167–1214.
4. Herth FJ, Eberhardt R, Vilmann P, Krasnik M, Ernst A: **Real-time endobronchial ultrasound guided transbronchial needle aspiration for sampling mediastinal lymph nodes.** *Thorax* 2006, **61**:795–798.
5. Yasufuku K, Chiyo M, Sekine Y, Chhajed PN, Shibuya K, Iizasa T, Fujisawa T: **Real- time endobronchial ultrasound-guided transbronchial needle aspiration of mediastinal and hilar lymph nodes.** *Chest* 2004, **126**:122–128.
6. Ernst AAD, Eberhardt R, Krasnik M, Herth FJ: **Diagnosis of mediastinal adenopathy- real-time endobronchial ultrasound guided needle aspiration versus mediastinoscopy.** *J Thorac Oncol* 2008, **3**:577–582.
7. Yasufuku K, Pierre A, Darling G, de Perrot M, Waddell T, Johnston M, da Cunha Santos G, Geddie W, Boerner S, Le LW, Keshavjee S: **A prospective controlled trial of endobronchial ultrasound-guided transbronchial needle aspiration compared with mediastinoscopy for mediastinal lymph node staging of lung cancer.** *J Thorac Cardiovasc Surg* 2011, **142**:1393–1400. e1391.
8. Eapen GA, Shah AM, Lei X, Jimenez CA, Morice RC, Yarmus L, Filner J, Ray C, Michaud G, Greenhill SR, Sarkiss M, Casal R, Rice D: **Complications, consequences, and practice patterns of endobronchial ultrasound-guided transbronchial needle aspiration: results of the AQuIRE registry.** *Chest* 2013, **143**:1044–1053.
9. Chalhoub MHK: **The use of endobronchial ultrasonography with transbronchial needle aspiration to sample a solitary substernal thyroid nodule.** *Chest* 2010, **137**:1435–1436.
10. Jeebun VNS, Harrison R: **Diagnosis of a posterior mediastinal goitre via endobronchial ultrasound-guided transbronchial needle aspiration.** *Eur Respir J* 2009, **34**:773–775.
11. Chalhoub M, Harris K: **Endobronchial ultrasonography with transbronchial needle aspiration to sample a solitary substernal thyroid nodule: a new approach.** *Heart Lung Circ* 2012, **21**:761–762.
12. La Rosa GL, Belfiore A, Giuffrida D, Sicurella C, Ippolito O, Russo G, Vigneri R: **Evaluation of the fine needle aspiration biopsy in the preoperative selection of cold thyroid nodules.** *Cancer* 1991, **67**:2137–2141.
13. Burch HB: **Evaluation and management of the solid thyroid nodule.** *Endocrinol Metab Clin North Am* 1995, **24**:663–710.
14. Tan GH, Gharib H: **Thyroid incidentalomas: management approaches to nonpalpable nodules discovered incidentally on thyroid imaging.** *Ann Intern Med* 1997, **126**:226–231.
15. Shie P, Cardarelli R, Sprawls K, Fulda KG, Taur A: **Systematic review: prevalence of malignant incidental thyroid nodules identified on**

fluorine18 fluorodeoxyglucose positron emission tomography. *Nucl Med Commun* 2009, **30:**742–748.
16. Wakely CPG, Mulvaney JH: **Intrathoracic goiter.** *SGO* 1940, **70:**703.
17. Shields TW: *General Thoracic Surgery. Sixth Edition. Chapter 168.* 2005:2500–2512.
18. Kennedy MP, Breen M, O'Regan K, McCarthy J, Horgan M, Henry MT: **Endobronchial ultrasound-guided transbronchial needle aspiration of thyroid nodules: pushing the boundary too far?** *Chest* 2012, **142:**1690–1691.

8

Takotsubo cardiomyopathy and transient thyrotoxicosis during combination therapy with interferon-alpha and ribavirin for chronic hepatitis C

Carmen Sorina Martin[1], Luminita Nicoleta Ionescu[2], Carmen Gabriela Barbu[1], Anca Elena Sirbu[1], Ioana Maria Lambrescu[3], Ioana Smarandita Lacau[4], Doina Ruxandra Dimulescu[5] and Simona Vasilica Fica[1*]

Abstract

Background: Thyroid dysfunction is a common complication of chronic hepatitis C (CHC) and its therapy. Takotsubo cardiomyopathy (TCM) is a multifactorial, stress related cardiomyopathy, rarely reported in association with thyrotoxicosis. Simultaneous occurrence of TCM and thyrotoxicosis due to hepatitis C and its treatment has never been reported.

Case presentation: A 47-year-old woman was admitted for acute chest pain, dyspnea, palpitations and diaphoresis. She had been diagnosed with CHC and had undergone 7 months of IFNα and Ribavirin therapy. At admission electrocardiogram (ECG) showed ST segment elevation, negative T waves and troponin was elevated suggesting ST segment elevation myocardial infarction (STEMI). Echocardiography demonstrated left ventricular apical akinesia and ballooning, with a left ventricular ejection fraction (LVEF) of 35%. Contrast angiography showed normal epicardial coronaries, yet a ventriculogram revealed left ventricular apical ballooning, consistent with TCM. Cardiac MRI showed left ventricle apical ballooning and no late enhancement suggesting the absence of any edema, scar or fibrosis in the left myocardium. She was diagnosed with non-autoimmune destructive thyroiditis: TSH=0.001 mU/L, free T4=2.41 ng/dl, total T3=199 ng/dl and negative thyroid antibodies. The thyroid ultrasonography showed a diffuse small goiter, no nodules and normal vascularization of the parenchyma. Following supportive treatment she experienced a complete recovery after a few weeks and she successfully completed her antiviral treatment, with no thyroid or cardiovascular dysfunction ever since. In patients treated with IFNα for CHC, the prevalence of thyroid dysfunction varies between 2.5–45.3% of cases. TCM is a stress related cardiomyopathy characterized by elevated cardiac enzymes, normal coronary angiography and an acute, transient, left ventricular apical dysfunction that mimics myocardial infarction. Most of the patients survive the initial acute event, typically recover normal ventricular function within one to four weeks and have a favorable outcome, as was the case with our patient. Thyrotoxicosis induced stress cardiomyopathy is rare and has been mostly reported in association with Graves' disease, thyroid storm, thyrotoxicosis factitia or following radioiodine therapy for toxic multinodular goiter.

Conclusion: Routine thyroid screening should be done in patients receiving IFN-alpha and Ribavirin for CHC and thyrotoxicosis should be considered as a possible and treatable underlying cause of TCM.

Keywords: Takotsubo cardiomyopathy, Thyrotoxicosis, Chronic hepatitis C, Interferon-alpha, Ribavirin

* Correspondence: simonafica@yahoo.com
[1]Endocrinology Department, Carol Davila University of Medicine and Pharmacy, Elias University Hospital, 17 Marasti Blvd, sector 1, 011461 Bucharest, Romania
Full list of author information is available at the end of the article

Background

Every year, 3–4 million people are infected with the hepatitis C virus (HCV) and about 150 million people are nowadays chronically infected worldwide [1]. Thyroid dysfunction represents the most common endocrine manifestation of chronic hepatitis C (CHC). Combination therapy with Interferon-alpha (IFNα) and Ribavirin represents the standard treatment for CHC [2]. In patients treated with IFNα for CHC, the prevalence of thyroid dysfunction varies between 2.5–45.3% of cases [3], depending on the study and diagnostic criteria applied. The main types of interferon induced thyroiditis are: autoimmune thyroiditis (Hashimoto's thyroiditis, Graves' disease or the development of thyroid antibodies) and non-autoimmune thyroiditis (destructive thyroiditis or non-autoimmune hypothyroidism) [4]. Furthermore, thyroid dysfunction is more prevalent in patients treated with IFN-α and Ribavirin combination therapy (12.1%) than in patients treated with IFN-α alone (6.6%) [5].

Takotsubo cardiomyopathy (TCM) is a multifactorial, stress related cardiomyopathy characterized by elevated cardiac enzymes, normal coronary angiography and an acute, transient, left ventricular apical dysfunction that mimics myocardial infarction. TCM caused by thyrotoxicosis has previously been reported in about 12 cases since 2004 [6].

We report a rare case of TCM associated with transient thyrotoxicosis, in a female patient treated with IFN-α and Ribavirin for CHC, in order to highlight an unusual complication of thyrotoxicosis and the difficulties associated with the management of CHC.

Case presentation

In 2007, a 47- year- old Caucasian woman was admitted for acute chest pain, dyspnea, palpitations and diaphoresis. The symptoms had started 3 days prior to admission, after experiencing emotional stress related to public lecture. Metoprolol 100 mg/day had been started. The patient was a nonsmoker and had no personal history of cardiovascular disorders. She had been diagnosed with CHC in 2006 and had undergone 7 months of pegylate-IFN-alpha (180 μg/week) and Ribavirin (1000 mg/day) therapy. Physical examination on admission revealed a heart rate of 85 beats/min and blood pressure of 160/80 mmHg. Routine biochemical and hematological tests were normal, except for the presence of anemia (hemoglobin = 9.74 g/dl, hematocrit = 31.4%), leucopenia (white blood cell count = 4290/mm3, neutrophils = 2250/mm3), hypocholesterolemia (123 mg/dl) and mild increase in liver enzymes (ALT = 53, AST = 55UI/L). C reactive protein was negative. Plasma free metanephrines = 68 pg/ml (<90) and normetanephrines = 126 pg/ml (<180) were in the normal range. ECG at admission showed sinus rhythm 85 beats/min, ST segment elevation and negative T waves in DI, DII, aVF, aVL, V2-V6 leads (Figure 1). The peak troponin was 2 ng/ml (<0.29). Echocardiography showed normal cardiac cavities, left ventricular apical akinesia and ballooning, septal hypokinesia and a LVEF of 35% (Figure 2). Contrast angiography showed normal epicardial coronaries (Figure 3), yet a ventriculogram revealed left ventricular apical hypokinesis and ballooning, consistent with TCM. For differential diagnosis and tissue characterization, cardiac MRI was performed, showing apical ballooning of the left ventricle. There were no bright areas in T2 sequence with fat suppression and no late enhancement suggesting the absence of any edema, scar or fibrosis in the left myocardium (Figure 4).

During the first days the patient received supportive therapy with angiotensin converting enzyme inhibitors, beta-blockers (metoprolol 200 mg/day), platelet aggregation inhibitors, statin, low molecular weight heparin, nitrates and anxiolytics, with favorable resolution of dyspnea and no chest pain. The troponin returned rapidly to normal within 72 hours (0.044 ng/ml). Despite high dose beta-blockers she was persistently tachycardic. The endocrinological evaluation highlighted: patient with no family or personal history of thyroid disorders, without fever, pain in the cervical region or ophthalmopathy; she had palpitations, excessive sweating, intolerance to heat, nervousness, easy fatigability, hyperkinesia; TSH = 0.001 mU/L, free T4 = 2.41 ng/dl (0.71-1.85), total T3 = 199 ng/dl (81–178), anti-thyroid peroxidase antibodies (TPOAb) = 3.8 IU/ml (0–12), antithyroglobulin antibodies = 56 UI/ml (<115) and anti-thyrotropin receptor antibodies (TRAb) = 1.05 IU/L (<1.75). The thyroid ultrasonography showed a diffuse heterogenic small goiter, no nodules and normal vascularization of the parenchyma. Non-autoimmune destructive thyroiditis was diagnosed and the patient continued treatment with beta-blockers and anxiolytics for the transient thyrotoxic phase of the thyroiditis. Antiviral treatment for CHC was stopped about 4 weeks and afterwards resumed, with the same dosages, for another 11 month.

Dynamic ECG over the first 10 days revealed regression and disappearance of the ST segment elevation, with persistently negative T waves, which normalized 2 weeks later. Repeat echocardiography performed 2 weeks after the admission showed a normal LVEF, with apical hypokinesia and 4 weeks later showed complete recovery of the apical akinesia. The clinical picture with the absence of late angina, the normalization of the ECG, associated with normal epicardial coronaries at angiography and the transient, acute, left ventricular apical ballooning, enabled us to diagnose a stress-related, reversible, ventricular apical dysfunction.

In the next 3 months she developed transient hypothyroidism and then became euthyroid (Figure 5). She successfully completed her antiviral treatment and she

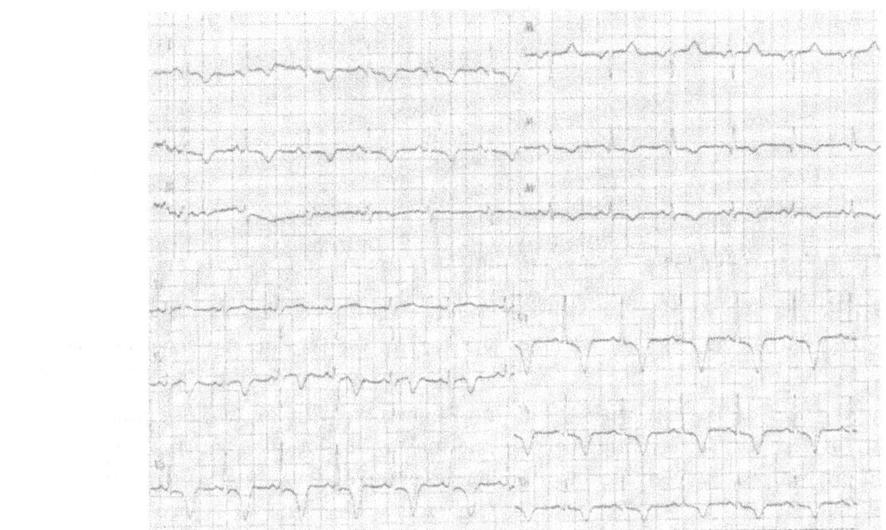

Figure 1 ECG at admission showing sinus rhythm 85 beats/min, ST segment elevation and negative T wave in DI, DII, aVF, aVL, V2-V6 leads.

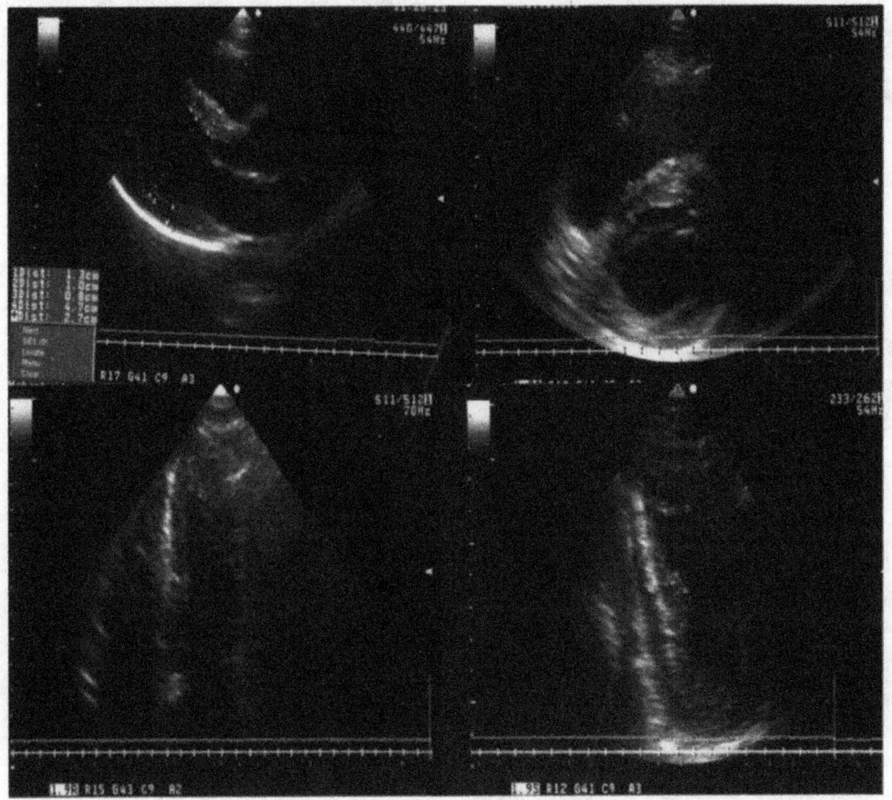

Figure 2 Baseline echocardiography showing normal cardiac cavities, septal hypokinesia, left ventricular apical akinesia and ballooning.

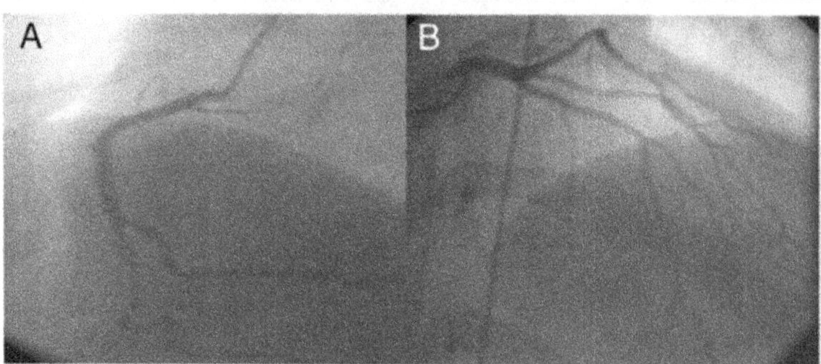

Figure 3 Right (A) and left (B) coronary arteriograms with normal coronary arteries without vasospastic phenomenon.

continues to be monitored as an outpatient with thyroid function tests and cardiac echocardiography every 6 month, with no thyroid or cardiovascular dysfunction ever since.

Discussion

TCM is an acute impairment of the cardiac function, named after the Japanese fishing pot used for trapping octopus, because of the peculiar left ventricle apical ballooning on left ventriculogram. The modified Mayo Clinic criteria for the diagnosis of TCM are: 1) transient hypokinesis, dyskinesis or akinesis of the left ventricular midsegments, with or without apical involvement; the regional wall-motion abnormalities extend beyond a single epicardial vascular distribution, and a stressful trigger is often, but not always, present; 2) absence of obstructive coronary disease or angiographic evidence of acute plaque rupture; 3) new electrocardiographic abnormalities (either ST-segment elevation and/or T-wave inversion) or modest elevation in cardiac troponin level; 4) absence of pheochromocytoma or myocarditis [7].

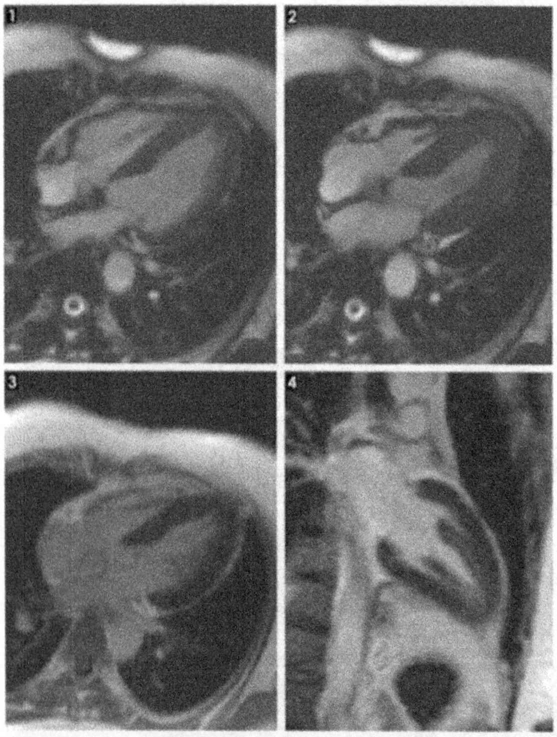

Figure 4 Cardiac MRI: 1,2 cine steady state free precession (SSFP) in four chambers view with apical ballooning; 3,4 triple inversion-recovery post injection of contrast agent with no late enhancement in the left myocardium.

Our case is a typical non-autoimmune destructive thyroiditis, in a woman with no personal history of thyroid or cardiovascular disorders, but with known history of CHC for which she was receiving IFNα and Ribavirin therapy for 7 months prior to the diagnosis. A higher prevalence of thyroid disorders has been reported in HCV-infected patients than in the general population [8]. Antiviral therapy of CHC possibly induces de novo or exacerbates pre-existing silent thyroid disorders [9]. Thyroid diseases may occur anytime during therapy and

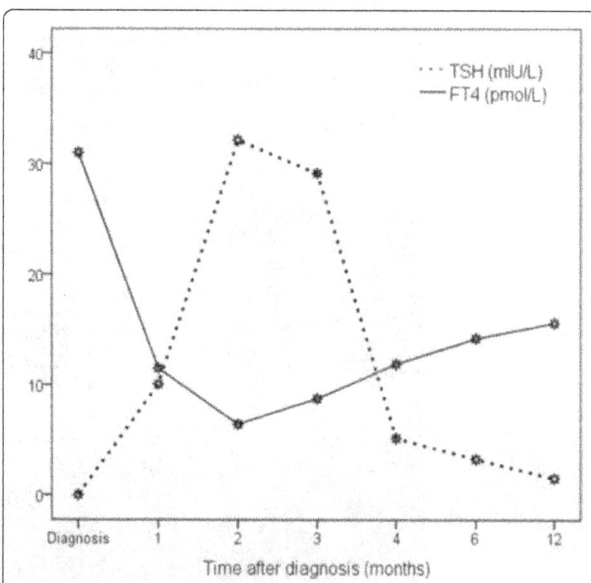

Figure 5 Thyroid function tests in the first year following the diagnosis.

are not absolute contraindications for IFNα or Ribavirin therapy. Furthermore, IFN-α dosage or treatment duration and the virological response to the treatment with IFN-α and Ribavirin seem not to be related to the incidence of thyroid dysfunction [10].

This case is special because of the unusual concomitant association of two transient illnesses: IFN-α induced thyroiditis and acute left ventricular apical ballooning. The association between thyrotoxicosis and cardiac complications is well known, yet thyrotoxicosis induced stress cardiomyopathy is rare [11]. TCM was reported in association with varied thyroid functional status, ranging from severe hypothyroidism [12], apathetic [13] or subclinical hyperthyroidism [14], endogenous or exogenous thyrotoxicosis [15,16], transient hyperthyroidism [17], thyroid storm [11,18] to even normal thyroid function [19]. TCM was also reported following radioiodine therapy [20] or surgical treatment for thyroid disorders [21]. To the best of our knowledge, until now, thyrotoxicosis induced stress cardiomyopathy has never been reported in association with thyroiditis precipitated by IFNα and Ribavirin therapy for CHC.

The patient was initially admitted for symptoms suggesting STEMI. However, echocardiography showing left ventricle apical ballooning, correlated to the coronary angiography that revealed no significant blockage and the absence of late enhancement on cardiac MRI, enabled us to diagnose a stress related reversible ventricular apical dysfunction. Stress-induced cardiomyopathy is an increasingly reported syndrome and it may account for approximately 2% of suspected acute coronary syndromes [22]. Left ventriculography is perhaps the best imaging modality to demonstrate the pathognomonic wall motion disturbance and to evaluate LVEF [23]. Cardiac MRI is, also, an important diagnostic modality for TCM, that can evaluate the regional wall motion abnormalities, can quantify ventricular function and identify the presence of edema/inflammation and the absence of necrosis/fibrosis [24]. Furthermore, cardiac MRI can differentiate TCM, characterized by the absence of delayed gadolinium hyperenhancement, from myocardial infarction and myocarditis, in which the opposite occurs. Both left ventriculography and cardiac MRI supported the TCM diagnosis in our case. Yet, myocarditis could not be ruled out by immunohistological examination of endomyocardial biopsies (EMB) or virus PCR, as proposed by the fourth Mayo criteria. However, in the reported case series of TCM, endomyocardial biopsy, the gold standard diagnostic for myocarditis, has not been systematically performed [25]. In a recent review, which included 286 patients from 14 studies, only 15 patients from 4 studies underwent EMB, with no evidence of myocarditis in any of them [26].

Postulated mechanisms for TCM pathogenesis include: direct cardiotoxicity of catecholamine excess, epicardial coronary vasospasm, micro-vascular dysfunction, in situ coronary thromboembolus with complete later recanalization, shifts in cardiac metabolism from fatty acids towards carbohydrates and left ventricular outflow tract obstruction, resulting in myocardial stunning [27]. Inflammation and oxidative stress might also play a role [28].

75% of patients with TCM have elevated serum catecholamine levels, even higher than patients with STEMI [29], which may explain the hypothesis of vascular dysfunction due to micro-vascular spasm. Supraphysiologic levels of catecholamines could trigger a switch in the coupling of β-2 adrenoreceptors from Gs to Gi protein, leading to decreased contractility. The left ventricular apex may be more vulnerable to catecholamine excess due to greater β-adrenergic receptor density and/or increased myocardial responsiveness [30]. This catecholamine hypotesis is also supported by the rat models, where Takostubo has been prevented with adrenergic blockade, by sampling of cardiac catecholamine levels in TCM [31] and by the reported cases in association with pheochromocytoma [32] and use of exogenous sympathomimetics.

The cause of myocardial stunning in thyrotoxic patients with normal coronary arteries is still unknown. Thyroid hormones have both direct and indirect actions on the cardiovascular system, can alter cardiovascular hemodynamics and represent a cause of cardiomyopathy. In thyrotoxic patients myocardial ischemia may occur due to coronary vasospasm [33], in situ coronary thromboembolus or direct metabolic effects of thyroid hormones.

The thyroid and adrenergic axes are closely interrelated, and pathologically high levels of thyroid hormones cause exaggerated chronotropic and contractile responses to catecholamines. Thyroid hormones modulate the transcription of multiple genes and also have extranuclear actions in cardiac myocytes, leading to various cardiovascular effects, similar to catecholamine-mediated stimulation of β-adrenergic receptors [34]. Thyroid hormones upregulate β-adrenergic receptors in many tissues, including the heart [35], thus, increasing sensitivity to catecholamines and potentiating catecholamine action. Furthermore, experimental animal data have shown that cardiovascular responses to hyperthyroidism are preserved in mice lacking all three β adrenergic receptors compared with wild-type mice [36]. An additional direct action of thyroid hormones at the intracellular level has been suggested based on the finding of thyroid hormone receptor expression on cardiac myocytes [37]. Hyperthyroidism can also mimic a state of catecholamine excess, mediated through a change in the balance between sympathetic and vagal innervation [38].

On the other hand, some studies have shown that plasma catecholamine levels, as in our case, are usually normal in TCM [6] and that the increase in β-adrenergic receptors is not always accompanied by a corresponding increase in cardiovascular sensitivity to catecholamines [39,40]. Some authors have even suggested that TCM might not be related to thyrotoxicosis, per se, but it could be a specific complication of autoimmune thyrotoxicosis [41]. Yet, the publication of TCM associated with exogenous thyrotoxicosis and radioiodine-induced thyroiditis argues against this theory.

Anyway, even if catecholamine levels are not increased in hyperthyroidism, their action seems to be amplified resulting in a hyper-responsive state to a minimal stimulation. Thyroid hormones can induce a catecholamine-mediated cardiotoxicity, which remains the most commonly proposed mechanism in TCM.

Despite the potential severe presentation, most of the patients survive the initial acute event, typically recover normal ventricular function within one to four weeks and have a favorable outcome, as was the case with our patient. Since TCM usually progresses to a full recovery, the question of whether patients with hyperthyroidism induced TCM would have recovered even without the correction of the thyroid function remains to be answered. Although infrequent, recurrence of the syndrome has been reported and seems to depend on the nature of the trigger [42]. Our patient has been followed for nearly 5 and a half years, with no recurrence of the TCM nor the thyroid dysfunction.

Conclusion

As previously suggested [4], we believe that TSH and thyroid antibody levels should be measured in all hepatitis C patients prior to starting IFNα therapy and TSH levels should be monitored every three months until completion of IFNα course. In hepatitis C patients treated with IFNα, multidisciplinary teams (gastroenterologist, endocrinologist, cardiologist) should be aware that thyrotoxicosis could be a possible and treatable underlying cause of TCM.

Consent

Written informed consent was obtained from the patient for publication of this Case report and any accompanying images. A copy of the written consent is available for review by the Editor of this journal.

Abbreviations

TCM: Takotsubo cardiomyopathy; IFN α: Interferon-alpha; CHC: Chronic hepatitis C; HCV: Hepatitis C virus; ECG: Electrocardiogram; STEMI: ST segment elevation myocardial infarction; LVEF: Left ventricular ejection fraction; TSH: Thyroid stimulating hormone; TPOAb: Anti-thyroid peroxidase antibodies; TRAb: Anti-thyrotropin receptor antibodies.

Competing interests

The authors declare that they have no competing interests.

Authors' contributions

CSM led the composition of this case report, acquisition of data and drafted the manuscript. IML performed literature review. CGB and AES participated in the endocrinological management and reviewed the manuscript. LNI participated in the cardiological treatment and performed echocardiography interpretation. ISL performed radiological interpretation. DRD and CSM continue clinical follow up of the patient to date. DRD and SVF critically reviewed the manuscript. All authors read and approved the manuscript.

Acknowledgements

The authors would like to thank Prof. Dr. Mircea Diculescu from Fundeni Clinical Institute of Gastroenterology and Dr. Florin Matache Duna from "Prof. Dr. Matei Balş" National Institute of Infectious Diseases, who conducted the gastroenterological treatment for our patient. We also thank Dr. Rodica Rotaru and Mrs. Suzana Florea from Elias University Hospital for their help with lab tests and Dr. Dan Deleanu from "C. C. Iliescu" Institute of Cardiovascular Diseases who performed the coronary angiography.

Funding

This research did not receive any specific grant from any funding agency in the public, commercial, or not-for-profit sector.

Author details

[1]Endocrinology Department, Carol Davila University of Medicine and Pharmacy, Elias University Hospital, 17 Marasti Blvd, sector 1, 011461 Bucharest, Romania. [2]Cardiology Department, Elias University Hospital, 17 Marasti Blvd, sector 1, Bucharest, Romania. [3]Endocrinology Department, Elias University Hospital, 17 Marasti Blvd, sector 1, Bucharest, Romania. [4]Radiology Department, Hiperdia, 17 Marasti Blvd, sector 1, Bucharest, Romania. [5]Cardiology Department, Carol Davila University of Medicine and Pharmacy, Elias University Hospital, 17 Marasti Blvd, sector 1, Bucharest, Romania.

References

1. World health organization, "hepatitis C. Fact sheet number 164," 2012. [http://www.who.int/mediacentre/factsheets/fs164/en]
2. Fried MW, Shiffman ML, Reddy KR, Smith C, Marinos G, Gonçales FL Jr, Häussinger D, Diago M, Carosi G, Dhumeaux D, Craxi A, Lin A, Hoffman J, Yu J: **Peginterferon alfa-2a plus ribavirin for chronic hepatitis C virus infection.** *N Engl J Med* 2002, **347**(13):975–982.
3. Carella C, Mazziotti G, Morisco F, Manganella G, Rotondi M, Tuccillo C, Sorvillo F, Caporaso N, Amato G: **Long-term outcome of interferon-Alfa induced thyroid autoimmunity and prognostic influence of thyroid autoantibody pattern at the end of treatment.** *J Clin Endocrinol Metab* 2001, **86**(5):1925–1929.
4. Tomer Y, Peters JJ, Menconi F: **Interferon induced thyroiditis.** *Best Pract Res Clin Endocrinol Metab* 2009, **23**(6):703–712.
5. Koh LK, Greenspan FS, Yeo PP: **Interferon-alpha induced thyroid dysfunction: three clinical presentations and a review of the literature.** *Thyroid* 1997, **7**:891–896.
6. Miyazaki S, Kamiishi T, Hosokawa N, Komura M, Konagai H, Sagai H, Takamoto T: **Reversible left ventricular dysfunction "takotsubo" cardiomyopathy associated with hyperthyroidism.** *Jpn Heart J* 2004, **45**(5):889–894.
7. Kawai S, Kitabatake A, Tomoike H: **Guidelines for diagnosis of takotsubo (ampulla) cardiomyopathy.** *Circ J* 2007, **71**(6):990–992.
8. Antonelli A, Ferri C, Pampana A, Fallahi P, Nesti C, Pasquini M, Marchi S, Ferrannini E: **Thyroid disorders in chronic hepatitis C.** *Am J Med* 2004, **117**(1):10–13.
9. Vezali E, Elefsiniotis I, Mihas C, Konstantinou E, Saroglou G: **Thyroid dysfunction in patients with chronic hepatitis C: virus- or therapy-related?** *J Gastroenterol Hepatol* 2009, **24**(6):1024–1029.
10. Dalgard O, Bjøro K, Hellum K, Myrvang B, Bjøro T, Haug E, Bel H: **Thyroid dysfunction during treatment of chronic hepatitis C with interferon**

alpha: no association with either interferon dosage or efficacy of therapy. *J Intern Med* 2002, **251**:400–406.
11. Eliades M, El-Maouche D, Choudhary C, Zinsmeister B, Burman KD: **Takotsubo cardiomyopathy associated with thyrotoxicosis: a case report and review of the literature.** *Thyroid* 2013, Not available-, ahead of print. doi:10.1089/thy.2012.0384.
12. Micallef T, Gruppetta M, Cassar A, Fava S: **Takotsubo cardiomyopathy and severe hypothyroidism.** *J Cardiovasc Med (Hagerstown)* 2011, **12**(11):824–827.
13. Al-Salameh A, Allain J, Meimoun P, Benali T, Desailloud R: **Takotsubo cardiomyopathy could occur in patients with apathetic hyperthyroidism.** *Thyroid* 2013, -Not available-, ahead of print. doi:10.1089/thy.2013.0354.
14. Dahdouh Z, Roule V, Bignon M, Grollier G: **Recurrent tako tsubo related to subclinical hyperthyroidism.** *Rev Esp Cardiol* 2011, **64**(11):1069–1071.
15. Alidjan F, Ezzhati M, Bruggeling W, van Guldener C: **Takotsubo cardiomyopathy precipitated by thyrotoxicosis.** *Thyroid* 2010, **20**(12):1427–1428.
16. Hutchings DC, Adlam D, Ferreira V, Karamitsos TD, Channon KM: **Takotsubo cardiomyopathy in association with endogenous and exogenous thyrotoxicosis.** *QJM* 2011, **104**(5):433–435.
17. Sarullo FM, Americo L, Accardo S, Cicero S, Schicchi R, Schirò M, Castello A: **Tako-tsubo cardiomyopathy observed in a patient with sepsis and transient hyperthyroidism.** *Monaldi Arch Chest Dis* 2009, **72**(1):33–36.
18. Radhakrishnan A, Granato JE: **An association between takotsubo cardiomyopathy and thyroid storm.** *Postgrad Med* 2009, **121**(3):126–130.
19. Hatzakorzian R, Bui H, Schricker T, Backman SB: **Broken heart syndrome triggered by an obstructive goiter not associated with thyrotoxicosis.** *Can J Anaesth* 2013, **60**(8):808–812.
20. van de Donk NW, America YG, Zelissen PM, Hamer BJ: **Takotsubo cardiomyopathy following radioiodine therapy for toxic multinodular goitre.** *Neth J Med* 2009, **67**(10):350–352.
21. Gundara JS, Lee JC, Ip J, Sidhu SB: **Takotsubo cardiomyopathy complicating thyroidectomy for Graves' disease.** *Thyroid* 2012, **22**(9):975–976.
22. Kurowski V, Kaiser A, von Hof K, Killermann DP, Mayer B, Hartmann F, Schunkert H, Radke PW: **Apical and midventricular transient left ventricular dysfunction syndrome (tako-tsubo cardiomyopathy): frequency, mechanisms, and prognosis.** *Chest* 2007, **132**(3):809–816.
23. Pilgrim TM, Wyss TR: **Takotsubo cardiomyopathy or transient left ventricular apical ballooning syndrome: a systematic review.** *Int J Cardiol* 2008, **124**(3):283–292.
24. Eitel I, von Knobelsdorff-Brenkenhoff F, Bernhardt P, Carbone I, Muellerleile K, Aldrovandi A, Francone M, Desch S, Gutberlet M, Strohm O, Schuler G, Schulz-Menger J, Thiele H, Friedrich MG: **Clinical characteristics and cardiovascular magnetic resonance findings in stress (takotsubo) cardiomyopathy.** *JAMA* 2011, **306**(3):277–286.
25. Caforio AL, Tona F, Vinci A, Calabrese F, Ramondo A, Cacciavillani L, Corbetti F, Leoni L, Thiene G, Iliceto S, Angelini A: **Acute biopsy-proven lymphocytic myocarditis mimicking takotsubo cardiomyopathy.** *Eur J Heart Fail* 2009, **11**(4):428–431.
26. Gianni M, Dentali F, Grandi AM, Sumner G, Hiralal R, Lonn E: **Apical ballooning syndrome or tako-tsubo cardiomyopathy: a systematic review.** *Eur Heart J* 2006, **27**:1523–1529.
27. Prasad A, Lerman A, Rihal CS: **Apical ballooning syndrome (tako-tsubo or stress cardiomyopathy): a mimic of acute myocardial infarction.** *Am Heart J* 2008, **155**:408–417.
28. Nef HM, Möllmann H, Kostin S, Troidl C, Voss S, Weber M, Dill T, Rolf A, Brandt R, Hamm CW, Elsässer A: **Tako-Tsubo cardiomyopathy: intraindividual structural analysis in the acute phase and after functional recovery.** *Eur Heart J* 2007, **28**:2456–2464.
29. Nef HM, Mo¨llmann H, Akashi YJ, Hamm CW: **Mechanisms of stress (takotsubo) cardiomyopathy.** *Nat Rev Cardiol* 2010, **7**:187–193.
30. Khallafi H, Chacko V, Varveralis N, Elmi F: **Broken heart syndrome: catecholamine surge or aborted myocardial infarction?** *J Invasive Cardiol* 2008, **20E**:9–13.
31. Sharkey SW, Lesser JR, Menon M, Parpart M, Maron MS, Maron BJ: **Spectrum and significance of electrocardiographic patterns, troponin levels, and thrombolysis in myocardial infarction frame count in patients with stress (tako-tsubo) cardiomyopathy and comparison to those in patients with ST-elevation anterior wall myocardial infarction.** *Am J Cardiol* 2008, **101**(12):1723–1728.
32. Kassim TA, Clarke DD, Mai VQ, Clyde PW, Mohamed Shakir KM: **Catecholamine-induced cardiomyopathy.** *Endocr Pract* 2008, **14**(9):1137–1149.
33. Masani ND, Northridge DB, Hall RJ: **Severe coronary vasospasm associated with hyperthyroidism causing myocardial infarction.** *Br Heart J* 1995, **74**:700–771.
34. Klein I, Ojamaa K: **Thyroid hormone and the cardiovascular system.** *N Engl J Med* 2001, **344**(7):501–509.
35. Bahouth SW: **Thyroid hormones transcriptionally regulate the beta 1-adrenergic receptor gene in cultured ventricular myocytes.** *J Biol Chem* 1991, **266**:15863–15869.
36. Silva JE, Bianco SD: **Thyroid-adrenergic interactions: physiological and clinical implications.** *Thyroid* 2008, **18**:157–165.
37. Dillmann WH: **Cellular action of thyroid hormone on the heart.** *Thyroid* 2002, **12**:447–452.
38. Chen JL, Chiu HW, Tseng YJ, Chu WC: **Hyperthyroidism is characterized by both increased sympathetic and decreased vagal modulation of heart rate: evidence from spectral analysis of heart rate variability.** *Clin Endocrinol* 2006, **64**:611–616.
39. Bachman ES, Hampton TG, Dhillon H, Amende I, Wang J, Morgan JP, Hollenberg AN: **The metabolic and cardiovascular effects of hyperthyroidism are largely independent of beta-adrenergic stimulation.** *Endocrinology* 2004, **145**(6):2767–2774.
40. Crozatier B, Su JB, Corsin A, Bouanani N-H: **Species differences in myocardial beta-adrenergic receptor regulation in response to hyperthyroidism.** *Circ Res* 1991, **69**:1234–1243.
41. Cakir M: **Takotsubo cardiomyopathy in thyrotoxicosis.** *Int J Cardiol* 2010, **145**:499–500.
42. Elesber AA, Prasad A, Lennon RJ, Wright RS, Lerman A, Rihal CS: **Four-year recurrence rate and prognosis of the apical ballooning syndrome.** *J Am Coll Cardiol* 2007, **50**(5):448–452.

9

Transient hypercortisolism and symptomatic hyperthyroidism associated to primary hyperparathyroidism in an elderly patient

Chiara Sabbadin[1*], Gabriella Donà[2], Luciana Bordin[2], Maurizio Iacobone[3], Valentina Camozzi[1], Caterina Mian[1] and Decio Armanini[1]

Abstract

Background: Primary hyperparathyroidism (PHPT) is often found on routine blood tests, at a relatively asymptomatic stage. However many studies suggest different systemic effects related to PHPT, which could be enhanced by an abnormal cortisol release due to chronic stress of hyperparathyroidism. Being PHPT frequently found in the 6th to 7th decade of life, a careful and multifaceted approach should be taken.

Case presentation: We report the case of an elderly patient with symptomatic PHPT and incidental pulmonary embolism. He was treated with hydration, zoledronic acid, cinacalcet and high-dose unfractionated heparin. Parathyroid surgery was successfully performed, but patient's conditions suddenly worsened because of a transient thyrotoxicosis, probably induced by a previous exposure to iodine load and/or thyroid surgical manipulation. A short-term treatment with beta-blockers was introduced for symptomatic relief. The patient also presented a transient hypercortisolism with elevated ACTH, likely due to stress related not only to aging and hospitalization but also to PHPT, resolved only four months after parathyroid surgery.

Conclusion: Chronic hyperparathyroidism has been linked with increased all-cause mortality. A functional chronic hypercortisolism could be established, enhancing PHPT related disorders. Only parathyroid surgery has been demonstrated to cure PHPT and complications related, showing similar outcome between older and younger patients. However, the management of post-operative period should be more careful in fragile patients. In particular, the early diagnosis and treatment of a transient post-operative thyrotoxicosis could improve recovery. Due to the increase in prevalence and the evidence of many related complications even in asymptomatic PHPT, expert opinion-based guidelines for surgical treatment of PHPT should be developed especially for elderly patients.

Keywords: Primary hyperparathyroidism, Elderly, Transient hyperthyroidism, Iodinated-contrast induced thyrotoxicosis, Functional hypercortisolism

Background

Primary hyperparathyroidism (PHPT) is the third most common endocrinopathy seen today, frequently found in the 6th to 7th decade of life. PHPT mainly is a sporadic disorder, caused in 85% of the cases by a single adenoma, in 15% by multi-gland disease and rarely by parathyroid carcinoma. Less than 10% of cases are inheritable, often associated with multi-gland hyperplasia. The most common presentation of PHPT is an asymptomatic hypercalcemia, incidentally found on routine blood tests. However, many patients may suffer from minimal symptoms such as asthenia, constipation, polyuria, hypertension and neuro-psychiatric complications [1]. In some cases a renal colic is the first presentation of the disease. In older patients, concomitant morbidity and

* Correspondence: chiara.sabbadin.1@studenti.unipd.it
[1]Department of Medicine-Endocrinology, University of Padua, Via Ospedale 105, 35128 Padua, Italy

poly-pharmacotherapy may worsen symptoms and complications, and impact the management of PHPT [2].

In this paper we report a complex case of an elderly patient with symptomatic PHPT associated with a functional transient hypercortisolism, resolved only after parathyroid surgery. The post-operative period was also characterized by a symptomatic transient thyrotoxicosis, probably induced by previous exposure to iodine load and/or thyroid surgical manipulation. The early diagnosis and treatment of this condition improved final outcome.

Case presentation

An 80-year old man was admitted to a general hospital for polyuria, vomiting, weight loss, worsening asthenia, myalgia and progressive cognitive impairment. He had a personal history of hypertension and type 2 diabetes, treated with losartan and metformin respectively. On physical examination he was sleepy, apyretic, hypertensive (upright blood pressure 150/100 mmHg) and tachycardic (100 beats for minute). He did complain of dyspnea, dry skin and mucosa and muscle weakness, without bone pain and neurological alterations. Biochemical assays revealed hypernatremia (149 mmol/L), severe hypercalcemia (4.08 mmol/L), hypophosfatemia (0.62 mmol/L), elevated levels of PTH (252 ng/L), reduced vitamin D (32 nmol/L) and slight renal failure (urea 8.7 mmol/L, creatinine 112 μmol/L). Blood count, liver and thyroid function were normal (Table 1). The electrocardiogram did not show remarkable signs of hypercalcemia. A cranial computed tomography (CT) scan excluded acute cerebrovascular events. A CT pulmonary angiography detected partial thrombosis in three segmental branches of the right upper lobe pulmonary artery. Doppler ultrasound (US) revealed a deep vein thrombosis of the left posterior tibial vein. The patient was treated with isotonic saline hydration, furosemide, supplementation of vitamin D and an injection of zoledronate 4 mg, with a mild improvement of hypercalcemia and related symptoms. Daily high-dose unfractionated heparin was also administered. The patient was then transferred to our Endocrine Unit and treated with cinacalcet, with decrease of PTH, calcemia and calciuria values. Amlodipine and insulin were also added for worsening hypertension and diabetes. Neck US revealed an enlarged thyroid with normal vascular pattern and at the lower pole of the left thyroid lobe a hypoechoic vascular nodule (14.7×10.5×9 mm), consistent with enlarged parathyroid. A sesta-MIBI scintigraphy showed a homogeneous tracer uptake over the thyroid in the early images and a remaining modest uptake in the lower left thyroid lobe in the later images; no other abnormal or ectopic uptake was found. Dual-energy x-ray absorptiometry revealed an osteopenia; all the radiological exams did not find brown tumors. Because of multiple co-morbidities, further investigations were performed to exclude other endocrine disorders: urinary metanephrine and normetanephrine values were normal, while plasma morning ACTH and daily urinary free cortisol were increased with impaired circadian cortisol rhythm, evaluated in two different measurements; serum cortisol after 1 mg overnight dexamethasone administration was not suppressed (Table 1). Direct abdomen CT was negative for adrenal diseases. Pituitary magnetic resonance imaging (MRI) evidenced a round mass, about 4 mm, without enhancement after gadolinium injection, in the left lateral portion of adenohypophysis, consistent with microadenoma. Screening for mutations of MEN genes was negative. The other pituitary hormones were normal. Because of the patient's general conditions and a probably stress-induced hypercortisolism, no other investigations were performed, giving priority to the surgical resolution of PHPT. Bilateral neck exploration was performed with removal of the upper right parathyroid and both the lower and the upper left parathyroid gland,

Table 1 Principal biochemical parameters of the patient before and after surgery for primary hyperparathyroidism

Parameter	Normal range	1 month before surgery	4 days after surgery	4 months after surgery
Ca (mmol/L)	2,1-2,5	4,2	2,5	2,2
P (mmol/L)	0,8-1,4	0,6	0,7	1,1
PTH (ng/L)	5-27	252	<4	12
ACTH (ng/L)	10-50	128	126	38
Morning salivary cortisol (ng/mL)	2,6-15,3	13,1	-	12,2
Late-night salivary cortisol (ng/mL)	0,1-5,2	15,8	-	3,4
Daily urinary cortisol (nmol/24 h)	30-193	557	281	80
Serum cortisol after 1 mg DST (nmol/L)	<50	223	-	30
TSH (mIU/L)	0,2-4	1,04	0,03	1,17
FT4 (pmol/L)	9-22	19,9	26,9	18,7
FT3 (pmol/L)	3,9-6,8	3,9	10,4	4,1

DST: dexamethasone soppression test.

with quick decrease of intra-operative PTH (from 1296 to 39 ng/L). The histological diagnosis was consistent with multi-glandular hyperplasia. Laboratory tests showed a decrease of calcium and PTH levels, treated with oral calcium and calcitriol. However, four days after surgery the patient developed a sinusal tachycardia, mild heart failure and agitation alternating with stupor, without evidence of infection nor of volemic imbalance. Further investigation revealed suppressed TSH, elevated free T4 and T3 values (Table 1), with undetectable anti-thyroid and TSH receptor antibodies. Thyroid palpation was not painful. The post-operatory 99mTcO4 scintigraphy showed a reduced tracer uptake over the thyroid, especially in the lower left thyroid lobe, consistent with an inflammatory area (Figure 1). Suspecting interference by the iodinated contrast used for pulmonary angio-CT about a month before, urinary iodine excretion was measured, resulting elevated (935 μg/L, normal range 100–200). Considering a possible dual pathogenesis of thyrotoxicosis, both destructive and iodine-induced, the patient was treated with atenolol for symptomatic relief. Two months after surgery, thyroid function and ioduria were normal and beta-blocker was progressively stopped; 1 mg overnight dexamethasone test (DST) was still pathological. After other two months, calcium-phosphate balance was normal and serum PTH was near the lower limit of normal, therefore calcium and calcitriol supplementation were continued. Adrenal function was finally normalized with adequate cortisol suppression after 1 mg overnight DST (Table 1). Pituitary MRI confirmed the presence of a microadenoma, compatible with a non-secretory incidentaloma, in careful biochemical and radiological follow-up.

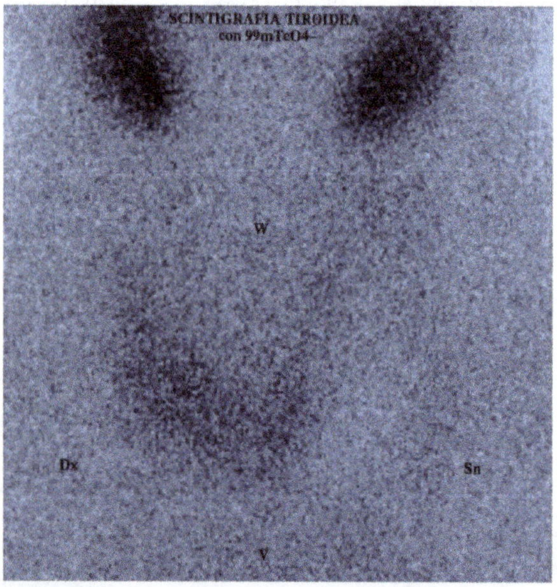

Figure 1 99mTcO4 scintigraphy, performed 4 days after parathyroid surgery, evidences a reduced uptake in total thyroid tissue, especially in the lower left lobe.

Discussion

We report an elderly patient presenting symptomatic hypercalcemia with moderate hemodynamic and neuropsychiatric failure. The detection of hypercalcemia and elevated PTH levels was diagnostic of PHPT. The biochemical/clinical presentation could also raise the suspicion of parathyroid carcinoma, which was excluded by the histological examinations. Rehydration was the first measure to take in this patient, not only to correct dehydration and improve renal failure, but also to dilute calcium excretion. Bisphosphonate administration was effective in reducing calcium levels and bone resorption, in particular recent controlled trials demonstrated the superiority of zoledronate compared with previous treatments [3]. The addition of cinacalcet may be useful in the elderly or in not-surgical candidates, being well tolerated [4]. Parathyroid surgery is the only definite cure for PHPT, but the risks and benefits of surgery should be extensively considered in the elderly, given their more fragile state and co-morbidities [5]. Preoperative imaging with ultrasonography and scintigraphy may be helpful before elective surgery and in suspected parathyroid carcinoma, even if their sensitivity drops in detecting multiglandular disease, as happened in our case report.

Our finding of a transient thyrotoxicosis after parathyroid surgery could be due to a dual pathogenesis: a destructive thyroiditis and/or an iodine-induced hyperthyroidism. The first condition is fairly unknown and underestimated since the symptoms could be masked by other postoperative events [6]. Thyrotoxicosis seems to be related to an increased release of thyroid hormones and/or autoantigen during surgical manipulation, which could reactivate underlying autoimmune thyroiditis [7]. It could be influenced by other mechanisms, like preoperative hypercalcemic setting, pre-existing goiter and difficult parathyroid glands identification during surgical exploration [8]. Our patient had an euthyroid goiter, without abnormal MIBI-uptake in preoperative investigations nor previous or underlying autoimmune thyroiditis. Retrospectively, the only apparent risk factors were the goiter, the previous pronounced hypercalcemic condition and the occasional finding of a multi-gland disease.

The second possible cause of transient thyrotoxicosis could be related to the previous iodinated contrast media exposure, leading to hypersecretion of thyroid hormones. This phenomenon, known as the Jod-Basedow effect, usually develops over 2 to 12 weeks, typically in old patients with underlying thyroid disease or living in areas of iodine deficiency. Exposure to a large iodine load can also cause acute destructive thyroiditis in people without pre-existing thyroid disorders [9]. TcO4-scintigraphy could not discriminate the cause of hyperthyroidism, since pertechnetate is trapped by thyroid, but not organified and the resulting tracer uptake may be reduced. As happened in our case, the assessment of urinary iodine concentration may be helpful [10]. Some researchers have investigated the incidence and the role of prophylactic measures to reduce the risk of iodine-induced thyrotoxicosis, without conclusive findings [11]. In our case the concomitant neck surgery could have been a precipitating factor in the pathogenesis of hyperthyroidism.

Both these conditions are usually self-limited and antithyroid drugs are not indicated. However, a short-term treatment with beta-blockers could be required for symptomatic relief, especially in fragile patients.

Since chronic hyperparathyroidism has been linked with increased all-cause mortality, in asymptomatic and elderly patients the optimal timing for parathyroidectomy is controversial [12]. Cardiovascular complications are the leading cause of this increased mortality [13], linked not only to mineral homeostasis disruption but also to a direct effect of PTH on cardiovascular structures [14]. The complexity of PTH functions is further highlighted by data suggesting a bidirectional link between PTH and the renin-angiotensin-aldosterone-system, playing a synergic role in enhancing metabolic and cardiovascular complications [15]. Several studies have also evidenced an altered hypotalamic-pituitary-adrenal (HPA) axis in PHPT, potentially contributing to cortical bone damage [16]. In vitro evidence supports a stimulatory effect of PTH on cortisol secretion [17] and of calcemia on ACTH release [18]. In vivo data show a hypercortisolism, loss of circadian rhythm and lack of cortisol suppression after low-dose DST in PHPT [19], which are not always recovered after surgical cure, as happened in our case.

Alteration of cortisol expression and its circadian variability are also typical of aging, hospitalization, psychiatric and stress conditions [20]. False-positive results of the 1 mg DST could be influenced by absorption, liver or renal alterations and the use of alcohol or drugs inducing CYP3A4. Being PHPT a long-standing disease frequently affecting old patients, the activation of adrenal function seems to recall a functional hypercortisolism due to chronic stress, which could be preserved by aging and other co-morbidities, enhancing the damaging effects of prolonged exposure to stress hormones [21].

In our case, HPA axis was evaluated because of multiple co-morbidities of the patient. The data suggestive of Cushing's syndrome were the incidental pulmonary thrombo-embolism, the uncontrolled hypertension and diabetes and the evidence of a pituitary microadenoma; however, the absence of typical stigmata and the presence of many confounding factors made the diagnosis uncertain. After discharge, further investigations excluded a Cushing's syndrome, but the slow normalization of HPA axis only after four months seems to be related to the resolution not only of the acute stressful condition but also of PHPT.

This complex picture suggests that parathyroid surgery may improve the prognosis, normalizing also HPA axis, which could contribute to PHPT related pathologies, such as bone metabolism, psychiatric, metabolic and cardiovascular disorders [22].

Conclusions

There is ample evidence that PHPT is associated with HPA axis alterations, which could be involved in the increased metabolic, cardiovascular and neuropsychiatric complications. A wide variety of medical therapies are available; however, only parathyroid surgery has been demonstrated to cure PHPT and complications related, showing similar outcome between older and younger patients. A transient thyrotoxicosis is a fairly underestimated condition, which could be secondary to previous iodinated contrast media exposure or to thyroid manipulation during parathyroid surgery. The early diagnosis and treatment of this complication may increase a successful recovery, especially in fragile patients.

In conclusion, due to the increase in prevalence and the evidence of many related complications even in asymptomatic PHPT, expert opinion-based guidelines for surgical treatment of PHPT should be developed especially for elderly patients.

Consent

Written informed consent was obtained from the patient for publication of this Case report and any accompanying images. A copy of the written consent is available for review by the Editor of this journal.

Abbreviations

PHPT: Primary hyperparathyroidism; CT: Computed tomography; US: Ultrasound; MRI: Magnetic resonance imaging; DST: Dexamethasone test; HPA: Hypotalamic-pituitary-adrenal.

Competing interests

The authors declare that they have no competing interests.

Authors' contributions

CS and DA treated the patient and drafted the article. GD and LB participated in the analysis and interpretation of data. MI operated the patient and together with VC and CM critically revised the manuscript. All authors read and approved the final manuscript.

Acknowledgements

We acknowledge Ms. Sophie Armanini for English revision.

Author details

[1]Department of Medicine-Endocrinology, University of Padua, Via Ospedale 105, 35128 Padua, Italy. [2]Department of Molecular Medicine-Biological Chemistry, University of Padua, Padua, Italy. [3]Minimally Invasive Endocrine Surgery Unit, Department of Surgery, Oncology and Gastroenterology, University of Padua, Padua, Italy.

References

1. Pyram R, Mahajan G, Gliwa A. Primary hyperparathyroidism: skeletal and non-skeletal effects, diagnosis and management. Maturitas. 2011;70:246–55.
2. Conroy S, Moulias S, Wassif WS. Primary hyperparathyroidism in the older person. Age Ageing. 2003;32:571–8.
3. Smith MR. Zoledronic acid to prevent skeletal complications in cancer: corroborating the evidence. Cancer Treat Rev. 2005;31 Suppl 3:19–25.
4. Jacobs L, Samson MM, Verhaar HJ, Koek HL. Therapeutic challenges in elderly patients with symptomatic hypercalcaemia caused by primary hyperparathyroidism. Neth J Med. 2012;70:35–8.
5. Jannasch O, Voigt C, Reschke K, Lippert H, Mroczkowski P. Comparison of outcome between older and younger patients following surgery for primary hyperparathyroidism. Pol Przegl Chir. 2013;85:598–604.
6. Rudofsky Jr G, Grafe IA, Metzner C, Leowardi C, Fohr B. Transient post-operative thyrotoxicosis after parathyroidectomy. Med Sci Monit. 2009;15:CS41–3.
7. Walfish PG, Caplan D, Rosen B. Postparathyroidectomy transient thyrotoxicosis. J Clin Endocrinol Metab. 1992;75:224–7.
8. Lindblom P, Valdemarsson S, Westerdahl J, Tennval J, Bergenfelz A. Hyperthyroidism after surgery for primary hyperparathyroidism. Langenbeck's Arch Surg. 1999;384:568–75.
9. Calvi L, Daniels GH. Acute thyrotoxicosis secondary to destructive thyroiditis associated with cardiac catheterization contrast dye. Thyroid. 2011;21:443–9.
10. Bahn RS, Burch HB, Cooper DS, Garber JR, Greenlee MC, Klein I, et al. Hyperthyroidism and other causes of thyrotoxicosis: management guidelines of the American Thyroid Association and American Association of Clinical Endocrinologists. Endocr Pract. 2011;17:456–520. Erratum in: Endocr Pract. 2013;19:384.
11. Hintze G, Blombach O, Fink H, Burkhardt U, Kobberling J. Risk of iodine-induced thyrotoxicosis after coronary angiography: an investigation in 788 unselected subjects. Eur J Endocrinol. 1999;140:264–7.
12. Yu N, Donnan PT, Leese GP. A record linkage study outcomes in patients with mild primary hyperparathyroidism: The Parathyroid Epidemiology and Audit Research Study (PEARS). Clin Endocrinol (Oxf). 2011;75:169–76.
13. Pilz S, Tomaschitz A, Drechsler C, Ritz E, Boehm BO, Grammer TB, et al. Parathyroid hormone level is associated with mortality and cardiovascular events in patients undergoing coronary angiography. Eur Heart J. 2010;31:1591–8.
14. Osto E, Fallo F, Pelizzo MR, Maddalozzo A, Sorgato N, Corbetti F, et al. Coronary microvascular dysfunction induced by primary hyperparathyroidism is restored after parathyroidectomy. Circulation. 2012;126:1031–9.
15. Sabbadin C, Cavedon E, Zanon M, Iacobone M, Armanini D. Resolution of hypertension and secondary aldosteronism after surgical treatment of primary hyperaldosteronism. J Endocrinol Invest. 2013;36:665–6.
16. Gianotti L, Tassone F, Pia A, Bovio S, Reimondo G, Visconti G, et al. May an altered hypotalamo-pituitary-adrenal axis contribute to cortical bone damage in primary hyperparathyroidism? Calcif Tissue Int. 2009;84:425–9.
17. Mazzocchi G, Aragona F, Malendowicz LK, Nussdorfer GG. PTH and PTH-related peptide enhance steroid secretion from human adrenocortical cells. Am J Physiol Endocrinol Metab. 2001;280:E209–13.
18. Fuleihan GE-H, Brown EM, Gleason R, Scott J, Adler GK. Calcium modulation of adrenocorticotropin levels in women – a clinical research study. J Clin Endocrinol Metab. 1996;81:932–6.
19. Rajput R, Bhansali A, Bhadada SK, Behera A, Mittal BR, Sialy R, et al. A pilot study on hypothalamo-pituitary-adrenocortical axis in primary hyperparathyroidism. Indian J Med Res. 2009;130:418–22.
20. Armanini D. Corticosteroid receptors in lymphocytes: a possible marker of brain involution? J Steroid Biochem Mol Biol. 1994;49:429–34.
21. Aguilera G. HPA axis responsiveness to stress: implications for healthy aging. Exp Gerontol. 2011;46:90–5.
22. Tirabassi G, Boscaro M, Arnaldi G. Harmful effects of functional hypercortisolism: a working hypothesis. Endocrine. 2014;46:370–86.

10

A case of masked toxic adenoma in a patient with non-thyroidal illness

Eun Ae Cho[1], Jee Hee Yoon[1], Hee Kyung Kim[1,2*] and Ho-Cheol Kang[1]

Abstract

Background: Non-thyroidal illness (NTI) refers to changes in thyroid hormone levels in critically ill patients in the absence of primary hypothalamic-pituitary-thyroid dysfunction, and these abnormalities usually resolve after clinical recovery. However, NTI can be accompanied by primary thyroid dysfunction. We report herein a case of a woman with NTI accompanied by primary hyperthyroidism.

Case presentation: A 52-year-old female was admitted to the intensive care unit with heart failure and atrial fibrillation. She had a longstanding thyroid nodule, and a thyroid function test revealed low levels of triiodothyronine and free thyroxine as well as undetectable thyroid stimulating hormone (TSH). She was diagnosed with NTI, and her TSH level began to recover but not completely at discharge. The thyroid function test was repeated after 42 months to reveal primary hyperthyroidism, and a thyroid scan confirmed a toxic nodule.

Conclusion: This case suggests that although NTI was diagnosed, primary hyperthyroidism should be considered as another possible diagnosis if TSH is undetectable. Thyroid function tests should be repeated after clinical recovery from acute illness.

Keywords: Thyroid, Non-thyroidal illness, Hyperthyroidism, Toxic adenoma

Background

Non-thyroidal illness (NTI) or euthyroid sick syndrome (ESS) is defined as a change in thyroid function during starvation or illness including a central reduction in thyroid stimulating hormone (TSH) secretion, decreased plasma triiodothyronine (T_3) levels and decreased thyroxine (T_4) and T_3 binding in serum [1]. It is a relatively common syndrome, affecting about 70% of hospitalized patients [2] and may occur with virtually any illness [3]. Abnormalities in thyroid function can occur within hours of acute illness, and the magnitude of reduction in thyroid hormone levels correlates with disease severity and mortality. Serum T_3 and free T_4 levels are independent predictors of survival [4-6], and low levels of T_3 are a poor prognostic factor of short- and long-term survival in patients with heart failure, acute myocardial infarction or acute stroke outside the intensive care unit (ICU) setting [7,8]. The pathophysiological mechanism responsible for NTI is complex and changes in the hypothalamic–pituitary–thyroid axis are the effect of various factors. Treatment of NTI with thyroid hormone is controversial, and abnormalities in thyroid function tests usually resolve after clinical recovery [3]. Primary thyroid dysfunction can be accompanied by NIT, and a follow-up thyroid function test is essential after recovery from illness to ascertain normalization. Here, we present a case of a woman with NTI who was later diagnosed with primary hyperthyroidism.

* Correspondence: albeppy@gmail.com
[1]Department of Internal Medicine, Chonnam National University Medical School, Gwangju, South Korea
[2]Department of Internal Medicine, Chonnam National University Hwasun Hospital, Chonnam National University Medical School, 322 Seoyang-ro, Hwasun-eup, Hwasun-gun, Jeonnam 519-763, South Korea
Full list of author information is available at the end of the article

Case presentation

A 52-year-old woman was admitted to the cardiology department ICU with generalized edema and orthopnea in July 2008. She had no significant medical history and was not taking any medications. An electrocardiogram revealed atrial fibrillation with a heart rate of 178 beats per minute. A chest X-ray detected pulmonary edema and cardiomegaly. A two-dimensional echocardiogram showed an ejection fraction of 57%, an enlarged left atrium without thrombi and grade 3 diastolic dysfunction. Diltiazem was used for heart rate control, but amiodarone or dopamine was not used during the hospitalization. Thyroid function tests were ordered as part of the atrial fibrillation evaluation. Serum free T_4 level was 0.282 ng/dL (normal, 0.8–1.71 ng/dL), T_3 was 0.307 ng/mL (normal, 0.6–1.6 ng/mL), and TSH was < 0.005 μIU/mL (normal, 0.4–4.8 μIU/mL). A physical examination revealed no apparent thyroid associated orbitopathy, but a large asymmetrical goiter, which was easily visible and palpable, was observed. A thyroid ultrasonogram demonstrated a 4.6 × 5.1 × 2.3 cm cystic dominant nodule in the lower portion of the right thyroid lobe and atrophy of the contralateral lobe (Figure 1). Five milliliters of serous, thin fluid was aspirated from the cyst. Aspiration cytopathology of the solid portion of the nodule was consistent with adenomatous goiter. An endocrine consultation was sought to evaluate the possibility of thyroid disease. She was diagnosed with NTI accompanying heart failure and a decision was made not to replace thyroid hormones but to follow-up on the thyroid function testing. Her symptoms resolved after 2 weeks, and she was subsequently discharged with a calcium channel blocker, an angiotensin receptor antagonist, a diuretic and aspirin. Thyroid function tests demonstrated a free T_4 level of 0.860 ng/dL, and a TSH level of 0.017 μIU/mL at discharge.

The thyroid function tests were not followed up until February 2012 (42 months) when she consulted the endocrinology department again for follow-up of the thyroid nodule. Her free T_4 and T_3 levels had increased to 5.30 ng/dL and 4.80 ng/mL, respectively, and TSH was < 0.005 μIU/mL. Anti-thyroid antibodies including anti-TPO antibody, anti-thyroglobulin antibody and TSH-binding inhibitory immunoglobulin were all negative. A follow-up thyroid ultrasonogram revealed an increase in the size of the previously observed nodule in the right lobe to 6.4 × 7.8 × 3.2 cm with contralateral lobe atrophy. A ^{99m}-Technetium-pertechnetate thyroid scan demonstrated heterogeneous uptake in the large nodule of the right thyroid gland with no visibility in the remaining gland, suggesting a functioning toxic nodule (Figure 2). She refused an operation or radioactive iodine therapy; therefore, 10 mg methimazole twice per day was prescribed. Her free T_4 and T_3 levels normalised (0.873 ng/dL and 0.941 ng/mL, respectively) 2 weeks later, and TSH was 0.009 μIU/mL.

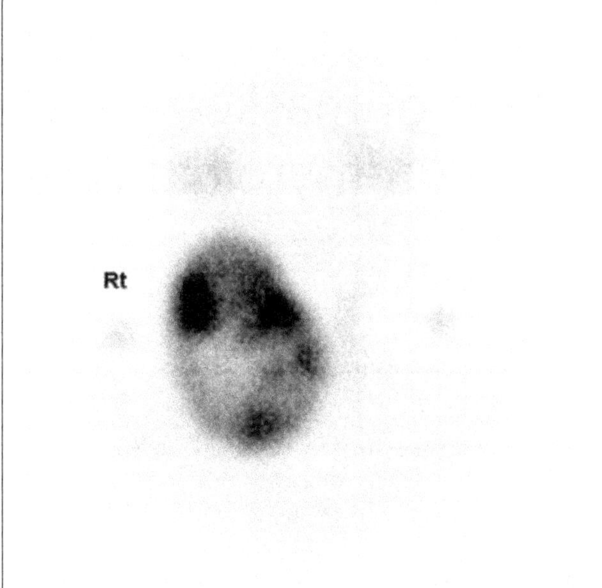

Figure 2 Thyroid scan. 99 m-Technetium pertechnetate thyroid scan reveals heterogeneously increased uptake in the large nodule of the right thyroid gland with decreased uptake by the remaining thyroid gland, suggesting a functioning nodule.

Discussion

Our patient had symptoms and signs of heart failure and atrial fibrillation. She had an asymmetric goiter, her T_3, free T_4 and TSH levels all decreased significantly; thus, she was diagnosed with NTI. TSH began to increase at discharge, but none of the thyroid hormone levels normalized. There was a follow-up loss of the thyroid function tests until 42 months after discharge. Testing revealed primary hyperthyroidism and a thyroid scan confirmed a functioning toxic nodule. Thus, primary hyperthyroidism, particularly toxic adenoma, should be considered in patients with NTI who have an undetectable level of TSH and a huge nodule with an atrophic remaining thyroid gland.

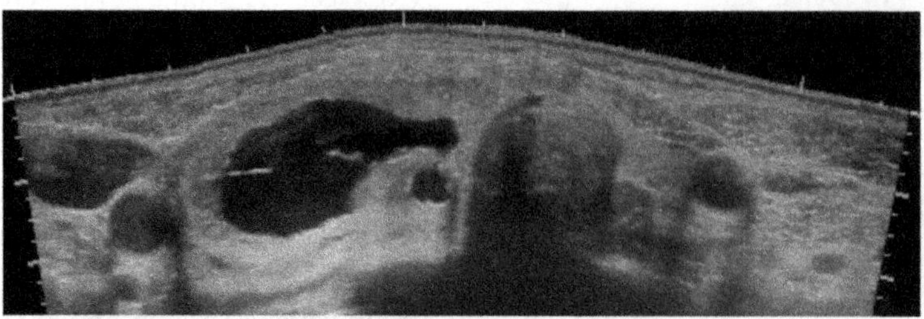

Figure 1 Ultrasonographic findings. Thyroid ultrasonogram demonstrates a 4.6 × 5.1 × 2.3 cm cystic dominant nodule in the lower portion of the right thyroid lobe and atrophy of the contralateral lobe.

NTI is a syndrome that reflects alterations in thyroid hormone levels during various illnesses [1]. Decreased total and free T_3 levels with normal levels of TSH can be observed in the acute phase of critical illness (low T_3 syndrome). Circulating T4 levels transiently rise during the acute phase of illness and normalize again when recovery follows quickly. However, patients who are severely ill and suffering from diseases that do not allow immediate recovery, present with reduced circulating total and free T4 concentrations. Reverse T_3 increases due to impaired T_4 conversion to T_3 via peripheral deiodination. As the disease progresses, a dramatic fall in total T_4 and T_3 occurs (low T_4 syndrome) [9], and about 50% of patients with NTI have decreased TSH levels, resulting from a reduction in thyroid releasing hormone secretion by the hypothalamus and indicating changes in hypothalamic–pituitary regulation [10]. Whether these changes are adaptive physiological mechanisms to conserve energy or consequences of the underlying illness is still a matter of debate [5,11]. However, treating NTI with thyroid hormones does not appear to be necessary, even though there is some controversy. For these reasons, routine thyroid function tests are not recommended in the intensive care setting unless a suspicion for thyroid dysfunction is based on history or a clinical evaluation. In the present case, a thyroid function test was ordered to evaluate atrial fibrillation and goiter.

The resolution of abnormal thyroid hormone levels after clinical recovery has been well documented. However, primary thyroid dysfunction can accompany NTI. TSH level may provide some clues for detecting underlying thyroid disease. Spencer et al. [12,13] reported that TSH can be low but detectable or high but < 20 μIU/mL in patients with NTI. The likelihood ratio for primary hyperthyroidism is 7.7 if TSH is undetectable, and the likelihood ratio is 11.1 for primary hypothyroidism if TSH > 20 μIU/mL [14]. Thus, TSH level should be considered in relation to the possibility of thyroid disease, and follow-up studies are mandatory, particularly if the value is not mildly abnormal. In our case, the patient had an undetectable level of TSH, and a thyroid ultrasonogram revealed a large cystic dominant nodule in the right thyroid lobe with atrophy of the opposite lobe. Although she was diagnosed with NTI, primary hyperthyroidism due to the toxic nodule should have been considered and a follow-up thyroid function test should have been performed after discharge.

Various drugs used in the hospital, particularly in the ICU, can alter thyroid function tests. Dopamine reduces serum TSH if used for a prolonged time [15]. Dobutamine, given in pharmacologic doses, also lowers TSH, even though TSH levels remain within the normal limits in subjects with a normal baseline TSH level [16]. Amiodarone is another drug that can cause alterations in thyroid function tests. Although most patients (>70%) on amiodarone remain euthyroid, the drug can lead to either amiodarone-induced hypothyroidism or amiodarone-induced thyrotoxicosis. High-dose glucocorticoids and octreotide also transiently suppress TSH, although central hypothyroidism does not appear to occur with these drugs [17,18]. Attention should be paid when interpreting thyroid function tests if any of these drugs have been used. Our patient never received any of these drugs.

A toxic nodule is a solitary, autonomously functioning thyroid nodule. The pathogenesis includes mutations in the TSH receptor leading to enhanced stimulation of thyroid follicular cell proliferation and function [19]. A thyroid nodule generally large enough to be palpable is present with suppressed TSH level, as in the present case. Patients initially have subclinical hyperthyroidism but when the adenoma grows to a significant size, frank hyperthyroidism develops, and elevated serum thyroid hormone levels accompany this condition [20]. Thyrotoxicosis is usually mild. A thyroid nodule appears on ultrasonography as a hypo-echogenic nodule with an atrophic thyroid gland. A thyroid scan is a definitive diagnostic test, demonstrating increased radioiodine uptake in the hyperfunctioning nodule and decreased uptake in the remaining gland. Radio-iodine ablation is usually the treatment of choice. Surgical resection of the adenoma or lobectomy to preserve thyroid function is another treatment option [1].

Conclusion

NTI is a very common syndrome in the intensive care setting, and routine thyroid function testing is generally not recommended. However, if there is a high suspicion for underlying thyroid disease, a thyroid function test should be performed and interpreted with caution. Thyroid function tests should be repeated after recovery from acute illness to ascertain euthyroid status. An evaluation for primary thyroid disease is essential, particularly when TSH is undetectable or >20 μIU/mL.

Consent

Written informed consent was obtained from the patient for publication of this case report and any accompanying images. A copy of the written consent is available for review by the Editor of this journal.

Competing interests

No potential conflict of interest relevant to this article was reported.

Authors' contributions

EAC – 1st author of case report. She involved in writing 1st draft. JHY – contributed by revision it critically for intellectual consent. HKK – diagnosed and treated the patient, and analyzed current literature on the topic to format a discussion, conclusion of the presented case. HCK – consultant physician overseeing the case of this patient. He had final approval of the case report to be submitted. All authors read and approved the final manuscript.

Author details

[1]Department of Internal Medicine, Chonnam National University Medical School, Gwangju, South Korea. [2]Department of Internal Medicine, Chonnam National University Hwasun Hospital, Chonnam National University Medical School, 322 Seoyang-ro, Hwasun-eup, Hwasun-gun, Jeonnam 519-763, South Korea.

References

1. Melmed SPK, Larsen PR, Kronenberg HM: *Williams Textbook of Endocrinology.* 12th edition. Philadelphia, PA: Saunders Elsevier; 2011:327–405.
2. Bermudez F, Surks MI, Oppenheimer JH: **High incidence of decreased serum triiodothyronine concentration in patients with nonthyroidal disease.** *J Clin Endocrinol Metab* 1975, **41**(1):27–40.
3. Adler SM, Wartofsky L: **The nonthyroidal illness syndrome.** *Endocrinol Metab Clin North Am* 2007, **36**(3):657–672. vi.
4. De Marinis L, Mancini A, Masala R, Torlontano M, Sandric S, Barbarino A: **Evaluation of pituitary-thyroid axis response to acute myocardial infarction.** *J Endocrinol Invest* 1985, **8**(6):507–511.
5. De Groot LJ: **Dangerous dogmas in medicine: the nonthyroidal illness syndrome.** *J Clin Endocrinol Metab* 1999, **84**(1):151–164.
6. Ray DC, Drummond GB, Wilkinson E, Beckett GJ: **Relationship of admission thyroid function tests to outcome in critical illness.** *Anaesthesia* 1995, **50**(12):1022–1025.
7. Iervasi G, Pingitore A, Landi P, Raciti M, Ripoli A, Scarlattini M, L'Abbate A, Donato L: **Low-T3 syndrome: a strong prognostic predictor of death in patients with heart disease.** *Circulation* 2003, **107**(5):708–713.
8. Iglesias P, Munoz A, Prado F, Guerrero MT, Macias MC, Ridruejo E, Tajada P, Diez JJ: **Alterations in thyroid function tests in aged hospitalized patients: prevalence, aetiology and clinical outcome.** *Clin Endocrinol (Oxf)* 2009, **70**(6):961–967.
9. Mebis L, Van den Berghe G: **Thyroid axis function and dysfunction in critical illness.** *Best Pract Res Clin Endocrinol Metab* 2011, **25**(5):745–757.
10. Plikat K, Langgartner J, Buettner R, Bollheimer LC, Woenckhaus U, Scholmerich J, Wrede CE: **Frequency and outcome of patients with nonthyroidal illness syndrome in a medical intensive care unit.** *Metabolism* 2007, **56**(2):239–244.
11. Wartofsky L, Burman KD, Ringel MD: **Trading one "dangerous dogma" for another? Thyroid hormone treatment of the "euthyroid sick syndrome".** *J Clin Endocrinol Metab* 1999, **84**(5):1759–1760.
12. Spencer C, Eigen A, Shen D, Duda M, Qualls S, Weiss S, Nicoloff J: **Specificity of sensitive assays of thyrotropin (TSH) used to screen for thyroid disease in hospitalized patients.** *Clin Chem* 1987, **33**(8):1391–1396.
13. Spencer CA, LoPresti JS, Patel A, Guttler RB, Eigen A, Shen D, Gray D, Nicoloff JT: **Applications of a new chemiluminometric thyrotropin assay to subnormal measurement.** *J Clin Endocrinol Metab* 1990, **70**(2):453–460.
14. Attia J, Margetts P, Guyatt G: **Diagnosis of thyroid disease in hospitalized patients: a systematic review.** *Arch Intern Med* 1999, **159**(7):658–665.
15. Kaptein EM, Spencer CA, Kamiel MB, Nicoloff JT: **Prolonged dopamine administration and thyroid hormone economy in normal and critically ill subjects.** *J Clin Endocrinol Metab* 1980, **51**(2):387–393.
16. Lee E, Chen P, Rao H, Lee J, Burmeister LA: **Effect of acute high dose dobutamine administration on serum thyrotrophin (TSH).** *Clin Endocrinol (Oxf)* 1999, **50**(4):487–492.
17. Nicoloff JT, Fisher DA, Appleman MD Jr: **The role of glucocorticoids in the regulation of thyroid function in man.** *J Clin Invest* 1970, **49**(10):1922–1929.
18. Colao A, Merola B, Ferone D, Marzullo P, Cerbone G, Longobardi S, Di Somma C, Lombardi G: **Acute and chronic effects of octreotide on thyroid axis in growth hormone-secreting and clinically non-functioning pituitary adenomas.** *Eur J Endocrinol* 1995, **133**(2):189–194.
19. Parma J, Duprez L, Van Sande J, Cochaux P, Gervy C, Mockel J, Dumont J, Vassart G: **Somatic mutations in the thyrotropin receptor gene cause hyperfunctioning thyroid adenomas.** *Nature* 1993, **365**(6447):649–651.
20. Hegedus L, Bonnema SJ, Bennedbaek FN: **Management of simple nodular goiter: current status and future perspectives.** *Endocr Rev* 2003, **24**(1):102–132.

11

Right thyroid hemiagenesis with adenoma and hyperplasia of parathyroid glands

Merima Oruci[1,6*], Yasuhiro Ito[2], Marko Buta[1], Ziv Radisavljevic[3], Gordana Pupic[4], Igor Djurisic[1] and Radan Dzodic[1,5]

Abstract

Background: Thyroid hemiagenesis is a rare anomaly, more commonly seen on the left side (ratio 4:1) and in females (ratio 3:1). The first to describe this anomaly was Handfield Jones in 1852.

Case presentation: We present a 66 year old female patient with right thyroid hemiagenesis, parathyroid adenoma on the side of hemiagenesis and parathyroid hyperplasia on the contralateral side. The patient had neck pain and was diagnosed as Hashimto thyroiditis with hyperparathyroidism. Parathyroid hormone, thyroglobulin antibodies (Tg-Ab) and thyroid peroxidase antibodies (TPO-Ab) were elevated. Neck ultrasound and technetium 99mTc-methoxyisobutyl isonitrile (MIBI) scintigraphy confirmed the right thyroid hemiagenesis, but not adenoma of parathyroid glands. Intraoperatively, right thyroid hemiagenesis was confirmed and left loboistmectomy was performed with removal of left inferior hyperplastic parathyroid gland. Postoperative PTH (parathyroid hormone) levels were within normal range. Five months after the operation PTH level was elevated again with calcium values at the upper limit. MIBI scintigraphy was performed again which showed increased accumulation of MIBI in the projection of the right parathyroid gland. Surgical reexploration of the neck and excision of the right upper parathyroid adenoma was performed which was located behind cricoid laryngeal cartilage. After surgery a normalization of calcium and PTH occured.

Conclusion: From available literature we have not found the case that described parathyroid adenoma on the side of thyroid hemiagenesis,with parathyroid hyperplasia on the contralateral side.

Keywords: Right thyroid hemiagenesis, Parathyroid adenoma, Parathyroid hyperplasia, Hyperparathyroidism

Background

Thyroid hemiagenesis is a rare anomaly, more commonly seen on the left side (ratio 4:1) and in females (ratio 3:1) [1]. The true incidence of hemiagenesis is not known because it is usually asymptomatic and it is incidentaly revealed due to certain pathologic conditions of the contralateral lobe. The prevalance of thyroid hemiagenesis in the literature varies between 0,2% to 0,025% [2-5]. The largest series of 40 thyroid hemiagenesis was published by Ruchala et al. [6]. The same author also performed a study showing that thyroid hemiagenesia was associated with slightly enhanced C cells hyperplasia compared to controls, which might indicate compensatory proliferation, however, the calcium-phosphate balance did not seem to be significantly affected [7].

Thyroid hemiagenesis anomaly was described for the first time in Europe 1852 by Handfield-Jones [8] and later in U.S.A. by Marshall in 1895 [9]. The absence of one thyroid lobe is usually asymptomatic and is often being diagnosed incidentally or during assessment for thyroid related or non-related conditions.

Maganini and Narendran were the first to decribe in the year 1977. case of upper left adenoma of the parathyroid gland in a patient with left thyroid hemiagenesia [10]. Teresa Kroeker published the case report of left lobe hemiagenesia and ipsilateral parathyroid adenoma [11]. Mydlarz et al. published in 2010.case report of ipsilateral doouble parathyroid adenoma and left thyoroid hemiagenesia [12]. The case report of parathyroid adenoma on the contralateral side of hemiagenesis was published by Sakurai et al. And they described the absence of parathyroid glands on the side of hemiagenesis [13].

* Correspondence: merimaoruci@hotmail.com
[1]Surgical Oncology clinic, Institute for Oncology and Radiology of Serbia, Pasterova 14, Belgrade 11000, Serbia
[6]Institute for Oncology and Radiology of Serbia, Pasterova 14, Belgrade 11000, Serbia

Duh et al. described thyroid hemiagenesis, together with parathyroid hyperplasia [14].

We report a case of parathyroid hyperplasia and adenoma, hyperparathyroidism, Hashimoto thyroiditis, and rare right thyroid hemiagenesis.

Case presentation

A 66-year-old woman was diagnosed with primary hyperparathyroidism, Hashimoto thyroiditis, and tumor in the left thyroid lobe in July 2009. There was no family history of thyroid and parathyroid disease. The parathyroid hormone (PTH) was elevated (136.2 pg/ml vs. normal value of 15–65 pg/ml) as well as calcium (Ca) level (2.73 mmol/L vs.normal value of 2.15-2.55 mmol/L). Also, thyroglobulin antibodes (TG-Ab), thyroid peroxidase antibodies (TPO-Ab) and thyroid stimulating hormone (TSH) (17.58 microU/ml vs. normal value of 0.27-4.2) were elevated, but L-thyroxine (T4) level was decreased (64.89 nmol/L vs. normal of 66–181 nmol/L). The patient was treated by L-thyroxine50 μg daily. The patient did not have nephrolithiasis or osteoporosis. Ultrasound of the neck verified absence of right thyroid lobe with heterogeneous structure size of 23x45 mm in the left lobe and enlarged lower left parathyroid gland size of 8x6 mm (Figure 1). Fine needle aspiration biopsy (FNAb) was not performed and the decision for the operation has been made only based on clinical and ultrasonographic findings. Technetium 99mTc-methoxyisobutyl isonitrile (MIBI) scintigraphy of parathyroid glands initially showed no pathological accumulation and only the left thyroid lobe could be visualized. (Figure 2). Tc99 was injected at the day of surgery. A left thyroid lobectomy and left lower parathyroidectomy were performed, both showing increased Tc99 accumulation. Exploratory surgery confirmed agenesis of the right thyroid lobe. Histopathologic examination confirmed Hashimoto thyroiditis of left lobe (Figure 3) and hyperplasia of the lower left parathyroid gland (Figure 4). Postoperative levels of calcium, PTH and phosphorus were normal. Five months later PTH level was increased again to 145 pg/mL. MIBI scintigraphy of parathyroid glands was performed again and pathologic accumulation was seen in the right parathyroid gland. Patient was reoperated and adenoma of the upper right parathyroid gland was removed size of 15x8 mm, located behind the crycoid cartilage (Figure 5). The right lower parathyroid gland was found and was normal in size and structure. Postoperative PTH, serum Ca and phosphorus (P) levels were normalized and their values still remain within normal range two years after the surgery.

Discussion

Here we report a rare case of right thyroid hemiagenesis, Hashimoto thyroiditis, hyperparathyroidism due to parathyroid hyperplasia and adenoma. Thyroid hemiagenesis was described previously with hyperparathyroidism [14], Hashimoto thyroiditis [15], thyroglossal duct cyst [16], follicular and papillary neoplasms [17,18]. Diagnosis of thyroid hemiagenesis can be easily accomplished by Tc-99m MIBI scintigraphy and ultrasonographic examination. In our case Tc-99m MIBI scintigraphy did not detect parathyroid adenoma before the left thyroid lobe

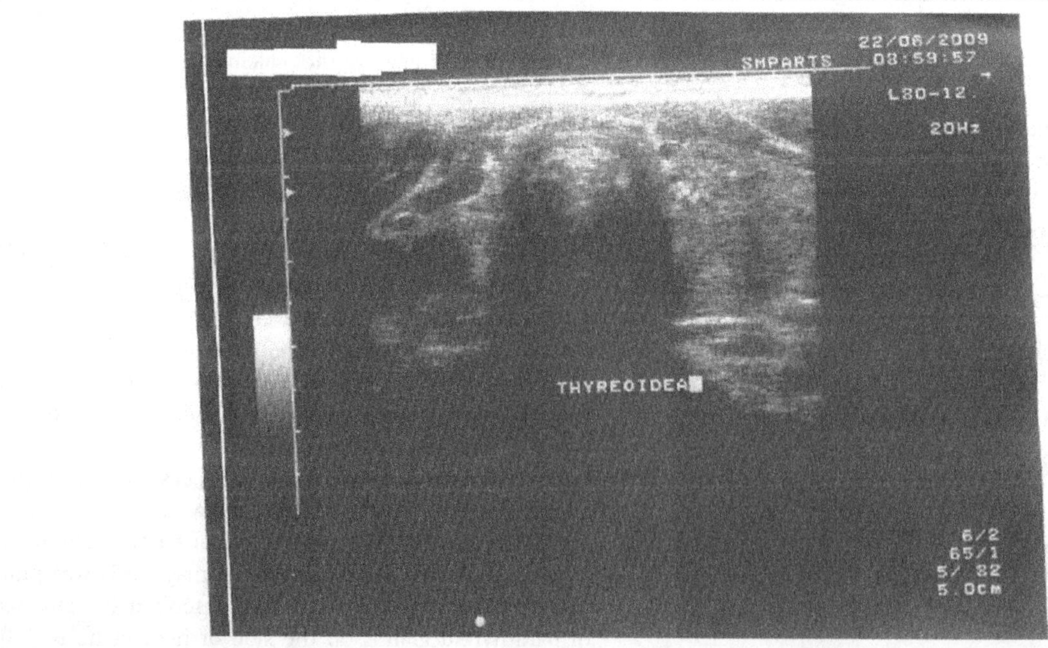

Figure 1 Neck ultrasound.

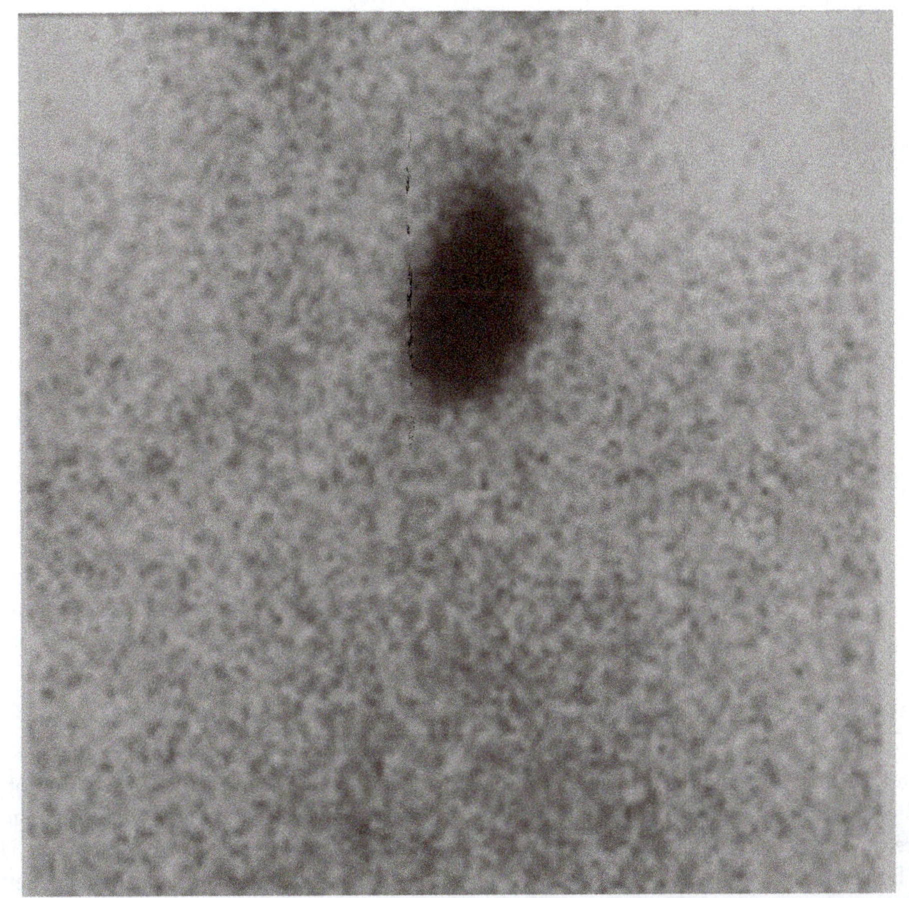

Figure 2 Neck scintigraphy (MIBI).

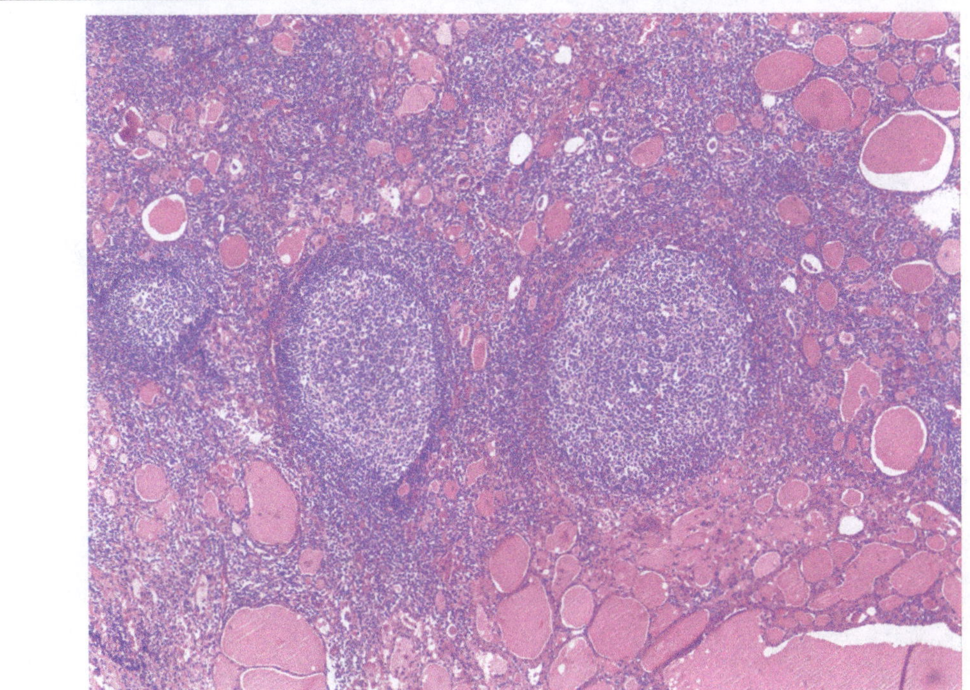

Figure 3 Hashimoto thyroiditis HE-staining, 20× magnification.

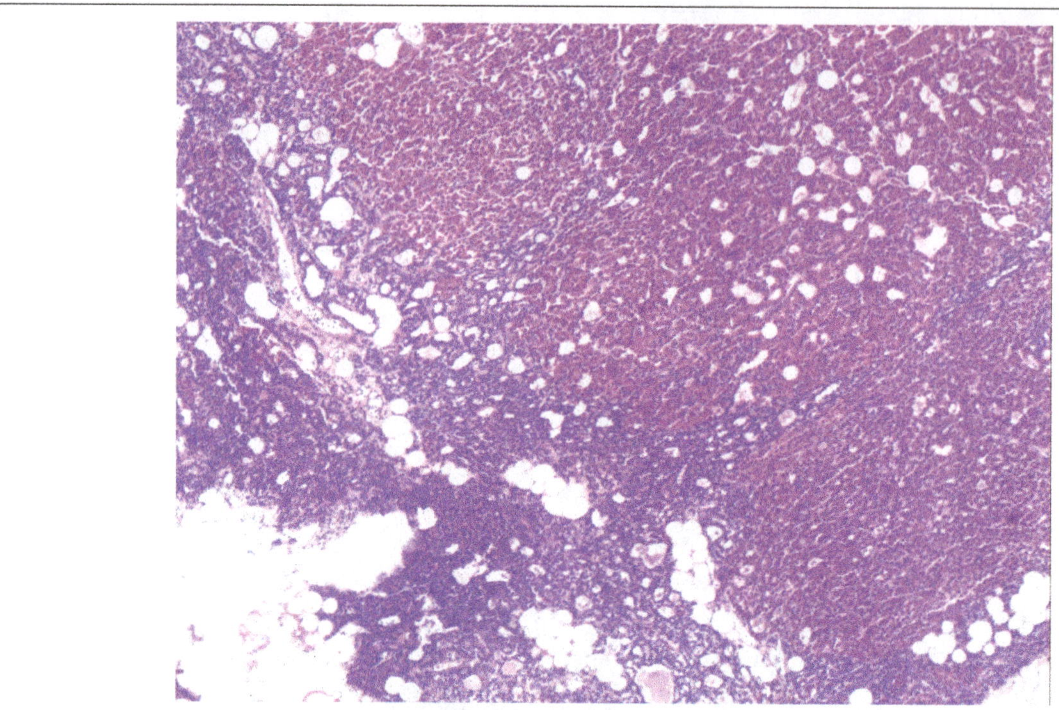

Figure 4 Hyperplasia of parathyroid gland HE-staining, 20× magnification.

was removed and we can speculate that the left lobe absorbed all radioactivity. Only after totalisation of thyroidectomy by removing the left lobe, right parathyroid adenoma could be seen. Explorative surgery was necessary for the final diagnosis and treatment.

Between 1970 and 2010, 329 cases of thyroid hemiagenesis have been reported. Left lobe agenesia was more frequent with female's predominance [19]. In humans the thyroid rudiment during thyroid development starts to acquire a bilobed structure at the end of the second

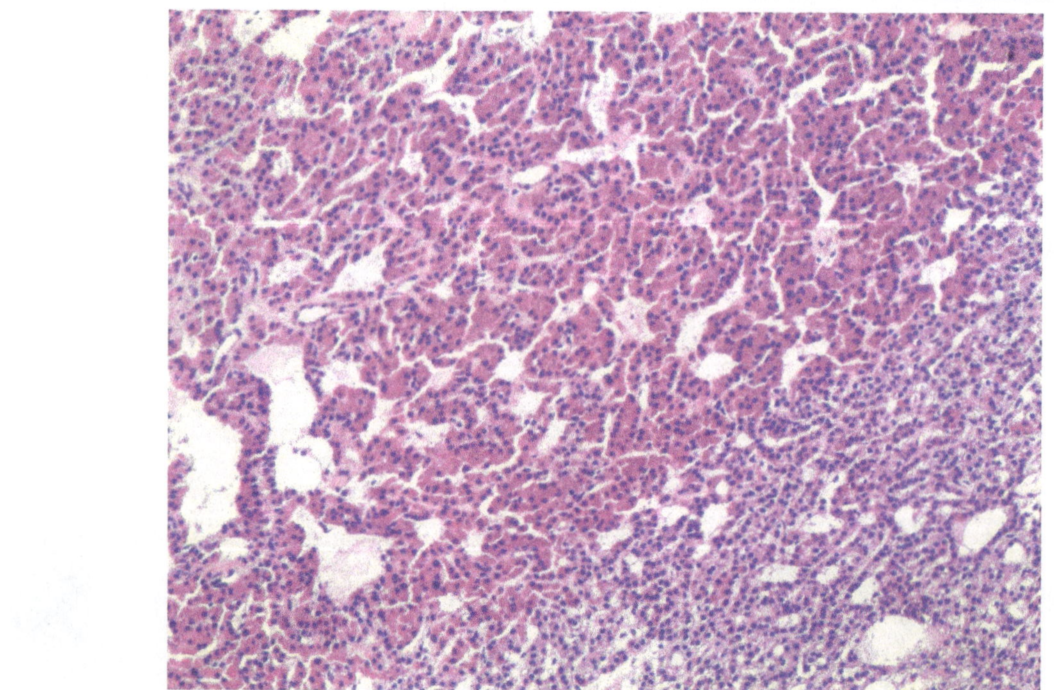

Figure 5 Adenoma of paratyroid gland HE-staining, 20× magnification.

month [20]. There are several known genes that control development and embryogenesis of thyroid gland but their role was not proven in hemiagenesis. In 1984 the case of thyroid hemiagenesis in two sisters was published [21]. Thyroid hemiagenesis could be found in some families suggesting genetic cause [22]. Certain familial hemiagenesis are caused by the transcriptional mutations of factors involved in embryogenesis.such as PAX8, TTF1,FOXE1, NKX2-5) [23]. In fact, only minority of cases of congenital hypothyroidism could be explained with such changes and it predominantly concerns cases of thyroid ectopy and agenesis, while in vast majority of patients with hemiagenesis the genetic background is unknown. GCMB gene is important for normal synthesis of parathyroid hormone in humans and could be involved in parathyroid adenoma genesis [24].

Conclusion

Until now there was no case of thyroid hemiagenesis together with parathyroid adenoma and hyperplasia described in the literature. The case description proves that in a patient with thyroid hemiagenesis, despite unilaterally abnormal development of the thyroid gland, the parathyroid glands are present on the side of agenesis. The connection between parathyroid hyperplasia and adenoma and genetic triggers in their development needs to be clarified. The destiny of parafollicular C cells on the side of hemiagenesis is still unknown.

Consent

Written informed consent was obtained from the patient for publication of this Case report and any accompanying images. A copy of the written consent is available for review by the Series Editor of this journal.

Competing interests

The autors declare that they have no competing interests.

Authors' contributions

MO designed the manuscript, interpreted data and revised the manuscript. YI revised the manuscript and pointed out certain genetic links. MB and ID collected data, revised the manuscript. RD made diagnosis, operated the patient, followed up the patient, interpreted data and designed the manuscript. ZR discussed molecular basis of this unusual case and helped in revision and interpretation of data. GP made pathological diagnosis and photos of histopathological slides. All authors read and approved the final manuscript.

Acknowledgement

The study was supported by Grant III41031 from the Ministry of Education and Science, Republic of Serbia.

Author details

[1]Surgical Oncology clinic, Institute for Oncology and Radiology of Serbia, Pasterova 14, Belgrade 11000, Serbia. [2]Department of Surgery, Kuma Hospital, 8-2-35, Shimoyamate-dori, Chuo-ku, Kobe 650-0011, Japan. [3]Department of Clinical Research, Brigham and Women's Hospital, Harvard Medical School, Boston, MA, USA. [4]Department of Pathology, Institute for Oncology and Radiology of Serbia, Pasterova 14, Belgrade 11000, Serbia. [5]University of Belgrade School of Medicine, Belgrade 11000, Serbia. [6]Institute for Oncology and Radiology of Serbia, Pasterova 14, Belgrade 11000, Serbia.

References

1. Melnik JC, Stemkowski PE: **Thyroid hemiagenesis(hockey stick sign): a review of the world literature and a report of four cases.** *J Clin Endocrinol Metab* 1981, **52**(2):247–251.
2. Shabana W, Delange F, Freson M, Osteaux M, De Schepper J: **Prevalence of thyroid hemiagenesis: ultrasound screening in normal children.** *Eur J Pediatr* 2000, **159**(6):456–458.
3. Maiorana R, Carta A, Floriddia G, Leonardi D, Buscema M, Sava L, Calaciura F, Vigneri R: **Thyroid hemiagenesis: prevalence in normal children and effect on thyroid function.** *J Clin Endocrinol Metab* 2003, **88**(4):1534–1536.
4. Korpal-Szczyrska M, Kosiak W, Swietom D: **Prevalence of thyroid hemiagenesis in an asymptomatic schoolchildren population.** *Thyroid* 2008, **18**(6):637–639.
5. Gursoy A, Anil C, Unal AD, Demirer AN, Tutuncu NB, Erdogan MF: **Clinical and epidemiological caracteristics of thyroid hemiagenesis: ultrasaund screening in patients with thyroid disease and normal population.** *Endocrine* 2008, **33**(3):338–341.
6. Ruchala M, Szczepanek E, Szaflarski W, Moczko J, Czarnywojtek A, Pietz L, Nowicki M, Niedziela M, Zabel M, Kohrle J, Sowinski J: **Increased risk of thyroid pathology in patient with thyroid hemiagenesis:results of a large cohort case-control study.** *Eur J Endocrinol* 2010, **162**:153–160.
7. Ruchala M, Szczepanek E, Sujka-Kordovska P, Zabel M, Biczysko M, Sowinski J: **The immunohistochemical demonstration of parafollicular cells and evaluation of calcium-phosphate balance in patients with thyroid hemiagenesis.** *Folia Histochem Cytobiol* 2011, **49**(2):299–305.
8. Handfield Jones C: **Thyroid gland.** In *The cyclopedia of anatomy and psihology*. Edited by Todd RB. London: Longman,Brown,Green, Longmans&Roberts; 1852:1103.
9. Marshall CF: **Variations in the form of the thyroid gland in man.** *J Anat Physiol* 1895, **29**(Pt2):234–239.
10. Maganini RJ, Narendran K: **Hyperparathyroidism in a patient with a parathyroid adenoma.** *IMJ Ill MED J* 1977, **151**(5):368–370.
11. Kroecker T, Stancoven K, Preskitt J: **Parathyroid adenoma on the ipsilateral side of thyroid hemiagenesis.** *Bayl Univ Med Cent* 2011, **24**(2):92–93.
12. Mydlarz WK, Zhang K, Micchelli ST, Kim M, Tufano RP: **Ipsilateral double parathyroid adenoma and thyroid hemiagenesis.** *ORL* 2010, **72**(5):272–274.
13. Sakurai K, Amano S, Enomoto K, Matsuo S, Kitajima A: **Primary hiperparathyroidism with thyroid hemiagenesis.** *Asian J Surg* 2007, **30**(2):151–153.
14. Duh QY, Ciulla TA, Clark OH: **Primary parathyroid hyperplasia associated with thyroid hemiagenesis and agenesis of the isthmus.** *Surgery* 1994, **115**:257–263.
15. Lazzarin M, Benati F, Menini C: **Agenesis of the thyroid lobe associated with Hashimoto's thyroiditis.** *Minerva Endocrinol* 1997, **22**:75–77.
16. Tsang SK, Maher J: **Thyroid hemiagenesis accompanying a thyroglossal duct cyst: a case report.** *Clin Nucl Med* 1998, **23**:229–232.
17. Khatri VP, Espinosa MH, Harada WA: **Papillary adenocarcinoma in thyroid hemiagenesis.** *Head Neck* 1992, **14**:312–315.
18. Huang SM, Chen HD, Wen TY, Kun MS: **Right thyroid hemiagenesis associated with papillary thyroid cancer and an ectopic prelaryngeal thyroid; a case report.** *J Formos Med Assoc* 2002, **101**:368–371.
19. Wu YH, Wein RO, Carter B: **Thyroid hemiagenesis: a case series and review of the literature.** *Am J Otolaryngol* 2012, **33**(3):299–302.
20. Fagman H, Nilsson M: **Morphogenesis of the thyroid gland.** *Mol Cell Endocrinol* 2010, **323**:35–54.

21. Rajmil HO, Rodriguez-Espinosa J, Soldevila J, Ordonez-Llanos J: **Thyroid hemiagenesis in two sistres.** *J Endocrinol Invest* 1984, **7**(4):393–394.
22. Castanet M, Leenhardt L, Ledger J, *et al*: **Thyroid hemiagenesis is a rare variant of thyroid dysgenesis with a familial component but without Pax8 mutations in a cohort of 22 cases.** *Pediatr Res* 2005, **57**:908–913.
23. Montanelli L, Tonacchera M: **Genetics and phenomics and hypothyroidism and thyroid dys- and agenesis due to PAX8 and TTF1mutations.** *Mol Cell Endocrinol* 2010, **322**:64–71.
24. Ding C, Buckingham B, Levine MA: **Familial isolated hypoparathyroidism caused by a mutation in the gene for the transcription factor GCMB.** *J Clin Invest* 2001, **108**:1215–1220.

12

High prevalence of metabolic syndrome in a mestizo group of adult patients with primary hyperparathyroidism (PHPT)

Victoria Mendoza-Zubieta[1*], Gloria A Gonzalez-Villaseñor[1], Guadalupe Vargas-Ortega[1], Baldomero Gonzalez[1], Claudia Ramirez-Renteria[2], Moises Mercado[2], Mario A Molina-Ayala[1] and Aldo Ferreira-Hermosillo[1]

Abstract

Background: Primary hyperparathyroidism (PHPT) and metabolic syndrome (MS) have been independently related to cardiovascular morbidities, however this association is still controversial. Mexican population has a high prevalence of metabolic syndrome, however its frequency seems to be even higher than expected in patients with PHPT.

Methods: We retrospectively reviewed the charts of patients that underwent parathyroidectomy for PHPT in a referral center and used the criteria from the National Cholesterol Educational Program (NCEP)/Adult Treatment Panel III (ATP III) to define MS before surgery. We compared the characteristics between the patients with and without MS.

Results: 60 patients were analyzed, 77% were female and 72% had a single parathyroid adenoma. MS was present in 59% of the patients, this group was significantly older (57 vs. 48 years, p = 0.01) and they had lower iPTH (115 vs. 161 ng/ml, p = 0.017). Other parameters did not show differences.

Conclusions: MS is frequent in our population diagnosed with primary hyperparathyroidism, adverse cardiovascular parameters are common and significant differences in calcium metabolism compared to the non-MS group are present.

Keywords: Primary hyperparathyroidism, Metabolic syndrome, Central obesity, Parathyroid hormone

Background

Primary hyperparathyroidism (PHPT) is a common endocrine disease, particularly in postmenopausal women. It is the main cause of hypercalcemia in outpatient settings and its prevalence is estimated to be 1 to 4 per 1000 people in the general population and 21 per 1000 in postmenopausal women [1]. The estimated incidence is 15.7/100.000 people /year in the USA [2].

PHPT is also associated with an increased risk of cardiovascular mortality [3-5]. Recent evidence shows that it is also associated with metabolic disorders and other components of metabolic syndrome (MS) such as hypertension (HTN), dyslipidemia, glucose intolerance, obesity, insulin resistance and reduced insulin secretion [6-8]. The ethiopathogenic mechanisms of MS are not completely understood and the association with calcium metabolism is being studied, since calcium is essential for many metabolic processes. Additionally, changes in vitamin D levels and other hormones in obese populations and patients with PHPT could be involved in the pathogenesis of cardiovascular and metabolic comorbidities. The association between these entities is complex and may be a source of additional morbidity and mortality.

The prevalence of MS, obesity and insulin resistance have increased continuously all around the world. Each one of them have been well documented as causes of increased cardiovascular morbidity and mortality [9-11]. However, the prevalence of MS varies according to definition criteria, age, sex and population studied. Between 1999–2010 the National Health and Nutrition Examination Survey (NAHNES) in USA reported an accumulated prevalence of 25.5% in adults older than 20 years of age; this prevalence decreased to 22.9% in 2010 [12]. In Europe the Diabetes Epidemiology: Collaborative Analysis of Diagnostic Criteria in Europe (DECODE)

* Correspondence: vmendozazu@yahoo.com
[1]Endocrinology Departament Hospital de Especialidades Centro Médico Nacional Siglo XXI, Instituto Mexicano del Seguro Social (IMSS), Cuauhtemoc N° 330, Colonia Doctores, México City, DF, Mexico

reported a prevalence of MS of 41% for male population and 38% for female population according to International Diabetes Federation (IDF) criteria [13]. In Mexico, the prevalence in adults older than 20 years of age is 41.6% according to the criteria proposed by the American Heart Association/National Heart Blood and Lung Institute (AHA/NHLBI) and 42% using the (NCEP:ATPIII) criteria [14]. Some polymorphisms associated altered lipid metabolism pathways are frequent in Mexico, which may be associated with the higher prevalence of MS in this mestizo population [15,16], however, other components of the MS are also frequent in these population. These data suggests that MS is twice as prevalent in our population compared to other countries, which also may have an influence on the calcium and vitamin D metabolism in both physiological and pathological states. The ethiopathogenic relationship between PHPT and MS is currently being investigated, it's unclear if the association of these two entities will affect mortality in the long term. Since Hispanic populations seem to be especially prone to high risk profiles for cardiovascular disease, specific analysis of these groups may help determine which patients require special diagnostic or treatment algorithms.

The purpose of this study was to evaluate the prevalence of MS in patients with PHPT and to compare the clinical and biochemical characteristics of patients with and without MS.

Methods

This cross-sectional study included patients from the Bone and Calcium Metabolism Clinic of the Hospital de Especialidades Centro Medico Nacional Siglo XXI diagnosed with PHPT during a 3 year-period between 2006 and 2009. A general evaluation including anthropometry was performed in all patients before surgery. We evaluated the signs and symptoms related to hypercalcemia (repeated nephrolithiasis, gastritis, polyuria, muscle weakness, osteosteoporosis or psychiatric disorders), personal history of bone fractures and we assessed biochemically for hypercalcemia, high blood level of intact parathyroid hormone (iPTH) and hypophosphatemia. Nephrolithiasis diagnosis was assessed through kidney ultrasonography only in patients with related symptoms. We also performed a bone densitometry through DEXA (dual-energy X-ray absorptiometry) to evaluate osteopenia or osteoporosis. We performed calcium:creatinine clearance ratio only in asymptomatic patients with a family history of hypercalcemia in order to differentiate between PHPT and familial hypocalciuric hypercalcemia (data not shown). Patients were subjected to localization studies such as neck ultrasonography and Tc99-sestamibi scintigraphy. Only the patients with confirmed PHPT (symptomatic or asymptomatic), which had an indication for surgery (serum calcium > 1.0 mg/dl above upper limit of normal range, BMD T score ≤ −2.5 at any site or fragility fracture, calculated glomerular filtration rate below 60 ml/min and age ≤ 50 years, according the Third International Workshop [17]), were included in the final analysis. After surgery, histopathology report was also reviewed. Subjects with incomplete clinical, pathology or biochemical evaluation were eliminated. Sixty patients fulfilled these criteria and were included for analysis. Information about demographic characteristics, previous diseases as hypertension, impairment of glucose metabolism (defined as impaired glucose tolerance in an oral glucose tolerance test or impaired fasting glucose) T2DM, dyslipidemia or obesity, diet and exercise habits were obtained from medical records.

The study was performed according to Declaration of Helsinki II and completed all the requirements of the local ethics committee (Comité Local de Investigación y Ética en Investigación en Salud). The protocol and the aim of the study were fully explained to the subjects, who gave their written consent.

Diagnostic criteria of the metabolic syndrome

Metabolic syndrome was defined according to the NCEP: ATPIII criteria as the presence of three or more of following components: waist circumference (WC) ≥102 cm in men and 88 cm in women, triglycerides > 150 mg/dl, c-HDL < 40 mg/dl in men and <50 mg/dl in women or a previously treated dyslipidemia, Systolic Blood Pressure of 130 mmHg or Diastolic Blood Pressure of 85 mm Hg or physician's diagnosis of hypertension or patients receiving treatment with antihypertensive drugs and fasting glucose >100 mg/dl or physician's diagnosis of diabetes [18].

Anthropometric measurements

At the time of evaluation we registered weight (kilograms) and height (meters), as well as waist circumference [WC] (centimeters). A single investigator, using the same calibrated scale with an integrated stadiometer, performed all the anthropometric measurements. WC was determined at the middle point between the inferior rim of the last costal arch and the superior rim of the anterosuperior iliac spine. Central obesity was defined using WC as previously mentioned. Body mass index (BMI) was calculated as the weight divided by height to the square. Those patients with BMI between 25–29.9 kg/m^2 were considered overweight and the ones with a BMI ≥30 kg/m^2 were considered obese according to World Health Organization (WHO) criteria. Blood pressure was determined in the left arm, after 10 minutes in a resting position, during a fasting state, without coffee or tobacco ingestion in the last week. The sphygmomanometer was calibrated and values were averaged after 2 different measurements with a 5-minute difference between them.

Biochemical determinations

For biochemical determinations all patients fulfilled a fasting state of 12 hours. Laboratory results were obtained with a 6 mL sample in BD Vacutainer (BD Franklin Lakes, New Jersey USA), centrifuged at 3150 *x g* for 15 minutes and serum was then analyzed with a kit for glucose, cholesterol, c-HDL and triglycerides (COBAS 2010 Roche Diagnostics, Indianapolis USA) using photocolorimetry with spectrophotometer Roche Modular P800 (2010 Roche Diagnostics, Indianapolis USA). c-HDL samples were treated with enzymes modified with polyethileneglycol and dextrane sulphate, analyzed with the same photocolorimetric technique. We used a specific chemioluminiscent assay to measure iPTH (DiaSorin Inc, Stillwater, Minnesota) with a sensitivity of 1 pg/ml and inter- and intra-assay coefficient of variation (CV) of 5.3% and 3.5%, respectively. Serum calcium (Ca) and phosphate (P) were tested using automated methods based on colorimetric and enzymatic assays (COBAS, Roche).

Statistical analysis

Results are expressed according to sample distribution with means and standard deviations (SD) or medians and interquartile ranges (IQR). Kolmogorov-Smirnov test was used to determine normality. To establish associations between quantitative variables, Student's *t* test or Mann–Whitney *U* test were used. Qualitative variables were associated with χ^2 or Fisher tests. Correlations between quantitative variables were tested with Pearson or Spearman test. A $p < 0.05$ was considered to be significant. Data were analyzed with SPSS v.16.

Results

Anthropometrical and clinical characteristics

Sixty patients with an average age of 53 years, completed clinical and biochemical assessment: 46 female and 14 male with a proportion of 3:1. According to our data, 65% of patients have a family history for T2DM and 48.3% for hypertension (data not shown). We found that 60% of patients (n = 36) had impaired glucose metabolism, 30% of patients had T2DM (n = 18), 68% (n = 41) had hypertriglyceridemia, 62% (n = 37) had central obesity, 40% (n = 24) had hypertension and 52% (n = 31) had low c-HDL concentration. In total, 60% (n = 36) of the patients with PHPT fulfilled MS diagnostic criteria according to the NCEP:ATPIII definition. Baseline characteristics of population are referred in Table 1.

Table 1 Baseline characteristics of patients with PHPT

Parameter	n = 60
Age (years), mean ± SD	53.5 ± 13.9
Female (%)	77
Weight (kg), median (IR)	68.2 (61.1-81.4)
Height (m), mean ± SD	1.57 ± 0.09
BMI (kg/m²), mean ± SD	29.08 ± 4.9
Waist (cm), median (IR)	91.5 (82.5-106.5)
Female	90.5 (83.5-105.5)
Male	97 (82–109)
Glucose (mg/dl), median (IR)	103 (87–115)
Calcium (mg/dl), mean ± SD	11.1 ± 1.09
Phosphorus (mg/dl), mean ± SD	3.08 ± 0.68
iPTH (ng/ml), median (RI)	127.5 (84.5-185)
Triglycerides (mg/dl), median (IR)	189.5 (130–269)
c-HDL (mg/dl), mean ± SD	47.3 ± 11.8
Female	48.7 ± 12.27
Male	42.7 ± 9.23
Clinical manifestations	
Pancreatitis	1%
Osteopenia	33%
Gastritis	37%
Osteoporosis	45%
Nephrolithiasis	52%
Muscular weakness	58%
Histopathology report	
Cancer	2%
Double adenoma	3%
Hyperplasia	23%
Single adenoma	72%

Abbreviations: BMI = body mass index, iPTH = intact parathyroid hormone, SD = standard deviation, IR = interquartile range.

When we compared patients with PHPT and MS (n = 36) and without MS (n = 24), we found that 89% had hypertriglyceridemia, 78% had alterations of glucose metabolism, 44% had T2DM, 83% had central obesity (according to sex), 58% had hypertension and 64% had low c-HDL concentration. In the group of patients that did not fulfill the MS criteria 29% (n = 7) had central obesity, 13% (n = 3) had HTN, 38% (n = 9) had hypertriglyceridemia, 33% (n = 8) had low c-HDL concentration, 33% (n = 8) had alterations on glucose metabolism and 8% (n = 2) had T2DM. It is noteworthy that not one of the patients in this study had completely normal metabolic parameters. Table 2 depicts other clinical and biochemical differences between groups. Considering that the age between groups was statistically different, we performed a stratified analysis dividing patients by age and sex. Most clinical and laboratory parameters were similar between these groups except for hypertension. Hypertensive patients were significantly older than the normotensive ones in both genders (66 + 20.2 years of age vs. 43 + 15.9, p = 0.037 for males and 60.7 + 9.8 vs. 49.7 + 10.7, p = 0.001 for females).

Table 2 Baseline clinical and biochemical characteristics of patients with PHPT with and without MS

	With MS	Without MS	*p*
Age (y), mean ± SD	57.2 ± 12.6	48 ± 14.2	0.014[a]
Female, n (%)	27 (75)	19 (79)	0.78
Weight (kg), median (IR)	73 (63–85)	63.5 (54–71)	0.010[b]
Height (m), mean ± SD	1.57 ± 0.09	1.56 ± 0.09	0.65
BMI (kg/m^2), mean ± SD	30.3 ± 4.58	27.1 ± 5.02	0.017[a]
Glucose (mg/dl), median (IR)	107 (96.7-126.5)	90 (84.5-102.7)	0.006[b]
Calcium (mg/dl), mean ± SD	10.8 ± 0.93	11.43 ± 1.25	0.07[a]
Phosphorus (mg/dl), mean ± SD	3.2 ± 0.60	2.9 ± 0.77	0.114
iPTH (ng/ml), median (IR)	115 (73.6-154.2)	161.5 (100.9-231.5)	0.017[b]
Triglycerides (mg/dl), median (IR)	231.5 (168.7-289.5)	133 (113.7-178.2)	<0.001[b]
c-HDL (mg/dl), mean ± SD			
Female			
Male	46.19 ± 12.6	52.42 ± 11.08	0.090
	41.78 ± 11.14	44.6 ± 4.72	0.604
Central obesity, n (%)	30(83)	7(29)	<0.001[c]
Hypertension, n(%)	21(58)	3(12.5)	<0.001[c]
Hypertriglyceridemia, n(%)	32(89)	9(38)	<0.001[c]
Low c-HDL concentration (%)	23(64)	8(33)	0.019[c]
Impairment of glucose metabolism, n(%)	28(78)	8(33)	0.001[c]
T2DM, n(%)	16(44)	2(8)	0.002[c]

Abbreviations: BMI = body mass index, T2DM = type 2 diabetes mellitus, IR = interquartile range, iPTH = intact parathyroid hormone. [a]Student *t* test, [b]Mann–Whitney *U* test, [c]Fisher's exact test.

We also found that 37% of total population was overweight and 33% were obese (according to BMI). In patients with MS the prevalence of obesity increased to 39% while overweight was present in 47%. In patients without MS the prevalence of excess weight and obesity was 21% and 25%, respectively; also, 87% of them had at least one component of MS.

We found that iPTH levels were higher in patients without MS (Table 2). Despite levels were not significant between groups, we found that phosphorus levels were negatively correlated with iPTH ($\rho = -0.416$, $p = 0.001$) and that calcium levels were higher in patients without MS. We did not find any correlation between iPTH, calcium and other metabolic parameters (data not shown).

Discussion

Our study shows that Mexican patients with PHPT have the highest prevalence of MS reported so far, reaching a staggering 60% of the cases. However, we should note that MS prevalence varies widely depending on diagnostic criteria used and the population studied. Nonetheless, other authors using the same criteria (NCEP:ATPIII criteria) reported lower prevalences; deLuis et al. reported a prevalence of MS of 32.3% in 62 patients with PHPT from Spain [19], Procopio et al. [20] found a prevalence of 47.6% in patients classified as low-risk asymptomatic, 8.7% in symptomatic patients and 8.3% in high-risk asymptomatic patients and Luigi et al. [21] reported a prevalence of 38% in 30 patients from University of Rome "Sapienza", Italy. In fact, according to our results, the presence of MS could be involved in the increased cardiovascular risk observed in patients with PHPT, which contrasts with Tassone et al. who reported that MS prevalence was similar between patients with PHPT and the general Italian population (Progetto Cuore Study) [22]. Unfortunately we don't have enough information comparing symptomatic or asymptomatic patients to compare with this group. At this point, we should consider that Mexico has one of the highest prevalences of obesity and hypoalphalipoproteinemia in the world (76.3% according to national health survey "ENSANUT 2006"), which may bias the whole sample and artificially increase the overall prevalence of MS. However the prevalence of MS is even higher in the patients with PHPT than in the general population of Mexico (36% according to ENSANUT 2006) [14]. More studies are required to assess if the presence of MS is involved in the higher frequency of cardiovascular risk factors associated with PHPT.

MS components are related to insulin resistance [10]. In our country, recent national health survey "ENSANUT 2012" reported that the prevalence of overweight and obesity is almost 73% [23], which is consistent with the 70% in our present findings. It seems that fatty acids released from adipose tissue in obese patients causes insulin resistance through disruption in insulin signaling cascade [24], increased inflammation, oxidative stress, coagulation abnormalities, endothelial damage, myocardial dysfunction and accelerated atherosclerosis [10,11]. We found that central obesity is one of the most frequent components of MS in this group (83% in MS group vs. 29% in the non-MS group, $p < 0.001$), just second to hypertriglyceridemia. The high prevalence of central obesity in these patients could be explored as the major cause of cardiovascular risk.

There are certain molecular associations between adipose tissue and PHTP. Some in vitro experiments showed that the increased levels of PTH rises intracellular calcium inside the adipocyte, promoting an increase in its activity for as much as 50-100%, and an increase in the expression of fatty acid synthetase, increase in the activity of glycerol-3-phosphate dehydrogenase and inhibition of basal lipolysis [25]. These changes could be associated to the increased lipogenesis and an increase in adipocyte volume and could contribute to hypertriglyceridemia, which was higher than reported for general population (31.4%) [14]. On other hand, it has also been demonstrated that PTH stimulates the adipose tissue differentiation and increases insulin resistance in these cells [26] in correlation to the adipose tissue mass. Finally, some studies suggest that increased fat mass induced by the increased concentrations of PTH acts as a leptin mediator [27]. Nonetheless de-Luis et al. [19] found that serum levels of leptin and adiponectin are not related to iPTH, vitamin D or calcium levels in patients with PHPT. Further data is required to clarify the inflammation component of PHPT in MS.

Other studies correlate the increased mass of adipose tissue with the decrease in the 25-hidroxyvitamin D concentration as well and a secondary form of hyperparathyroidism [28]. This deficiency in vitamin D seems to be associated to abnormalities in the carbohydrate metabolism but pharmacological approaches haven't shown favorable results [29]. Norenstedt et al. [30] studied 150 patients with PHPT after parathyroidectomy randomized in two groups, one with oral calcium carbonate and the other with calcium carbonate plus cholecalciferol. These authors found no improvement in metabolic parameters after one year of supplementation, despite the decrease in PTH levels. In the period where these patients were studied, vitamin D was not considered to be part of the diagnostic algorithm of PHPT and therefore was not available in our hospital. We consider that the low serum calcium reported in most of these patients, and even lower concentrations found in MS patients may have multiple causes. For once, it may be related to severe vitamin D deficiency, which is very frequent in the Mexican population (24% vs. 1% in other populations) [31] and has been reported to be even lower in obese patients [32]. The lower vitamin D concentrations usually seen in Mexican patients may have an impact in the calcium metabolism reported in our patients. Also, most of the patients were classified as having a relatively mild hyperparathyroidism, which is usually accompanied by lower serum calcium and PTH levels, unlike other reports were hyperparathyroidism was detected in more advanced stages. Other authors showed that obese patients with PHPT usually have higher PTHi levels than the ones in our report; however, all patients fulfilled diagnostic criteria for PHPT and had other indications for surgery, such as recurrent lithiasis or severe osteoporosis. Also, pathologic and imagenologic studies confirmed diagnosis. Clinical data associated with hyperparathyroidism may be an important consideration when a patient has a mildly altered laboratory results but damage to target organs such as bone or kidney are present.

Hyperparathyroidism (in any of its clinical presentations) is associated with altered carbohydrate metabolism and a disturbed insulin secretion or impaired cellular sensitivity [33,34]. In fact, Kumar et al. found that insulin sensitivity was lower in PHTP patients in comparison with a control group (60% vs. 113.7%) [35]. Procopio et al. found that almost 40% of patients with hyperparathyroidism have glucose intolerance in comparison with 25% found in healthy controls [33,34]. On the other hand, the prevalence of PHPT in patients with T2DM is 15%, (3 to 5 times higher than in patients without diabetes) [14]. According to data from ENSANUT 2012 the prevalence of T2DM in general population was 8.9% for patients between 40 to 49 years old and 19.2% for patients between 50 to 59 years old [36]. In our study, the prevalence of T2DM was 44%, twice than that reported for general population in any age group.

Regarding hypertension, we observed a prevalence of 40% in PHPT patients that is higher than in general population: 32.4% for male and 31.1% for female, [37,38]. A previous study has suggested that calcium levels are implicated in the pathogenesis of hypertension [39]. It seems that the increase in PTH levels promotes endothelial calcium influx and vasoconstriction. At this point, Petramala et al. found a positive correlation between iPTH levels and blood pressure [21]. However, in our study calcium and PTH levels were lower in patients with MS in comparison with patients without MS. This was also observed by Procopio et al. [20] and suggests that other metabolic a, such as vitamin D deficiency, could be involved.

Age and sex may be factors associated with the development of metabolic syndrome. In our study, the group with MS was statistically older than the group without it, which may reflect the evolution of MS trough time. Pairing patients by age or following them for several years, may reveal differences in the development of MS between patients treated surgically and the ones that haven't, however, this study may not be ethical in patients with overt or severe PHPT. Long term follow up studies have not been conclusive in terms of determining the usefulness of treating PHPT in order to improve cardiovascular risk profiles, since most of them have been followed for periods of around 1 year after surgery, which is not enough to correct some biochemical abnormalities and other confounding factors like diet and exercise which have not been controlled.

There are some limitations in our study that should also be considered. First, we studied a relatively small sample of PHPT patients, however we intended to have only patients whose diagnosis was confirmed by pathology and that had completed screening protocols. Second, the cross-sectional design of the study prevents us from comparing this group with a healthy control group. However this study is the first to describe the prevalence of MS in Mexican patients with PHPT, and the results suggest that MS may be more prevalent in some groups than previously expected. Populations where cardiovascular risk factors are frequent could be adversely affected if PHPT is also associated. Prospective studies of this population including wider searches for metabolic, inflammatory and cardiovascular parameters are warranted in order to properly assess their cardiovascular risk before and after surgery.

Conclusion

Our data shows the highest prevalence of MS in patients with PHPT ever reported. In our population, this could be related to the high prevalence of overweight and obesity. The most prevalent components of MS in PHPT are hypertriglyceridemia, central obesity and glucose metabolism impairment. These prevalences are even higher than reported in general population. We suggest that MS is involved in the cardiovascular risk associated to PHPT.

Ethical standards

The study was performed according to Declaration of Helsinki II and completed all the requirements of the local ethics committee (Comité Local de Investigación y Ética en Investigación en Salud). The protocol and the aim of the study were fully explained to the subjects, who gave their written consent.

Competing interests

The authors declare that they have no competing interests.

Authors' contributions

VMZ participated in the design of the study and helped to draft the manuscript. GAGV participated in collecting data and carried out information analysis. GVO participated in collecting data and carried out information analysis. BGV participated in collecting data and carried out information analysis. CRR helped write main draft, performed the final information and statistical analysis. MMA helped to draft the manuscript and carried out information analysis. MAMA participated in collecting data and helped to draft the manuscript. AFH helped write main draft, performed the final information and statistical analysis. All the authors read and approved the final manuscript.

Acknowledgements

The authors have no additional acknowledgements.

Author details

[1]Endocrinology Departament Hospital de Especialidades Centro Médico Nacional Siglo XXI, Instituto Mexicano del Seguro Social (IMSS), Cuauhtemoc N° 330, Colonia Doctores, México City, DF, Mexico. [2]Endocrinology Experimental Investigation Unit Hospital de Especialidades Centro Médico Nacional Siglo XXI, Instituto Mexicano del Seguro Social (IMSS), Cuauhtemoc N° 330, Colonia Doctores, México City, DF, Mexico.

References

1. Adami S, Marcocci C, Gatti D. Epidemiology of primary hyperparathyroidism in Europe. J Bone Miner Res. 2002;17 Suppl 2:N18–23.
2. Wermers RA, Khosla S, Atkinson EJ, Achenbach SJ, Oberg AL, Grant CS, et al. Incidence of primary hyperparathyroidism in Rochester, Minnesota, 1993–2001: an update on the changing epidemiology of the disease. J Bone Miner Res. 2006;21(1):171–7.
3. Hedback GM, Oden AS. Cardiovascular disease, hypertension and renal function in primary hyperparathyroidism. J Intern Med. 2002;251(6):476–83.
4. Nilsson IL, Yin L, Lundgren E, Rastad J, Ekbom A. Clinical presentation of primary hyperparathyroidism in Europe–nationwide cohort analysis on mortality from nonmalignant causes. J Bone Miner Res. 2002;17 Suppl 2:N68–74.
5. Silverberg SJ, Lewiecki EM, Mosekilde L, Peacock M, Rubin MR. Presentation of asymptomatic primary hyperparathyroidism: proceedings of the third international workshop. J Clin Endocrinol Metab. 2009;94(2):351–65.
6. Garcia de la Torre N, Wass JA, Turner HE. Parathyroid adenomas and cardiovascular risk. Endocr Relat Cancer. 2003;10(2):309–22.
7. Han D, Trooskin S, Wang X. Prevalence of cardiovascular risk factors in male and female patients with primary hyperparathyroidism. J Endocrinol Invest. 2012;35(6):548–52.
8. Bolland MJ, Grey AB, Gamble GD, Reid IR. Association between primary hyperparathyroidism and increased body weight: a meta-analysis. J Clin Endocrinol Metab. 2005;90(3):1525–30.
9. Oda E. Metabolic syndrome: its history, mechanisms, and limitations. Acta Diabetol. 2012;49(2):89–95.
10. Reaven GM. Banting lecture 1988. Role of insulin resistance in human disease. Diabetes. 1988;37(12):1595–607.
11. Samson SL, Garber AJ. Metabolic syndrome. Endocrinol Metab Clin North Am. 2014;43(1):1–23.
12. Beltran-Sanchez H, Harhay MO, Harhay MM, McElligott S. Prevalence and trends of metabolic syndrome in the adult U.S. population 1999–2010. J Am College of Cardiology. 2013;62(8):697–703.
13. Gao W. Does the constellation of risk factors with and without abdominal adiposity associate with different cardiovascular mortality risk? Int J Obes (Lond). 2008;32(5):757–62.
14. Rojas R, Aguilar-Salinas CA, Jimenez-Corona A, Shamah-Levy T, Rauda J, Avila-Burgos L, et al. Metabolic syndrome in Mexican adults: results from the National Health and Nutrition Survey 2006. Salud Publica Mex. 2010;52 Suppl 1:S11–8.
15. Acuna-Alonzo V, Flores-Dorantes T, Kruit JK, Villarreal-Molina T, Arellano-Campos O, Hunemeier T, et al. A functional ABCA1 gene variant is associated with low HDL-cholesterol levels and shows evidence of positive selection in Native Americans. Hum Mol Genet. 2010;19(14):2877–85.
16. Lopez-Reyes A, Rodriguez-Perez JM, Fernandez-Torres J, Martinez-Rodriguez N, Perez-Hernandez N, Fuentes-Gomez AJ, et al. The HIF1A rs2057482 polymorphism is associated with risk of developing premature coronary artery disease and with some metabolic and cardiovascular risk factors. The Genetics of Atherosclerotic Disease (GEA) Mexican Study. Exp Mol Pathol. 2014;96(3):405–10.

17. Bilezikian JP, Khan AA, Potts Jr JT. Guidelines for the management of asymptomatic primary hyperparathyroidism: summary statement from the third international workshop. J Clin Endocrinol Metab. 2009;94(2):335–9.
18. Expert Panel on Detection, Evaluation, and Treatment of High Blood Cholesterol in Adults. Executive Summary of The Third Report of The National Cholesterol Education Program (NCEP) Expert Panel on Detection, Evaluation, And Treatment of High Blood Cholesterol In Adults (Adult Treatment Panel III). JAMA. 2001;285(19):2486–97.
19. de Luis DA, Soto GD, Conde R, Izaola O, de la Fuente B. Relation of leptin and adiponectin with cardiovascular risk factors, intact parathormone, and vitamin D levels in patients with primary hyperparathyroidism. J Clin Lab Anal. 2012;26(5):398–402.
20. Procopio M, Barale M, Bertaina S, Sigrist S, Mazzetti R, Loiacono M, et al. Cardiovascular risk and metabolic syndrome in primary hyperparathyroidism and their correlation to different clinical forms. Endocrine. 2014;47(2):581–9.
21. Petramala L, Chiara FM, Laura Z, Cristiano M, Giuseppina C, Luciano C, et al. Arterial Hypertension. Metabolic Syndrome and Subclinical Cardiovascular Organ Damage in Patients with Asymptomatic Primary Hyperparathyroidism before and after Parathyroidectomy: Preliminary Results. Int J Endocrinol. 2012;2012:408295.
22. Tassone F, Gianotti L, Baffoni C, Cesario F, Magro G, Pellegrino M, et al. Prevalence and characteristics of metabolic syndrome in primary hyperparathyroidism. J Endocrinol Invest. 2012;35(9):841–6.
23. Barquera S, Campos-Nonato I, Hernandez-Barrera L, Pedroza A, Rivera-Dommarco JA. Prevalence of obesity in Mexican adults 2000–2012. Salud Publica Mex. 2013;55 Suppl 2:S151–60.
24. Gallagher EJ, LeRoith D, Karnieli E. The metabolic syndrome–from insulin resistance to obesity and diabetes. Endocrinol Metab Clin North Am. 2008;37(3):559–79. vii.
25. Dorheim MA, Sullivan M, Dandapani V, Wu X, Hudson J, Segarini PR, et al. Osteoblastic gene expression during adipogenesis in hematopoietic supporting murine bone marrow stromal cells. J Cell Physiol. 1993;154(2):317–28.
26. Raisz LG, Kream BE. Regulation of bone formation. N Engl J Med. 1983;309(1):29–35.
27. Grethen E, Hill KM, Jones R, Cacucci BM, Gupta CE, Acton A, et al. Serum leptin, parathyroid hormone, 1,25-dihydroxyvitamin D, fibroblast growth factor 23, bone alkaline phosphatase, and sclerostin relationships in obesity. J Clin Endocrinol Metab. 2012;97(5):1655–62.
28. Botella-Carretero JI, Alvarez-Blasco F, Villafruela JJ, Balsa JA, Vazquez C, Escobar-Morreale HF. Vitamin D deficiency is associated with the metabolic syndrome in morbid obesity. Clin Nutr. 2007;26(5):573–80.
29. de Boer IH, Tinker LF, Connelly S, Curb JD, Howard BV, Kestenbaum B, et al. Calcium plus vitamin D supplementation and the risk of incident diabetes in the Women's Health Initiative. Diabetes Care. 2008;31(4):701–7.
30. Norenstedt S, Pernow Y, Brismar K, Saaf M, Ekip A, Granath F, et al. Primary hyperparathyroidism and metabolic risk factors, impact of parathyroidectomy and vitamin D supplementation, and results of a randomized double-blind study. European J Endocrinology/European Federation of Endocrine Societies. 2013;169(6):795–804.
31. Brito A, Cori H, Olivares M, Fernanda Mujica M, Cediel G, Lopez de Romana D. Less than adequate vitamin D status and intake in Latin America and the Caribbean:a problem of unknown magnitude. Food Nutr Bull. 2013;34(1):52–64.
32. Elizondo-Montemayor L, Ugalde-Casas PA, Serrano-Gonzalez M, Cuello-Garcia CA, Borbolla-Escoboza JR. Serum 25-hydroxyvitamin d concentration, life factors and obesity in Mexican children. Obesity (Silver Spring). 2010;18(9):1805–11.
33. Procopio M, Magro G, Cesario F, Piovesan A, Pia A, Molineri N, et al. The oral glucose tolerance test reveals a high frequency of both impaired glucose tolerance and undiagnosed Type 2 diabetes mellitus in primary hyperparathyroidism. Diabet Med. 2002;19(11):958–61.
34. Taylor WH, Khaleeli AA. Coincident diabetes mellitus and primary hyperparathyroidism. Diabetes Metab Res Rev. 2001;17(3):175–80.
35. Kumar S, Olukoga AO, Gordon C, Mawer EB, France M, Hosker JP, et al. Impaired glucose tolerance and insulin insensitivity in primary hyperparathyroidism. Clin Endocrinol (Oxf). 1994;40(1):47–53.
36. Hernandez-Avila M, Gutierrez JP, Reynoso-Noveron N. Diabetes mellitus in Mexico. Status of the epidemic. Salud Publica Mex. 2013;55 Suppl 2:S129–36.
37. Campos-Nonato I, Hernandez-Barrera L, Rojas-Martinez R, Pedroza A, Medina-Garcia C, Barquera-Cervera S, et al. Hypertension: prevalence, early diagnosis, control and trends in Mexican adults. Salud Publica Mex. 2013;55 Suppl 2:S144–50.
38. Barquera S, Campos-Nonato I, Hernandez-Barrera L, Villalpando S, Rodriguez-Gilabert C, Durazo-Arvizu R, et al. Hypertension in Mexican adults: results from the National Health and Nutrition Survey 2006. Salud Publica Mex. 2010;52 Suppl 1:S63–71.
39. Fardella C, Rodriguez-Portales JA. Intracellular calcium and blood pressure: comparison between primary hyperparathyroidism and essential hypertension. J Endocrinol Invest. 1995;18(11):827–32.

13

Localized subacute thyroiditis presenting as a painful hot nodule

Lian-Xi Li[1*†], Xing Wu[2†], Bing Hu[2], Hui-Zhen Zhang[3] and Han-Kui Lu[4*]

Abstract

Background: A diagnosis of subacute thyroiditis is readily considered when patients present with a particular set of typical clinical characteristics. Subacute thyroiditis sometimes presents as a solitary cold nodule; however, the presence of a hot nodule in patients with subacute thyroiditis is exceedingly rare.

Case presentation: Here, the case of a 57-year-old woman complaining of pain in the left neck and fatigue for two weeks is presented. Physical examination revealed a painful and tender nodule with a diameter of approximately 1.5 cm in the left neck, although all laboratory tests, including white blood cell count, neutrophil percentage, erythrocyte sedimentation rate (ESR), thyroid function, and thyroglobin levels, were normal. A neck ultrasound revealed a hypoechoic mass (1.5 × 0.8 cm) in the left thyroid, and thyroid scintigraphy of the left thyroid with Technetium-99 m (99 m-Tc) demonstrated a focal accumulation of radiotracer. Furthermore, fine-needle aspiration biopsy from the nodule revealed the presence of multinuclear giant cells. The patient was well; there was no cervical mass detected upon palpation following two months of prednisone treatment, and follow-up ultrasound screening and scintigraphy demonstrated the disappearance of the nodule.

Conclusion: This case, presenting with a localized painful hot nodule, normal thyroid function, normal ESR, and normal serum thyroglobulin levels, is a rare case of subacute thyroiditis, which should be considered during differential diagnosis.

Keywords: Subacute thyroiditis, Thyroid nodule, Hot nodule

Background

Subacute thyroiditis, also known as de Quervain's thyroiditis, giant-cell thyroiditis, or subacute granulomatous thyroiditis, is a spontaneously remitting inflammatory disease of the thyroid gland [1,2]. Subacute thyroiditis is generally caused by viral infection and is the most common cause of a painful thyroid [1,3]. Patients with subacute thyroiditis usually have a history of antecedent viral infection and subsequently suffer from neck pain, thyroid tenderness, fever, and fatigue. Upon physical examination, the thyroid of the patient is often tender and diffusely enlarged.

In most cases, a diagnosis of subacute thyroiditis is usually self-evident and can be made based on patient history, physical and laboratory findings, and the clinical course of the disease. In some cases, in addition to the clinical course and features, fine needle aspiration cytology, ultrasound, and scintigraphy analyses may support the diagnosis of subacute thyroiditis. For example, thyroid radioisotope scanning generally demonstrates a low uptake of Technetium-99 m (99 m-Tc) or 131I [4]. However, patients with subacute thyroiditis sometimes present with puzzling clinical features that can escape early recognition [2,3,5,6]. Here, a patient with subacute thyroiditis, who presented with a solitary painful thyroid nodule in the absence of typical laboratory test characteristics that would suggest subacute thyroiditis and whose 99 m-Tc thyroid scan revealed a hot nodule in the left lobe of thyroid, is described. To the best of our knowledge, the presence of a hot nodule in a patient with subacute thyroiditis has not been previously reported.

* Correspondence: lilx@sjtu.edu.cn; luhankui@sina.com
†Equal contributors
[1]Department of Endocrinology and Metabolism, Shanghai Diabetes Institute; Shanghai Clinical Center for Diabetes; Shanghai key Laboratory of Diabetes Mellitus, Shanghai Jiao Tong University Affiliated Sixth People's Hospital, 600 Yishan Road, Shanghai 200233, China
[4]Department of Nuclear Medicine, Shanghai Jiao Tong University Affiliated Sixth People's Hospital, 600 Yishan Road, Shanghai 200233, China

Case presentation

A 57-year-old woman with no history of thyroid disease visited our outpatient endocrine clinic on July 27, 2012. Two weeks prior, she had developed symptoms of pain in the left neck and fatigue. Physical examination revealed a focal nodule of the left thyroid lobe that had a diameter of approximately 1.5 cm without local redness or lymph node enlargement, which was painful and tender upon examination. There was no fever or signs of hyperthyroidism such as tachycardia, insomnia, or tremors. The patient's thyroid function tests were normal (thyroid stimulating hormone = 1.25 mU/L, normal range: 0.27-4.2 mU/L; free triiodothyronine = 5.59 pmmol/L, normal range: 3.1-6.8 pmmol/L; free thyroxine = 18.80 pmmol/L, normal range: 12–22 pmmol/L) and tests for anti-thyroglobulin (<10 KIU/L, normal range: 0–115 KIU/L), anti-thyroid peroxidase (10.54 KIU/L, normal range: 0–35 KIU/L), and anti-thyrotropin-receptor antibodies (<1 U/L, normal range: 0–2 U/L) were negative. The patient's serum thyroglobulin levels were normal (61.32 ug/L, normal range: 1.40-78 ug/L); her white cell count was 5.2×10^9/L with a normal differential, and her erythrocyte sedimentation rate (ESR) was 20 mm/hour (normal range: 0–38 mm/h).

A thyroid ultrasound examination revealed a dyshomogeneous and hypoechoic mass (1.5 × 0.8 cm) in the left thyroid lobe that exhibited an irregular and poorly defined border (Figure 1A). Thyroid scintigraphy with 99 m-Tc demonstrated a focal accumulation of radiotracer uptake in the lower part of the left thyroid lobe but a normal uptake and configuration of the middle and upper portion of the left lobe and the right lobe (Figure 1B). Fine-needle aspiration biopsy from the nodule in the lower left lobe revealed multinuclear giant cells consistent with subacute thyroiditis (Figure 2). Subsequently, localized subacute thyroiditis was suspected and the patient was put on prednisone (30 mg/day) for 10 days, which resulted in a rapid resolution of the neck pain. Within a week, the patient's fatigue had disappeared and the tender thyroid nodule had regressed. Prednisone was gradually withdrawn and ultimately stopped after 2 months at which time palpation did not demonstrate a cervical mass. Repeated ultrasound screening revealed a disappearance of the hypoechoic nodule (Figure 3A) and follow-up scintigraphy analysis found the thyroid exhibited an even distribution of radionuclide in both lobes (Figure 3B).

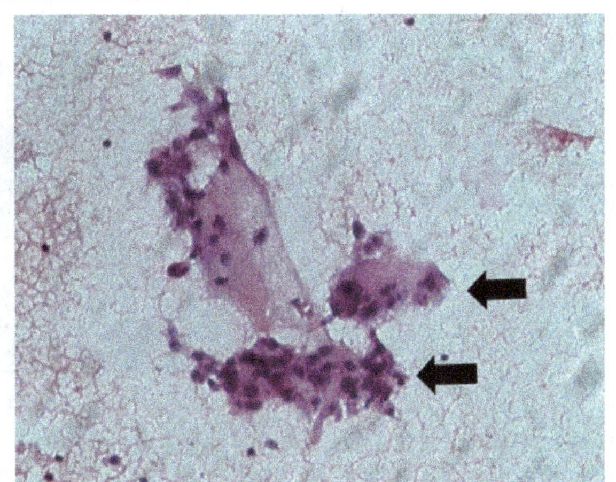

Figure 2 Fine-needle aspiration cytology of the left thyroid nodule. Fine-needle aspiration biopsy from the nodule in the left lobe revealed multinuclear giant cells in the thyroid nodule consistent with subacute thyroiditis (indicated by black arrows).

Conclusions

Subacute thyroiditis is the most common cause of non-autoimmune thyroiditis [7]. In addition to the typical clinical signs, characteristic ultrasound findings of subacute thyroiditis include the presence of an ill-defined hypoechoic area with a nonhomogeneous pattern [8]. Recently, Ruchala et al. [9] demonstrated the usefulness of

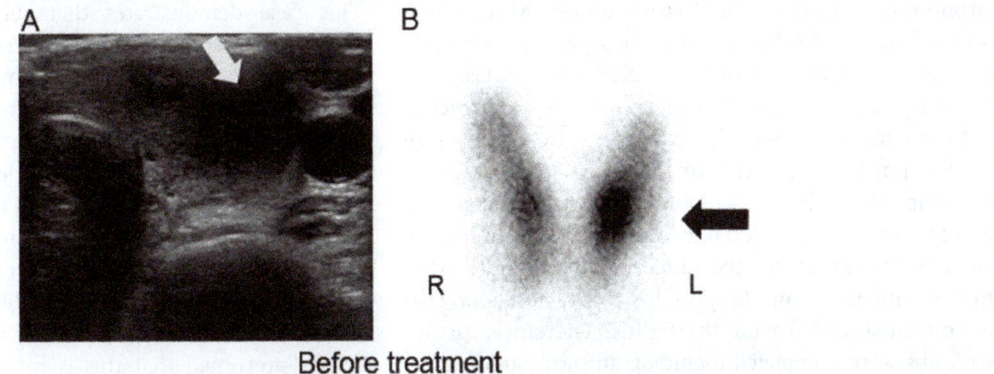

Figure 1 Initial thyroid ultrasound scanning and 99 m-Technetium scintiscan. A. Thyroid ultrasonography revealed a dyshomogeneous and hypoechoic nodule (15 × 0.8 mm) with an irregular and poorly defined border in the left thyroid lobe (indicated by a white arrow). **B.** Thyroid scintigraphy with 99 m-Tc showed a focal accumulation of radiotracer uptake in the lower lobe of the left thyroid, which represents the palpable tender nodule (indicated by a black arrow).

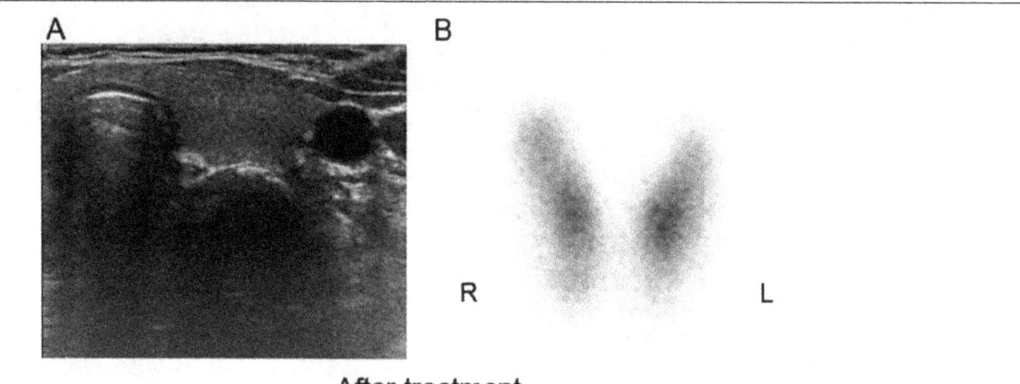

Figure 3 Follow-up ultrasound scanning and 99 m-Technetium scintiscan. A. Follow-up ultrasound scanning demonstrated the disappearance of the hypoechoic nodule in the left thyroid lobe. **B.** Follow-up scintigraphy showed the disappearance of the "hot" nodule in the left thyroid lobe and an even distribution of radionuclide in both lobes.

sonoelastography for the diagnosis of subacute thyroiditis. The cytological features found during thyroid fine-needle aspiration include the presence of large multinucleated giant cells or epithelioid granulomas, but the absence of these findings does not exclude the diagnosis of subacute thyroiditis [10,11]. Generally speaking, elevated serum thyroid hormones, a tender enlarged thyroid, and low radioiodine thyroid uptake are characteristic of subacute thyroiditis [12]. Although cases with these typical signs may present little difficulty for a diagnosis of subacute thyroiditis, this disorder does not always present in a classic fashion and may lead to difficulties during diagnosis [5,6]. Sometimes the diagnosis may be less clear, particularly when the primary presenting symptom is a solitary thyroid nodule in conjunction with normal thyroid function, thyroglobulin levels, and a normal ESR [13].

Previously, thyroid nodules have been identified in association with subacute thyroiditis and, in some patients with subacute thyroiditis, only one nodule is present [14,15]. For example, Liel [16] reported a case that presented with the coexistence of subacute thyroiditis and an autonomously functioning thyroid nodule. More often, localized forms of subacute thyroiditis present as painful and tender "cold" thyroid nodules, which disappear following recovery [14]. However, subacute thyroiditis that presents as a painful "hot" nodule is exceedingly rare and has not been reported. In this case, laboratory tests, including white blood cell count, neutrophil percentage, thyroid function, thyroglobin levels, and ESR, were normal and non-diagnostic but the clinical findings (neck pain, thyroid tenderness, and fatigue) led to the consideration of a diagnosis of subacute thyroiditis. Therefore, further work-ups were completed including an ultrasound examination of the neck, thyroid scintigraphy with 99 m-Tc, and fine needle aspiration cytology of the nodule. Ultrasound examination demonstrated a dyshomogeneous and hypoechoic mass in the thyroid, which was characteristic of subacute thyroiditis, and thyroid scintigraphy showed a focal accumulation of radiotracer uptake in the thyroid nodule. The histological features of the nodule were also typical of subacute thyroiditis. Therefore, a diagnosis of localized subacute thyroiditis was given and the patient was prescribed prednisone, which resulted in the disappearance of the hot thyroid nodule. The treatment of subacute thyroiditis is essentially symptomatic and includes non-steroidal anti-inflammatory agents or, occasionally, glucocorticoids if the symptoms are prolonged or severe. In the current case, treatment with steroids resulted in an amelioration of the patient's symptoms and the disappearance of the thyroid nodule after 2 months.

Based on the course and the clinical presentation of the present case, a diagnosis of subacute thyroiditis could be established. The disappearance of the thyroid nodule following prednisone treatment further confirms the diagnosis of subacute thyroiditis following presentation with a thyroid hot nodule. Here, the appearance of the hot thyroid nodule was unusual in that it did not show the usual pattern of low uptake during radioisotope scanning. This case demonstrates that subacute thyroiditis may present as a solitary painful hot nodule in conjunction with normal thyroid function, thyroglobulin levels, and ESR and should, therefore, be considered in the differential diagnosis of such lesions.

The mechanism of 99 mm-Tc localization in subacute thyroiditis is not known. Tonami et al. [17] reported two cases of subacute thyroiditis in which thyroid scintigrams with 201TI chloride showed increased radionuclide activity in the affected areas but decreased activity in the affected areas following thyroid scintigrams with 99 m-Tc. It was presumed that this is primarily due to increased membrane permeability in the inflammatory lesion without the apparent destruction of the thyroid gland, which is typically indicated by normal thyroglobulin levels and thyroid function in the patient. Therefore, the present case suggests the clinical and pathological heterogeneity of subacute thyroiditis.

In conclusion, this case demonstrates that subacute thyroiditis should be considered as a differential diagnosis following presentation with a solitary painful thyroid hot nodule in conjunction with normal thyroid function, thyroglobulin levels, and ESR. Additionally, this case emphasizes the heterogeneous pattern of thyroid imaging in subacute thyroiditis.

Consent

Written informed consent was obtained by the patient for the publication of this case report and any accompanying images.

Competing interests

The authors declare that they have no competing interests.

Authors' contributions

LL drafted the manuscript; WX collected all medical reports of the patients and LHK revised the manuscript critically. HB performed ultrasound examination and ZHZ carried out pathological examination. All authors read and approved the final manuscript.

Acknowledgments

This work was supported by grants from the National Natural Science Foundation of China (81170759) and Innovation Program of Shanghai Municipal Education Commission (1322015).

Author details

[1]Department of Endocrinology and Metabolism, Shanghai Diabetes Institute; Shanghai Clinical Center for Diabetes; Shanghai key Laboratory of Diabetes Mellitus, Shanghai Jiao Tong University Affiliated Sixth People's Hospital, 600 Yishan Road, Shanghai 200233, China. [2]Department of Ultrasonography, Shanghai Jiao Tong University Affiliated Sixth People's Hospital, 600 Yishan Road, Shanghai 200233, China. [3]Department of Pathology, Shanghai Jiao Tong University Affiliated Sixth People's Hospital, 600 Yishan Road, Shanghai 200233, China. [4]Department of Nuclear Medicine, Shanghai Jiao Tong University Affiliated Sixth People's Hospital, 600 Yishan Road, Shanghai 200233, China.

References

1. Pearce EN, Farwell AP, Braverman LE: **Thyroiditis.** *N Engl J Med* 2003, **348:**2646–2655.
2. Geva T, Theodor R: **Atypical presentation of subacute thyroiditis.** *Arch Dis Child* 1988, **63:**845–846.
3. Tsai CH, Lee JJ, Liu CL, Tzen CY, Cheng SP: **Atypical subacute thyroiditis.** *Surgery* 2010, **147:**461–462.
4. Kitchener MI, Chapman IM: **Subacute thyroiditis: a review of 105 cases.** *Clin Nucl Med* 1989, **14:**439–442.
5. Huang C, Wang X: **Subacute thyroiditis manifesting as a thyroid mass, vocal cord paralysis, and hypercalcemia.** *Endocr Pract* 2012, **18:**e17–e20.
6. Bartels PC, Boer RO: **Subacute thyroiditis (de Quervain) presenting as a painless "cold" nodule.** *J Nucl Med* 1987, **28:**1488–1490.
7. Bianda T, Schmid C: **De Quervain's subacute thyroiditis presenting as a painless solitary thyroid nodule.** *Postgrad Med J* 1998, **74:**602–603.
8. Park SY, Kim EK, Kim MJ, *et al*: **Ultrasonographic characteristics of subacute granulomatous thyroiditis.** *Korean J Radiol* 2006, **7:**229–234.
9. Ruchala M, Szczepanek E, Sowinski J: **Sonoelastography in de Quervain thyroiditis.** *J Clin Endocrinol Metab* 2011, **96:**289–290.
10. Mordes DA, Brachtel EF: **Cytopathology of subacute thyroiditis.** *Diagn Cytopathol* 2012, **40:**433–434.
11. Garcia SJ, Gimenez BA, Sola PJ, *et al*: **Fine-needle aspiration of subacute granulomatous thyroiditis (De Quervain's thyroiditis): a clinico-cytologic review of 36 cases.** *Diagn Cytopathol* 1997, **16:**214–220.
12. Sari O, Erbas B, Erbas T: **Subacute thyroiditis in a single lobe.** *Clin Nucl Med* 2001, **26:**400–401.
13. Szczepanek-Parulska E, Zybek A, Biczysko M, Majewski P, Ruchala M: **What might cause pain in the thyroid gland? Report of a patient with subacute thyroiditis of atypical presentation.** *Endokrynol Pol* 2012, **63:**138–142.
14. Hardoff R, Baron E, Sheinfeld M, Luboshitsky R: **Localized manifestations of subacute thyroiditis presenting as solitary transient cold thyroid nodules. A report of 11 patients.** *Clin Nucl Med* 1995, **20:**981–984.
15. Nygaard B, Jarlov AE, Hegedus L, Schaadt B, Kristensen LO, Hansen JM: **Long-term follow-up of thyroid scintigraphies after 131I therapy of solitary autonomous thyroid nodules.** *Thyroid* 1994, **4:**167–171.
16. Liel Y: **The survivor: association of an autonomously functioning thyroid nodule and subacute thyroiditis.** *Thyroid* 2007, **17:**183–184.
17. Tonami N, Bunko H, Kuwajima A, Hisada K: **Increased localization of 201 Tl-chloride in subacute thyroiditis.** *Clin Nucl Med* 1979, **4:**3–5.

14

Polymorphisms of interleukin-21 and interleukin-21-receptor genes confer risk for autoimmune thyroid diseases

Jian Zhang[1], Wan Xia Xiao[2], Yuan Feng Zhu[3,4], Fatuma Said Muhali[3], Ling Xiao[3], Wen Juan Jiang[3], Xiao Hong Shi[3], Lian Hua Zhou[3] and Jin An Zhang[3*]

Abstract

Background: The abnormality of interleukin-21 (IL-21)-IL-21-receptor (IL-21R) system has been found in many autoimmune diseases including autoimmune thyroid diseases (AITDs). In this study, we investigated whether polymorphisms of the IL-21 and IL-21R are associated with Graves' disease (GD) and Hashimoto's thyroiditis (HT), two major forms of AITDs, among a Chinese population.

Methods: Rs907715, rs4833837, rs2221903 and rs2055979 of the IL-21 gene and rs3093301 and rs2285452 of the IL-21R gene were explored in a case–control study including 405 GD, 228 HT patients and 242 controls. These genes were genotyped by the PCR and restriction fragment length polymorphism (RFLP) analysis and the MASS spectrometry method.

Results: For IL-21 gene, we identified and confirmed a higher prevalence of A alleles of rs2221903 (P = 0.018, OR = 1.50 95% CI = 1.07-2.09) in GD patients. We also found a significant association between rs2221903 and HT (allele: P = 0.009, OR = 1.69 95% CI = 1.13-2.51; genotype: recessive P = 0.021, OR = 11.72 95% CI = 1.46-94.13). For the IL-21R gene, compared with controls, the genotype frequencies of rs3093301 and rs2285452 were significantly different in HT patients using dominant genetic model (P = 0.023, OR = 1.61 95% CI = 1.07-2.42; P = 0.031, OR = 1.71 95% CI = 1.05-2.80, respectively). Furthermore, the haplotype AA containing the major alleles of rs4833837 and rs2221903 was associated with increased susceptibility to GD with an OR of 1.50(95% CI =1.08-2.09, P = 0.016), and to HT with an OR of 1.69(95% CI =1.14-2.52, P = 0.009).

Conclusion: Our results indicated that the SNPs of the IL-21 gene is associated with the development of GD. In addition, we found that individuals with the SNPs of the common IL-21 and IL-21R may have higher risk of HT.

Keywords: Interleukin-21 (IL-21), Interleukin-21 receptor (IL-21R), Graves' disease, Hashimoto's thyroiditis, Single nucleotide polymorphism (SNP)

Background

Autoimmune thyroid diseases (AITDs), the thyroid-specific autoimmune disorders, affect about 5% of the population. The etiology of AITDs includes genetic and environmental factors resulting in immune abnormality and the development of AITDs.

In 2000, the interleukin-21(IL-21)-IL21-receptor (IL-21R) system was discovered [1]. IL-21 and IL-21R are located on human chromosome 4q26-27 and 16p11, respectively. The IL-21, preferentially produced by CD4 + T cells, has various functions, such as driving B cells to differentiate into memory cells and ultimately plasma cells, augmenting T cells' proliferation, and promoting the activity of natural killer (NK) cells [2]. In accordance with these roles of IL-21, IL-21R is mainly expressed in B cells, T cells and NK cells, keratinocytes, and some of myeloid cells. Animal and clinical studies demonstrated the dysregulations of IL-21 and IL-21R in autoimmune diseases. For example, compared with IL-21R-competent BXSB-Yaa mice for multiple parameters of SLE, the

* Correspondence: zhangjinan@hotmail.com
[3]Endocrinology Department, Jinshan Hospital, Fudan University, 1508 Longhang Road, Shanghai 201508, China

IL-21R-deficient Yaa mice showed none of the abnormalities characteristic of systemic lupus erythematosus (SLE) [3]. IL-21R is overexpressed in the inflamed synovial membrane and in peripheral blood or synovial fluid leukocytes of rheumatoid arthritis (RA) patients [4]. And the evident increase of serum IL-21 level in primary Sjogren's syndrome (pSS) patients has positive correlation with the levels of gamma-globulin and erythrocyte sedimentation rate [5].These suggests that IL-21 and IL-21R may play a critical role in the pathogenesis of autoimmune diseases. Recently, H.Y. Jia [6] also reported that an increase of serum IL-21 level in patients with primary GD.

In recent years, the associations between the IL-21 gene or IL-21R gene polymorphisms and autoimmune diseases have been gradually reported. In a HapMap-CEU population, a large block (480 kb) of linkage disequilibrium encompassing KIAA1109/Tenr/IL2/IL21 showed genetic associations with type 1 diabetes mellitus (T1DM) [7,8], RA [8], juvenile idiopathic arthritis (JIA) [9], psoriasis and psoriatic arthritis(PA) [10]. Similarly, the polymorphisms of the IL2/IL21 gene region likely to confer to the susceptibility to coeliac disease in Scandinavia families [11] and a US population [12], to ulcerative colitis in a North American and an Italian cohort [13], and to multiple sclerosis in a Spanish population [14]. After the SNPs in the IL-21 gene were analyzed, the significant differences of rs907715 and rs2221903 allele and genotype frequencies were found between SLE and controls [15]. In addition to these reports, an association between microsatellite polymorphisms of the IL-21R and diabetes in Japanese patients, between rs3093301 and rs2285452 in the IL-21R gene region and SLE in the European-derived cohort were documented [16].

Therefore, it is reasonable to speculate that IL-21 and IL-21R are the candidate genes for AITDs. Plagnol [17] reported that the rs2069763 in chromosome 4q27 were associated with the GD susceptibility in a Caucasian cohort. And a recent study that indicated that rs907715 of IL-21 gene was associated with GD in a Chinese population [6].

In this study, additional variants of the IL-21 gene and two SNPs of the IL-21R gene in addition to previously reported variants were investigated in two subtypes of AITDs including GD and HT.

Methods

Patients and controls

AITDs patients and healthy controls were enrolled from the First Affiliated Hospital, Medical School of Xi'an Jiaotong University. A total of 633 independent patients with AITDs, including 405 GD and 228 HT, and 242 unrelated healthy controls were recruited. GD and HT were diagnosed based on clinical and laboratory evidence of hyperthyroidism and hypothyroidism respectively and diffuse goitre, supported by the presence of antithyroglobulin antibody (TgAb) and/or antithyroid peroxidase antibody (TPOAb) and/or exophthalmos. The controls were healthy subjects without clinical evidence or family history of any AITDs. This study was approved by the ethics committee of Jinshan hospital of Fudan University. All patients and control subjects were asked to sign an informed consent.

Genotyping

Genomic DNA was extracted from peripheral blood leukocytes using the Nucleon Bacc kit from TianGen Biotech CO. LTD (Beijing, China).

Rs907715, rs4833837, rs2221903 and rs2055979 spanning a large region which captured all common variation in the IL-21 gene and rs3093301 and rs2285452 which were only two tag-SNPs of IL-21R gene confirmed to be associated with SLE in European-derived cohort were selected from the published SNP database (http://www.ncbi.nlm.nih.gov/SNP). All of these SNPs were validated polymorphisms, and have a minor allele frequency(MAF) of more than 1%. Rs907715, rs4833837, and rs222190 are located on intron 2 of IL-21R and rs2055979 on intron 3. For IL-21R gene, rs3093301 is in intron 2 and rs2285452 in exon 10.

All of the four IL-21 SNPs and rs2285452 were typed using mass spectrometry method (Shanghai Benegene Biotechnologies CO. Ltd. Shanghai, China). Rs3093301 was typed using PCR-restriction fragment length polymorphism (PCR-RELP) method. The appropriate fragment of rs3093301 in the IL-21R gene was amplified using specific primers (forward: 5′-AATTGCTCCT CAGCAGATCC-3′, reverse: 5′-GCATCAGCCTCCC GAGTAG-3′). The PCR reaction was performed in a 25μl mixture, containing 100ng genomic DNA and 0.1 mM solution of each primer, 12.5 μl 2*Taq PCR MasterMix (TianGen Biotech CO. LTD, Beijing, China) and 9.5 μl ddH_2O. PCR was carried out with initial denaturation for 5 min at 95°C, followed by 37 cycles of annealing for 30 seconds at 60°C, extension for 30 seconds at 72°C and denaturation for 30 seconds, and a final extension for 5 min at 72°C. The product (383 bp) was digested with restriction enzyme NIaIII (Fermentas Life Sciences) at 37 centigrade for 10 hours, and analyzed on a 3% agarose gel. There were three profiles of the digested fragments: 210 bp, 44 bp, and 129 bp indicating the presence of TT, two fragments of 254 bp and 129 bp indicating the presence of CC, and four fragments of 254 bp, 210 bp, 129 bp and 44 bp representing TC genotype.

Statistical analysis

In this study, we used a population-based case–control method. Statistical analysis was performed using Haploview 4.1 and SPSS 11.0. Hardy-Weinberg equilibrium (HWE) of

Table 1 Allele distributions and HWE P value of the four SNPs in IL21 gene and two SNPs in IL-21R gene

SNP ID	HWE P value			Associated allele	Count (frequency %)			GD P value (OR,95% CI)	HT P value (OR,95% CI)
	Control	GD	HT		Control	GD	HT		
IL-21									
rs907715	0.634	0.968	0.085	A	208(44.6)	348(44.5)	210(46.9)	0.963	0.497
rs4833837	0.999	0.300	0.715	G	56(11.6)	86(10.6)	44(9.6)	0.606	0.340
rs2221903	0.055	0.329	0.715	A	405(84.7)	721(89.2)	412(90.4)	0.018 (1.50, 1.07-2.09)	0.009 (1.69,1.13-2.51)
rs2055979	0.507	0.999	0.484	T	186(38.9)	312(39.7)	160(36.5)	0.782	0.458
IL-21R									
rs3093301	0.427	0.732	0.172	T	228(47.1)	387(48.0)	192(42.3)	0.752	0.138
rs2285452	0.326	0.510	0.830	A	55(11.3)	89(11.0)	36(7.9)	0.797	0.068

each SNP was analyzed in controls using Goodness-of-fit test. Categorical data were analyzed by chi-square or Fisher's exact test. For continuous data, Student's t-test was used for the normalized data, and non-parametric test was used for non-normalized data. Furthermore, corrected P value and gene-gene interaction were analyzed using logistic regression analysis. In this study, a two-tailed P value less than 0.05 was considered to be significantly difference.

Results

Four SNPs (rs907715, rs4833837, rs2221903 and rs2055979) of the IL-21 gene and two SNPs (rs3093301 and rs2285452) of the IL-21R gene were typed in 405 GD and 228 HT patients and 242 controls. For the tested SNPs, genotyping successful rate was more than 96.9%. All of the 6 genotyped SNPs showed a MAF more than 7% and HWE analysis in the three groups showed P values of more than 0.05 (seen in Table 1). When comparing age and sex distributions between patients and controls, we found the control group matched well with the GD group, but not with HT group (seen in Table 2). The distributions of the SNPs genotypes in HT patients were analyzed using logistic regression analysis adjusted for sex and age when compared with the controls.

Association of the IL-21 gene polymorphisms with GD and HT

A genetic association between GD and HT and one of the four genotyped IL-21 SNPs was found in this study. For the SNP rs2221903 located in the intron 2 regions, the frequency of A allele was 89.2% in GD and 90.4% in HT, respectively, significantly higher than 84.7% in healthy controls (GD: P = 0.018, OR = 1.495 95% CI = 1.070-2.086; HT: P = 0.009, OR = 1.69 95% CI = 1.13-2.51). In contrast to these results, the allele frequencies of rs907715, rs4833837 and rs2055979 were similar between patients and controls (Table 1). As the distributions of rs907715, rs4833837, rs2221903 and rs2055979 genotypes in patients and controls are shown in Table 3. For rs2221903, the frequencies of the genotypes carrying risk allele (A) were higher both in GD (AA: 80.2%, GA: 18.1%) and HT (AA: 81.1%, GA:18.4%) patients than in controls (AA: 73.6%, GA: 22.2%), but statistical significance was only found when the recessive genetic model was used in HT patients (AA + GA vs. GG, P = 0.021, OR = 11.72 95% CI = 1.46-94.13), in comparison with the controls. In this study, no significant association was observed between GD or HT and rs907715, rs4833837 or rs2055979 genotypes while different genetic models were applied for analysis.

Association of the IL-21R gene polymorphisms with GD and HT

As shown in Table 1, the rs3093301 and rs2285452 SNPs in IL-21R showed no association with GD or HT (P = 0.797-0.068).

Nominal associations were found between rs3093301 and rs2285452 and HT when the dominant genetic model (CC *vs.* TC + TT, P = 0.023, OR = 1.61 95% CI = 1.070-2.42); GG *vs.* GT + TT, P = 0.031, OR = 1.71 95% CI = 1.05-2.80, respectively) was used for analysis. Genotype analysis of rs3093301 and rs2285452 using additive and recessive genetic model did not indicate

Table 2 Age and sex characteristics of GD and HT patients and controls

Group	Age			Sex		
	Kolmogorov - Smirnov P value	Z score	P value	Male/female counts	χ2	P value
control	<0.001	–	–	67/175	–	–
GD	<0.001	-0.487	0.626	114/291	0.016	0.899
HT	0.200	-2.599	0.009	27/201	18.410	1.7E-5

Table 3 Genotype distributions of the four SNPs of IL21 gene and two SNPs of IL-21R gene

SNP ID	Genotype	Control	GD				HT			
		Count (frequency %)	Count (frequency %)	Additive P value	Dominant P value	Recessive P value	Count (frequency %)	Additive P value	Dominant P value (OR,95% CI)	Recessive P value (OR,95% CI)
IL-21										
	GG	69(29.6)	121(30.9)				70(31.3)			
rs907715	GA	120(51.5)	192(49.1)	0.845	0.726	0.746	98(43.8)	0.334	0.568	0.264
	AA	44(18.9)	78(19.9)				56(25.0)			
	AA	189(78.1)	325(80.4)				185(81.1)			
rs4833837	GA	50(20.7)	72(17.8)	0.61	0.474	0.751	42(18.4)	0.67	0.667	0.401
	GG	3(1.2)	7(1.7)				1(0.4)			
	AA	176(73.6)	324(80.2)				185(81.1)			
rs2221903	GA	53(22.2)	73(18.1)	0.063	0.053	0.061	42(18.4)	0.07	0.132	0.021 (11.72,1.46-94.13)
	GG	10(4.2)	7(1.7)				1(0.4)			
	GG	92(38.5)	143(36.4)				91(41.6)			
rs2055979	GT	108(45.2)	188(47.8)	0.808	0.595	0.857	96(43.8)	0.731	0.455	0.572
	TT	39(16.3)	62(15.8)				32(14.6)			
IL-21R										
	CC	64(26.4)	111(27.5)				81(35.7)			
rs3093301	TC	128(52.9)	197(48.9)	0.571	0.762	0.391	100(44.1)	0.079	0.023 (1.61, 1.07-2.42)	0.896
	TT	50(20.7)	95(23.6)				46(20.3)			
	GG	185(77.7)	318(78.7)				193(85.0)			
rs2285452	GA	52(21.8)	83(20.5)	0.823	0.707	0.999	32(14.1)	0.051	0.031 (1.71, 1.05-2.80)	0.435
	AA	1(0.4)	3(0.7)				2(0.9)			

any significant difference between HT patients and controls (Table 3). For rs3093301 and rs2285452, no significant different distribution was found in GD patients and controls when different genetic models was used (showed by Table 3).

Haplotype analysis in GD and HT

As shown in Table 4, rs4833837 and rs2221903 (r-square = 0.901) were identified as an LD block using the Haploview 4.1. The total frequency of haplotypes listed in Table 5 was more than 99.0% in every group. AA containing major alleles of these two SNPs was associated with increased susceptibility to GD with an OR of 1.50 (95% CI =1.08-2.09, P = 0.016), and to HT with an OR of 1.69 (95% CI =1.14-2.52, P = 0.009) (Table 5).

Table 4 The linkage disequilibrium analysis of the SNPs in IL-21 and IL-21R gene

r-square			
IL-21	rs4833837	rs2221903	rs2055979
rs907715	0.099	0.090	0.493
rs4833837	–	0.901	0.067
rs2221903	–	–	0.059
IL-21R	rs2285452		
rs3093301	0.369(0.018)		

Discussion

IL-21 is a member of the common-gamma chain family of cytokines with immunoregulatory activity. IL-21R has been shown to form a heterodimeric receptor complex with the common gamma-chain. IL-21 binding with this receptor leads to the activation of multiple downstream signaling molecules, including JAK1, JAK3, STAT1 and STAT3, therefore affects the innate and adaptive immune responses by inducing the differentiation, proliferation and activity of multiple target cells. The dysregulation of IL-21 and IL-21R plays a role in multiple immune-mediated diseases, including SLE [3], psoriasis [5], RA [4] and other chronic inflammatory diseases [18]. Like other autoimmune diseases, GD and HT are chronic diseases initiated by the loss of immunological tolerance to self-antigens. Previous studies indicate that some immune-related genes may participate in the development of AITDs.

In this study, we found a significant association between GD or HT and rs2221903 located in the IL-21 gene region, and the frequencies of the haplotypes in the IL-21 gene that consists of rs4833837 and rs2221903 in GD and HT patients were significantly different from

Table 5 The frequencies of the haplotypes of IL-21 gene in patients and controls

Reference SNP		Frequency %			GD		HT	
rs4833837	rs2221903	Control	GD	HT	p	OR (95% CI)	p	OR (95% CI)
A	A	84.7	89.3	90.4	0.016	1.500 (1.08-2.09)	0.009	1.694 (1.14-2.52)
G	G	11.6	10.7	9.6	0.640	0.92 (0.64-1.31)	0.340	0.816 (0.54-1.24)
A	G	3.7	0.0	0.0	4.0E-8	-	4.0E-4	-

controls. For rs3093301 and rs2285452 polymorphisms of the IL-21R gene, there were significantly different distributions of these genotypes between HT patients and the controls.

In different from Jia's study [6], we did not find the rs907715 SNP linkage with GD. In Jia's report, the AA genotype frequency was lower in GD patients (19.4%) than in controls (30%). The gene frequency in patients of our study was similar to that of Jia's study, but different in the two control groups. In our study the frequency of AA genotype in the control group was 18.9%, which is similar to the frequency in the HapMap-CHB population. This may be the geographical or selection variation that results in this difference. It should be noted that the lack of association in our study does not completely exclude the possibility of IL-21R as a candidate gene for GD because of the following three reasons: 1) The average MAF of the six SNPs is 0.271, which gives our study genetic power of about 0.8 for GD and 0.7 for HT group with an OR of homozygote 2.0, and of heterozygote 1.5, therefore studies with a larger sample size are necessary to confirm whether patients with these SNPs have more risk for development of GD. 2) As many other immunologic disorders, AITDs is believed to derive from a multiple network of various susceptible loci, which exert synergic or additive effects, but each locus may play a small role [19]. 3) 13 tag-SNPs in the HapMap-CHB population and 17 in the HapMap-CEU population covered a 49.8 kb on 16p11, where IL-21R gene located. And we just explored the association between the two tag-SNPs of them and AITDs in Chinese cohort.

In genetics, a recessive gene is an allele that causes a phenotype (visible or detectable characteristic) that is only seen in a homozygous genotype (an organism that has two copies of the same allele) and never in a heterozygous genotype. While dominance is a relationship between alleles of a gene, in which one allele masks the expression (phenotype) of another allele at the same locus. Our study didn't find any synergistic effect of the risk genotype. And we were unable to conclude whether these two genes were either recessive or dominant over the other gene.

IL-21 is located on chromosome 4q26-27, which is close to IL-2, a region that has been linked to AITDs susceptibility [17]. Jia's et al. found rs907715 of IL-21 gene being associated with GD in a Chinese population while Plagnol found only rs2069763 and did not find association of rs2069762 and rs6822844 of IL-2 with GD, maybe there is ethnicity or regional effect contributing to these results differences. Therefore, we can not exclude that the SNPs of the IL-21 and IL-21R genes are only an indicator of a candidate gene contributing to AITDs. Further studies such as screening the rest common variations in IL21R gene, identifying the causal SNP for this association, and exploring gene-environment interaction in GD and HT cohort studies are required to clarify the effect of IL-21 and IL-21R on AITDs susceptibility. Replication of these associations between IL-21 and IL-21R gene and AITDs is also required in larger independent databases of different cohorts.

Conclusion

In conclusion, our study confirmed the synergic effect of the IL-21 SNPs in the development of GD. In addition, to the best of our knowledge, we are the first to report the association of the IL-21 and IL-21R SNPs with an increased risk of HT.

Competing interests

The authors report no competing interests. The authors alone are responsible for the content and writing of the paper.

Authors' contributions

WXX and YFZ recruited the subjects and participated in the sequence alignment. LX and WJJ extracted genomic DNA from peripheral blood leukocytes. XHS carried out the molecular genetic studies, participated in the sequence alignment. JZ carried out the immunoassays and drafted the manuscript. SFM participated in the design of the study and performed the statistical analysis. JAZ and LHZ conceived of the study, and participated in its design and coordination. All authors read and approved the final manuscript.

Acknowledgments

This work was supported by grants from the National Natural Science Foundation of China (30871184, 81070627).

Author details

[1]Department of Clinical Laboratory, Jinshan Hospital of Fudan University, Shanghai 201508, China. [2]Internal Medicine Department, Xi'an Aviation Group Hospital, Xi'an 710021, China. [3]Endocrinology Department, Jinshan Hospital, Fudan University, 1508 Longhang Road, Shanghai 201508, China. [4]Endocrinology Department, Weinan Central Hospital, Weinan, Shaanxi 714000, China.

References

1. Ozaki K, Kikly K, Michalovich D, Young PR, Leonard WJ: **Cloning of a type I cytokine receptor most related to the IL-2 receptor beta chain.** *Proc Natl Acad Sci USA* 2000, **97**:1439–1444.

2. Parrish-Novak J, Dillon SR, Nelson A, Hammond A, Sprecher C, Gross JA, Johnston J, Madden K, Xu W, West J, Schrader S, Burkhead S, Heipel M, Brandt C, Kuijper JL, Kramer J, Conklin D, Presnell SR, Berry J, Shiota F, Bort S, Hambly K, Mudri S, Clegg C, Moore M, Grant FJ, Lofton-Day C, Gilbert T, Rayond F, Ching A, *et al*: **Interleukin 21 and its receptor are involved in NK cell expansion and regulation of lymphocyte function.** *Nature* 2000, **408:**57–63.
3. Bubier JA, Sproule TJ, Foreman O, Spolski R, Shaffer DJ, Morse HC 3rd, Leonard WJ, Roopenian DC: **A critical role for IL-21 receptor signaling in the pathogenesis of systemic lupus erythematosus in BXSB-Yaa mice.** *Proc Natl Acad Sci USA* 2009, **106:**1518–1523.
4. Li J, Shen W, Kong K, Liu Z: **Interleukin –21 induces T-cell activation and proinflammatory cytokine secretion in rheumatoid arthritis.** *Scand J Immunol* 2006, **64:**515–522.
5. Yuan SL, Jiang L, Zhang XL, Li SF, Duan HM, Wang XF: **Serum IL-21 level in patients with primary Sjogren's syndrome and clinical significance of IL-21.** *Xi Bao Yu Fen Zi Mian Yi Xue Za Zhi* 2007, **23:**124–126.
6. Jia HY, Zhang ZG, Gu XJ, Guo T, Cui B, Ning G, Zhao YJ: **Association between interleukin 21 and Graves' disease.** *Genet Mol Res* 2011, **10:**3338–3346.
7. Wellcome Trust Case Control Consortium: **Genome-wide association study of 14,000 cases of seven common diseases and 3,000 shared controls.** *Nature* 2007, **447:**661–678.
8. Zhernakova A, Alizadeh BZ, Bevova M, Van Leeuwen MA, Coenen MJ, Franke B, Franke L, Posthumus MD, Van Heel DA, Van der Steege G, Radstake TR, Barrera P, Roep BO, Koeleman BP, Wijmenga C: **Novel association in chromosome 4q27 region with rheumatoid arthritis and confirmation of type 1 diabetes point to a general risk locus for autoimmune diseases.** *Am J Hum Genet* 2007, **81:**1284–1288.
9. Hinks A, Eyre S, Ke X, Barton A, Martin P, Flynn E, Packham J, Worthington J, Thomson W: **Association of the AFF3 gene and IL2/IL21 gene region with juvenile idiopathic arthritis.** *Genes Immun* 2010, **11:**194–198.
10. Liu Y, Helms C, Liao W, Zaba LC, Duan S, Gardner J, Wise C, Miner A, Malloy MJ, Pullinger CR, Kane JP, Saccone S, Worthington J, Bruce I, Kwok PY, Menter A, Krueger J, Barton A, Saccone NL, Bowcock AM: **A genome-wide association study of psoriasis and psoriatic arthritis identifies new disease loci.** *PLoS Genet* 2008, **4:**e1000041.
11. Adamovic S, Amundsen SS, Lie BA, Gudjónsdóttir AH, Ascher H, Ek J, Van Heel DA, Nilsson S, Sollid LM, Torinsson Naluai A: **Association study of IL2/IL21 and FcgRIIa: significant association with the IL2/IL21 region in Scandinavian coeliac disease families.** *Genes Immun* 2008, **9:**364–367.
12. Garner CP, Murray JA, Ding YC, Tien Z, Van Heel DA, Neuhausen SL: **Replication of celiac disease UK genome-wide association study results in a US population.** *Hum Mol Genet* 2009, **18:**4219–4225.
13. Festen EA, Goyette P, Scott R, Annese V, Zhernakova A, Lian J, Lefèbvre C, Brant SR, Cho JH, Silverberg MS, Taylor KD, De Jong DJ, Stokkers PC, Mcgovern D, Palmieri O, Achkar JP, Xavier RJ, Daly MJ, Duerr RH, Wijmenga C, Weersma RK, Rioux JD: **Genetic variants in the region harbouring IL2/IL21 associated with ulcerative colitis.** *Gut* 2009, **5:**799–804.
14. Fedetz M, Ndagire D, Fernandez O, Leyva L, Guerrero M, Arnal C, Lucas M, Izquierdo G, Delgado C, Alcina A, Matesanz F: **Multiple sclerosis association study with the TENR-IL2-IL21 region in a Spanish population.** *Tissue Antigens* 2009, **74:**244–247.
15. Sawalha AH, Kaufman KM, Kelly JA, Adler AJ, Aberle T, Kilpatrick J, Wakeland EK, Li QZ, Wandstrat AE, Karp DR, James JA, Merrill JT, Lipsky P, Harley JB: **Genetic association of interleukin-21 polymorphisms with systemic lupus erythematosus.** *Ann Rheum Dis* 2008, **67:**458–461.
16. Webb R, Merrill JT, Kelly JA, Sestak A, Kaufman KM, Langefeld CD, Ziegler J, Kimberly RP, Edberg JC, Ramsey-Goldman R, Petri M, Reveille JD, Alarcón GS, Vilá LM, Alarcón-Riquelme ME, James JA, Gilkeson GS, Jacob CO, Moser KL, Gaffney PM, Vyse TJ, Nath SK, Lipsky P, Harley JB, Sawalha AH: **A polymorphism within IL21R confers risk for systemic lupus erythematosus.** *Arthritis Rheum* 2009, **60:**2402–2407.
17. Plagnol V, Howson JM, Smyth DJ, Walker N, Hafler JP, Wallace C, Stevens H, Jackson L, Simmonds MJ, Type 1 Diabetes Genetics Consortium, Bingley PJ, Gough SC, Todd JA: **Genome-wide association analysis of autoantibody positivity in type 1 diabetes cases.** *PLoS Genet* 2011, **7:**e1002216.
18. De Nitto D, Sarra M, Pallone F, Monteleone G: **Interleukin-21 triggers effector cell responses in the gut.** *World J Gastroenterol* 2010, **16:**3638–3641.
19. Leonard WJ, Spolski R: **Interleukin-21: a modulator of lymphoid proliferation, apoptosis and differentiation.** *Nat Rev Immunol* 2005, **5:**688–698.

15

Increased waist circumference is independently associated with hypothyroidism in Mexican Americans: replicative evidence from two large, population-based studies

Manju Mamtani[1*], Hemant Kulkarni[1], Thomas D Dyer[1], Laura Almasy[1], Michael C Mahaney[1], Ravindranath Duggirala[1], Anthony G Comuzzie[1], Paul B Samollow[2], John Blangero[1] and Joanne E Curran[1]

Abstract

Background: Mexican Americans are at an increased risk of both thyroid dysfunction and metabolic syndrome (MS). Thus it is conceivable that some components of the MS may be associated with the risk of thyroid dysfunction in these individuals. Our objective was to investigate and replicate the potential association of MS traits with thyroid dysfunction in Mexican Americans.

Methods: We conducted association testing for 18 MS traits in two large studies on Mexican Americans – the San Antonio Family Heart Study (SAFHS) and the National Health and Nutrition Examination Survey (NHANES) 2007–10. A total of 907 participants from 42 families in SAFHS and 1633 unrelated participants from NHANES 2007–10 were included in this study. The outcome measures were prevalence of clinical and subclinical hypothyroidism and thyroid function index (TFI) – a measure of thyroid function. For the SAFHS, we used polygenic regression analyses with multiple covariates to test associations in setting of family studies. For the NHANES 2007–10, we corrected for the survey design variables as needed for association analyses in survey data. In both datasets, we corrected for age, sex and their linear and quadratic interactions.

Results: TFI was an accurate indicator of clinical thyroid status (area under the receiver-operating-characteristic curve to detect clinical hypothyroidism, 0.98) in both SAFHS and NHANES 2007–10. Of the 18 MS traits, waist circumference (WC) showed the most consistent association with TFI in both studies independently of age, sex and body mass index (BMI). In the SAFHS and NHANES 2007–10 datasets, each standard deviation increase in WC was associated with 0.13 ($p < 0.001$) and 0.11 ($p < 0.001$) unit increase in the TFI, respectively. In a series of polygenic and linear regression models, central obesity (defined as WC ≥ 102 cm in men and ≥88 cm in women) was associated with clinical and subclinical hypothyroidism independent of age, sex, BMI and type 2 diabetes in both datasets. Estimated prevalence of hypothyroidism was consistently high in those with central obesity, especially below 45y of age.

Conclusions: WC independently associates with increased risk of thyroid dysfunction. Use of WC to identify Mexican American subjects at high risk of thyroid dysfunction should be investigated in future studies.

Keywords: Waist circumference, Central obesity, Thyroid dysfunction, Mexican Americans

* Correspondence: mmamtani@txbiomedgenetics.org
[1]Department of Genetics, Texas Biomedical Research Institute, 7620 NW Loop 410, San Antonio, TX, USA
Full list of author information is available at the end of the article

Background

Reportedly 5-10% of the United States population has subclinical or clinical hypothyroidism [1,2]. It is of clinical interest that differential prevalence estimates of hypothyroidism are influenced by age [3], sex , ethnicity [4] and other risk factors like presence of type 2 diabetes (T2D) [5,6]. Further, Mexican American and white ethnicity is associated with a high risk of thyroid dysfunction [3,7-9]. Knowledge of these risk factors is crucial to identify hypothyroidism in its nascent, subclinical stage since it is associated with preventable but dangerous complications like hyperlipidemia, insulin resistance, atherosclerosis and additional risks to mothers and infants [10]. The accuracy of traditional strategies to detect thyroid dysfunction that use a constellation of symptoms and signs has been greatly increased by recent improvements in the assays for thyroxine and thyroid stimulating hormone (TSH). For example, Helfand and Crapo [10] have described that the sensitivity and specificity of TSH to confirm thyroid disease is 98% and 92%, respectively. In primary care settings however, the observed accuracy is not as high. For example, the positive predictive value of a low TSH to detect hyperthyroidism has been reported to be only 24% while that of a high TSH to detect hypothyroidism is only 6% [10]. Improved screening programs for thyroid dysfunction will therefore need detection of differential thyroid dysfunction risks across epidemiologically diverse groups.

There is now burgeoning evidence that vindicates a potential link between thyroid dysfunction and metabolic syndrome (MS). Even in a euthyroid state, a high normal TSH is strongly associated with MS [11]. Similarly, in the National Health and Nutrition Examination Survey (NHANES) 2007–2008 data [4], body mass index (BMI) and waist circumference (WC) were associated with serum TSH levels. More recently, the Health, Ageing and Body Composition Study [12] reported that unit increase in TSH was associated with a 3% increase in the odds of MS. It is also instructive in this regard that mutations in the thyroid hormone receptor beta (THRB) gene are associated with increased energy intake, hyperphagia and resting energy expenditure [13]. It is noteworthy, however, that MS represents a constellation of correlated phenotypic traits that together capture a wide spectrum of metabolic disorders including prediabetes, type 2 diabetes, insulin resistance, hypertension, obesity and dyslipidemia [14]. However, the relative and comparative contribution of these individual components of MS to thyroid dysfunction is currently unknown.

Since Mexican Americans are at an increased risk of MS, here we investigated the associations of MS-related traits with indicators of thyroid dysfunction in Mexican Americans from two large studies – San Antonio Family Heart Study (SAFHS) [15,16] and NHANES 2007–10. The former study is uniquely suited to investigate the hypothesized association between MS and thyroid function in families who are at a high risk of both MS and thyroid abnormalities while the latter study provides a rich, nationally representative population based setting. We aimed to investigate and replicate the MS-thyroid function nexus in these epidemiologically distinct scenarios using an appropriate and robust analytical approach. Here we report our finding that central obesity – a component of MS – is additively, independently and significantly associated with altered thyroid function.

Methods

Study participants

San Antonio Family Heart Study (SAFHS)

The recruitment and ascertainment procedures used in the SAFHS have been described in details elsewhere [15-17]. Briefly, the study has now recruited over 1600 subjects from 42 large and extended families with a majority of these subjects having completed up to three additional follow-up visits spaced ~5 years apart. In the analyses presented here we used the data and samples collected during the first visit. Profiling of thyroid-related traits was available for 919 subjects (from 42 families). Informed consent was obtained from all participants before collection of samples. The Institutional Review Board of the University of Texas Health Sciences Center at San Antonio approved the study.

The National Health and Nutrition Examination Survey (NHANES) 2007–10

NHANES is a yearly survey conducted by the National Center of Health Statistics of the Centers for Disease Control and Prevention (CDC). These datasets are publicly available in a de-identified fashion. Detailed description of the NHANES 2007–10 survey and sampling strategies can be found online at http://www.cdc.gov/nchs/nhanes.htm. The NHANES 2007–10 dataset contained thyroid related components. From this multi-ethnic dataset, we selected Mexican American responders (n = 1636). Detailed characteristics of the SAFHS and NHANES 2007–10 participants are shown in Table 1.

Phenotypic traits related to thyroid function

Traits in SAFHS and NHANES 2007–10

In the SAFHS, available thyroid-related traits were total and free thyroxine (TT4 and FT4), total and free triiodothyronine (TT3 and FT3), reverse triiodothyronine (RT3C), thyroxine binding globulin (TBG), thyroglobulin (THG) and thyroid stimulating hormone (TSH). R3TC was available for only 451 (49.1%) subjects. The experimental methods used for measuring thyroid-related

Table 1 Characteristics of the study subjects

Characteristic	SAFHS (n = 919)		NHANES 2007–10 (n = 1636)	
	Value	N	Value	N
Demographics				
Age [mean (SE)] y	38.92 (0.54)	907	35.42 (0.81[†])	1636
Females [n (%)]	555 (61.19)	907	842 (47.98[††])	1636
Diabetes at enrolment [n (%)]	126 (13.91)	906	170 (7.35)	1635
Anthropometric indexes [mean (SE)]				
Waist cm	94.71 (0.58)	898	95.65 (0.68)	1589
BMI Kg/m^2	29.50 (0.23)	900	28.49 (0.27)	1618
WHR	0.89 (0.003)	897	-	-
Blood pressure [mean (SE)]				
Systolic mmHg	119.96 (0.61)	899	116.98 (0.75)	1504
Diastolic mmHg	70.56 (0.34)	899	66.84 (0.56)	1504
Biochemical indexes [mean (SE)]				
Fasting glucose mmol/L	5.59 (0.07)	907	6.00 (0.11)	805
Fasting insulin µU/mL	16.72 (0.65)	894	15.64 (0.63)	803
Total serum cholesterol mg/dl	189.06 (1.32)	906	190.35 (1.54)	1636
Serum triglycerides mg/dl	151.56 (4.40)	906	141.15 (3.31)	805
HDL cholesterol mg/dl	50.54 (0.43)	905	48.90 (0.31)	1636
LDL cholesterol mg/dl	109.92 (1.10)	906	112.42 (1.52)	785
Thyroid related traits [mean (SE)]				
Total thyroxine µg/dl	7.63 (0.07)	839	8.19 (0.08)	1628
Free thyroxine ng/dl	1.38 (0.01)	907	0.80 (0.01)	1636
Total triiodothyronine ng/dl	122.15 (0.92)	845	122.89 (1.03)	1635
Free triiodothyronine pg/ml	3.62 (0.04)	907	3.42 (0.03)	1634
Reverse triiodothyronine ng/dl	23.00 (0.30)	451	-	-
Thyroxine binding globulin µg/ml	19.84 (0.19)	856	-	-
Thyroglobulin ng/ml	11.56 (1.11)	879	11.27 (1.15)	1635
Thyroid stimulating hormone µU/ml	2.96 (0.14)	907	2.00 (0.14)	1635

[†]All proportions in NHANES samples are adjusted for survey design variables.
[††]For NHANES samples standard errors represent linearized standard errors.

traits in the SAFHS have been described previously [18]. Of these traits, data on R3TC and TBG was not available in the NHANES 2007–10 dataset. Thyroid profile data for both studies is shown in Table 1. Finally, to capture the information content of TSH, FT3 and FT4 in a single, composite and continuous measure we developed an index [which we termed the thyroid function index (TFI)] as: TFI = TSH/(FT3 × FT4). We conceptualized this index on the basis of the clinical expectation that high values of TSH combined with low values of FT3 and FT4 values would be indicative of hypothyroidism and, conversely, low value of TSH combined with high values of FT3 and FT4 would be indicative of hyperthyroidism. Before conducting any association analyses for the TFI trait, we first validated this index in both SAFHS and NHANES 2007–10 participants.

Clinical thyroid status

Based on the values of TSH, FT4 and FT3, we used the recommended definitions [19,20] of thyroid status as follows: clinical hypothyroidism (CO) – TSH ≥3.0 µIU/ml AND (FT3 < 3.5 pmol/L OR FT4 < 10 pmol/L); subclinical hypothyroidism (SO) – TSH ≥3.0 µIU/ml AND (FT3 ≥ 3.5 pmol/L OR FT4 ≥ 10 pmol/L); clinical hyperthyroidism (CR) – TSH <0.3 µIU/ml AND (FT3 ≥ 6.5 pmol/L OR FT4 ≥ 19 pmol/L); subclinical hyperthyroidism (SR) – TSH <0.3 µIU/ml AND (FT3 < 6.5 pmol/L OR FT4 < 19 pmol/L). Further, we defined hypothyroidism as presence of clinical or subclinical hypothyroidism.

Metabolic syndrome related traits

We used data on 18 phenotypic traits related to metabolic syndrome (12 continuous and six dichotomous).

The continuous traits included fasting and post-glucose load plasma levels of glucose and insulin (measured by 2-hour oral glucose tolerance test); two homeostasis model of assessment (HOMA) measures – HOMA-IR representing insulin resistance and HOMA-β representing β-cell function; three measures of obesity – body mass index (BMI), WC and waist-hip ratio (WHR); systolic and diastolic blood pressure; and three serum lipid measures – total cholesterol, triglycerides and high-density lipoprotein cholesterol (HDL-C). The methods of assessment for these traits in the SAFHS and NHANES 2007–10 participants have been extensively described. ([16,17,21] and http://wwwn.cdc.gov/nchs/nhanes/search/nhanes07_08.aspx/analyticnote_2007-2010.pdf. The definitions of the six dichotomous traits (central obesity, raised triglycerides, low HDL-C, T2D, high blood pressure and metabolic syndrome) are provided in Additional file 1: Table S1.

Statistical analyses

Inverse normalization of continuous traits

To ensure that i) inferences regarding association were not influenced by a potentially non-normal distribution of the continuous traits and ii) the results from the SAFHS and NHANES 2007–10 can be evaluated using a comparative metric, we inverse-normalized all continuous traits before conducting regression analyses. This transformation was used to generate inverse-normalized traits having a mean of 0 and a standard deviation of 1 which was then used in the regression analyses.

Validation of TFI

We validated the TFI using receiver operating characteristic (ROC) curves and estimating the comparative area under the ROC curve (AUC) for the individual components of TFI and TFI *per se*. To estimate AUC, we used the Wilcoxon statistic and its standard error as described by Hanley and McNeil [22]. We used the STATA 12.0 package and roctab program to estimate these statistics.

Polygenic regression analyses in SAFHS

We examined association between TFI and phenotypic traits related to MS in the SAFHS participants using polygenic regression models in a variance-components framework [23,24]. These models implicitly account for the genetic correlations and kinship structures and do not consider the individual subjects as an independent unit. The polygenic regression models were of the following form: $TFI_i = m + \Sigma\, b_k a_{ik} + g_i + e_i$ where, TFI is the inverse-normalized log-transformed thyroid function index; m is the trait mean; a is the covariate vector of dimension k with b as the corresponding regression coefficients; g is the polygenic effect and e is the residual error for an individual indexed by i. The term g was modeled as random effects based on the coefficients of relationship in the kinship matrix. All models were first run with only the MS-related trait as the covariate (unadjusted models) and then additionally included adjustments for age, age^2, sex, age x sex and age^2 x sex interactions as covariates (adjusted models). Further, we adjusted these models for the use of lipid lowering, antihypertensive and antidiabetic agents. Statistical significance of the association between a MS-related trait and TFI was tested by constraining the corresponding regression coefficient to zero and comparing the log-likelihoods of the constrained and unconstrained models in a likelihood ratio χ^2 test. These analyses were conducted using the SOLAR software package [25]. Statistical significance was tested at a global type I error rate of 0.05.

Survey design-corrected regression analyses in NHANES 2007–10 dataset

Since the NHANES dataset is based on a complex sampling strategy to recruit a nationally representative sample, we used appropriate survey based analytical methods as detailed on the Centers for Disease Control and Prevention website (http://www.cdc.gov/nchs/tutorials/nhanes/). Briefly, we corrected for the proportional sampling units and the sampling weights using the svyset command in STATA 12.0 (Stata Corp, College Station, TX) software package. Since it was likely that the subset of Mexican Americans included in this study could have come from some specific sampling units, we used the singleunit (scaled) option in the svyset command. All regression analyses were then conducted using the svy command and regress subcommand.

Correction for multiple testing

We used 18 MS traits that are conceptually correlated with each other to varying degrees. Therefore, these traits do not represent independent tests. To estimate the effective number of independent tests we used the method of Li and Ji [26] which relies upon the eigenvalues of the full correlation matrix for the traits and then uses a Sidak type correction to estimate the corrected type I error rate for a global alpha error of 0.05. Using this method we estimated that the corrected alpha for the SAFHS dataset was 0.0051 and for the NHANES dataset it was 0.0073.

Prevalence of hypothyroidism

In the SAFHS participants, we used a liability threshold model approach to determine the prevalence of hypothyroidism within combinatorial classes determined by age categories and presence or absence of central obesity. The polygenic regression models used in this scenario were specifically tailored for discrete traits and additively accounted for kinship structure. In the NHANES 2007–10 participants, we estimated the proportion of hypothyroidism within each class after correcting for the survey design variables (sampling weights, proportionality sampling units and strata) using the svy command in STATA software package.

Results

Study participants

Of the 919 SAFHS and 1636 NHANES 2007–10 participants who underwent thyroid profiling, we included 907 SAFHS and 1633 NHANES 2007–10 participants for whom data on FT3, FT4 and TSH were available. We observed (Table 1) that the SAFHS participants were slightly older (~3 y), had a higher proportion of females (~12%) and had a higher prevalence of diabetes (~2 times) as compared to the NHANES 2007–10 responders. However, the anthropometric indexes, blood pressure, oral glucose tolerance test results and serum lipid profiles were similar in both studies. With regard to the thyroid profile, the mean FT4 and TSH levels were higher in SAFHS participants but other thyroid-related traits were comparable across the two studies. Consequently, the prevalence of clinical hypothyroidism was comparable across the two studies but the prevalence of subclinical hypothyroidism was higher in the SAFHS participants than the NHANES responders (25.5% vs 6.7%, Figure 1A). For the SAFHS, informed consent was obtained from all participants before data and sample collection. The study was approved by the Institutional Review Board of the University of Texas Health Science Center at San Antonio. The NHANES study has been approved by the National Center of Health Statistics Institutional Review Board under protocols #98-12 and #2005-06. The study involved interviews, collection of biological samples after taking informed consent from all participants. All protocols used in the study are in accordance with the Declaration of Helsinki.

Validation of thyroid function index

The distribution of TFI was heavily skewed in both studies (Figure 1B, left panels). Therefore, we log-transformed the TFI and found that the log-transformed TFI was distributed symmetrically in both datasets (Figure 1B, right panels). However, we observed that the log-transformed TFI had a non-significant skew in the SAFHS dataset ($p = 0.168$) but not in the NHANES 2007–10 dataset ($p < 0.001$). Therefore, in all ensuing analyses we further corrected for this departure from normality by using an inverse-normalization method. From this point forward, TFI implies inverse-normalized, log-transformed TFI.

The TFI demonstrated (Figure 1C) a clear gradient of distribution with very low values corroborating clinical hyperthyroidism and high values characterizing clinical hypothyroidism. In a head to head comparative evaluation of TFI and its individual components to diagnose clinical hypothyroidism (Figure 1D), we observed that the TFI superseded all of its individual components in both studies. Specifically, the AUC for TFI was 98% while the AUCs for TSH, FT3 and FT4 were consistently below that of TFI in both the studies. These results therefore validated the potential use of TFI as a replicable and generalizable continuous measure of thyroid function.

MS-related traits and TFI: SAFHS participants

We studied the association of 18 MS-related traits with TFI in SAFHS participants after accounting for the kinship structure using a series of polygenic regression models (Table 2). Even after accounting for age, sex and their interactions in addition to the kinship structure, we found that WC ($\beta = 0.13$, $p = 0.0002$), BMI ($\beta = 0.11$, $p = 0.0015$), WHR ($\beta = 0.09$, $p = 0.0103$) and serum triglycerides ($\beta = 0.08$, $p = 0.0183$) were significantly associated with TFI. Consequently, central obesity (defined on the basis of WC) and metabolic syndrome were also significantly associated with TFI. In males, WHR ($\beta = 0.20$, $p = 0.008$) and metabolic syndrome ($\beta = 0.25$, $p = 0.0379$) were the only two traits significantly associated with TFI. However, in females WC ($\beta = 0.14$, $p = 0.001$), BMI ($\beta = 0.13$, $p = 0.0026$), WHR ($\beta = 0.10$, $p = 0.022$) and central obesity ($\beta = 0.20$, $p = 0.0247$) achieved statistical significance for association with TFI. Thus, these results indicated a consistent association of central obesity with TFI in the SAFHS participants.

MS-related traits and TFI: NHANES 2007–10

We conducted conceptually similar analyses in the NHANES 2007–10 participants. Here we used the appropriate survey design correction methods to statistically account for the potential confounding due to study design. We observed (Table 3) that after correcting for age, sex and their interactions, HOMA-IR ($\beta = 0.06$, $p = 0.0448$), WC ($\beta = 0.11$, $p = 0.0008$), BMI ($\beta = 0.12$, $p = 0.0004$), total serum cholesterol ($\beta = 0.11$, $p = 0.0014$) and serum triglycerides ($\beta = 0.09$, $p = 0.036$) were statistically significantly associated with TFI. In males, several traits were significantly associated with TFI but the strongest associations were again observed for WC ($\beta = 0.20$, $p = 7.6 \times 10^{-8}$), BMI ($\beta = 0.20$, $p = 1.3 \times 10^{-7}$) and central obesity ($\beta = 0.30$, $p = 5.0 \times 10^{-5}$). However, in females only total serum cholesterol ($\beta = 0.11$, $p = 0.0437$) was statistically significantly associated.

Association of WC with TFI is independent of BMI

Since both WC and BMI were positively associated with TFI in both studies, we compared the strength of association of these two traits with TFI using interactive models (Additional file 1: Table S2). Our results indicated that in both the studies WC was significantly associated with TFI

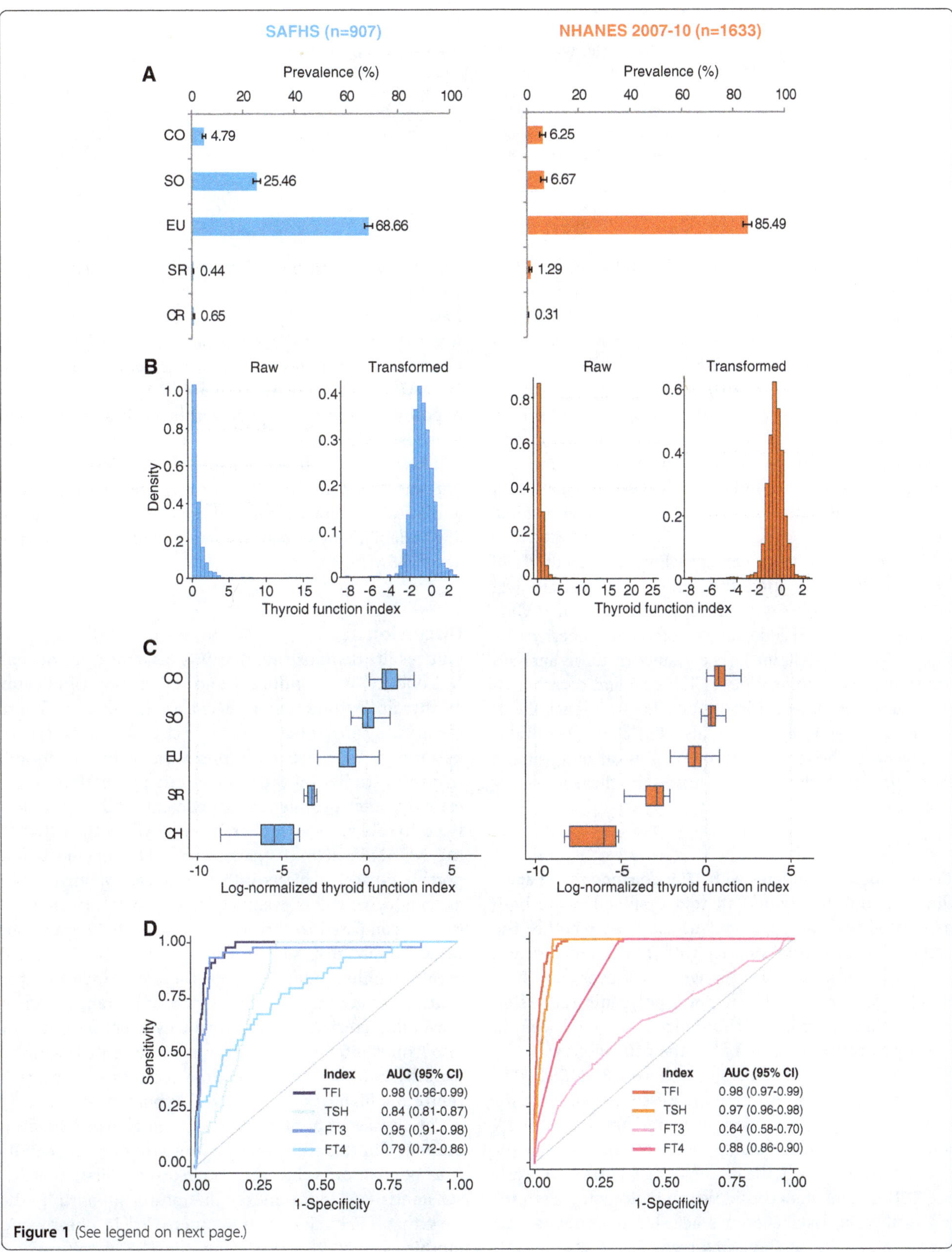

Figure 1 (See legend on next page.)

(See figure on previous page.)

Figure 1 Development and validation of thyroid function index (TFI) as a marker of thyroid function. Results are color coded as blue for SAFHS and red for NHANES 2007–10 participants. **(A)** Spectrum of clinical thyroid status. Bars represent prevalence (%) while error bars represent 95% confidence interval. CO, clinical hypothyroidism; SO, subclinical hypothyroidism; EU, euthyroid; SR, subclinical hyperthyroidism; CR, clinical hyperthyroidism. **(B)** Effect of log-transformation on distribution of TFI. Left and right panels show histograms for raw and log-transformed TFI, respectively. **(C)** Box and whisker plots showing distribution of log-normalized TFI by thyroid status. **(D)** Receiver operating characteristics (ROC) curves comparing the discriminatory performance of TFI, TSH, FT3 and FT4 to detect clinical hypothyroidism. AUC, area under the ROC curve; CI, confidence interval.

whether analyzed separately in males ($\beta = 0.40$, $p = 0.001$ in SAFHS and $\beta = 0.28$, $p = 0.004$ in NHANES 2007–10) and females ($\beta = 0.19$, $p = 0.018$ in SAFHS and $\beta = 0.19$, $p = 0.07$ in NHANES 2007–10) or in all participants together ($\beta = 0.22$, $p = 0.001$ in SAFHS and $\beta = 0.13$, $p = 0.066$ in NHANES 2007–10). Interestingly, a stronger association signal between WC and TFI was observed in males as compared to females in both SAFHS and NAHNES 2007–10 participants in interactive models. These results together indicated that the association of WC with TFI is independent of the potential confounding due to BMI.

Since it is clinically more appealing to use cutoffs of WC and BMI, we used the similar approach to test whether central obesity (defined on the basis of WC) is associated with TFI independent of general obesity (defined as BMI ≥ 30 kg/m^2). The results of these analyses are shown in Additional file 1: Table S3 and corroborate the inferences drawn from results in Additional file 1: Table S2. Therefore, to facilitate clinical use we evaluated central obesity (instead of WC) as an independent determinant of thyroid dysfunction in the succeeding analyses.

Central obesity associates with TFI independently of age

Since central obesity and thyroid dysfunction are both associated with age, we next investigated whether the association of central obesity with TFI is independent of age. For this, we slid the age cutoff over the range 30-60 y and at each cutoff ran a polygenic regression model that included dichotomized age and central obesity as covariates and TFI as the dependent variable. We observed that in SAFHS as well as NHANES 2007–10 participants, the estimated regression coefficient for central obesity (green diamonds and bars in Figure 2A and 2B) was robustly stable and hovered between 0.2 and 0.3 irrespective of the cutoff for age. Further, as existing T2D is sometimes considered an indication for screening of thyroid dysfunction, we adjusted these models for presence of T2D also. We observed (Figure 2C and 2D) that the significant and independent association of central obesity with TFI was sustained even after accounting for age and presence of T2D.

Prevalence of hypothyroidism based on central obesity and age

Lastly, we estimated prevalence of clinical and subclinical hypothyroidism in subgroups defined by 5-yearly age intervals and presence or absence of central obesity. In SAFHS participants (Figure 3A), prevalence of hypothyroidism was higher within each age subgroup in those with central obesity than without. In the NHANES 2007–10 participants (Figure 3B), this finding was replicated in all age categories except 45–49 and 55-59 y. Thus, central obesity showed an additive and independent screening benefit especially below the age of 45 y.

Discussion

Our results demonstrate that WC, as a measure of central obesity, is a significant and independent indicator of thyroid dysfunction in Mexican Americans. These results are substantiated by the fact that the associative patterns were consistently observed in two large and disparate studies on the same ethnic population. Interestingly, the prevalence of clinical and subclinical hypothyroidism was higher in the SAFHS than that in the NHANES 2007–10 participants. This finding is important because subjects with subclinical hypothyroidism are at a higher risk of eventual overt hypothyroidism in future as compared to the euthyroid subjects [27] and our results imply that such subjects may be concentrated within families. Our findings therefore indicate that central obesity may be not only an important player in the multifactorial web of thyroid dysfunction but may also contribute to the development of future clinical hypothyroidism by predicting the subjects who are currently at a high risk of subclinical hypothyroidism.

The prevalence of subclinical and clinical hypothyroidism estimated in this study may be somewhat higher than its true population value for two reasons. First, there is substantial evidence in the literature supporting the view that TSH values may be increased in obesity and morbid obesity [28-31]. Second, the TSH cutoff used to define hypothyroidism here is restrictive. It is not uncommon to use 5 μU/ml as the upper limit of normal TSH [19,32,33]. If this high cutoff value is used then

Table 2 Association of metabolic syndrome related traits with thyroid function index in the SAFHS participants

Metabolic syndrome-related trait	All subjects				Males				Females			
	Unadjusted		Adjusted†		Unadjusted		Adjusted††		Unadjusted		Adjusted††	
	β	p	β	p	β	p	β	p	β	P	β	p
Fasting glucose	0.08	0.03	−0.02	0.62	0.07	0.19	0.01	0.91	0.07	0.14	−0.03	0.53
2-hour glucose	0.14	<0.0001	0.05	0.15	0.16	<0.01	0.11	0.05	0.09	0.06	−0.01	0.82
Fasting insulin	0.04	0.27	0.00	0.96	0.03	0.62	0.01	0.78	0.03	0.52	−0.01	0.77
2-hour insulin	0.08	0.02	0.04	0.22	0.07	0.18	0.04	0.43	0.07	0.13	0.03	0.47
HOMA-IR	0.06	0.12	0.00	0.94	0.04	0.41	0.02	0.78	0.05	0.33	−0.02	0.68
HOMA-β	−0.07	0.06	0.02	0.58	−0.05	0.38	0.01	0.86	−0.06	0.1763	0.04	0.47
WC	0.19	<0.0001	**0.13**	**<0.001**	0.12	0.04	0.08	0.18	0.20	<0.0001	**0.14**	**0.001**
BMI	0.15	<0.0001	**0.11**	**<0.01**	0.04	0.45	0.02	0.76	0.18	<0.0001	**0.13**	**<0.01**
WHR	0.15	<0.0001	0.09	0.01	0.23	<0.001	0.20	<0.01	0.16	0.0001	0.10	0.02
Total serum cholesterol	0.12	0.0001	0.06	0.06	0.08	0.10	0.07	0.19	0.11	0.0101	0.03	0.46
Serum triglycerides	0.15	<0.0001	0.08	0.02	0.12	0.02	0.09	0.07	0.14	<0.01	0.07	0.14
Serum HDL cholesterol	0.05	0.11	0.06	0.06	0.05	0.32	0.07	0.15	0.02	0.67	0.02	0.69
Central obesity	0.30	<0.0001	**0.20**	**<0.01**	0.16	0.14	0.13	0.26	0.33	0.0001	0.20	0.02
Raised triglycerides	0.16	0.02	0.05	0.42	0.13	0.19	0.09	0.39	0.19	0.03	0.06	0.49
Low HDL cholesterol	−0.02	0.81	−0.05	0.46	0.12	0.28	0.08	0.49	−0.11	0.20	−0.11	0.17
High blood pressure	−0.25	<0.01	−0.05	0.61	−0.10	0.44	0.06	0.65	−0.26	0.01	−0.06	0.61
Type 2 diabetes	0.15	0.04	−0.04	0.60	0.14	0.22	−0.01	0.95	0.15	0.14	−0.04	0.70
Metabolic syndrome	0.27	<0.0001	0.16	0.02	0.28	0.02	0.25	0.04	0.24	<0.01	0.11	0.24

†Adjusted for age, age^2, sex, age x sex interaction and age^2 x sex interaction; ††, adjusted for age and age^2; numbers in bold face indicate statistically significant associations after correcting for multiple testing.

Table 3 Association of metabolic syndrome related traits with thyroid function index in NHANES 2007–2010 participants*

Metabolic syndrome-related trait	All subjects				Males				Females			
	Unadjusted		Adjusted†		Unadjusted		Adjusted††		Unadjusted		Adjusted††	
	β	p	β	P	β	p	β	p	β	P	β	P
Fasting glucose	0.09	0.08	0.01	0.78	0.15	<0.01	0.12	0.03	0.08	0.25	−0.02	0.76
Fasting insulin	0.05	0.13	0.06	0.07	0.12	<0.01	0.12	<0.01	−0.05	0.32	−0.03	0.56
HOMA-IR	0.07	0.02	0.06	0.04	0.15	<0.001	0.14	<0.001	−0.02	0.70	−0.03	0.52
HOMA-β	0.00	0.98	0.05	0.20	0.05	0.30	0.08	0.12	−0.09	0.16	0.00	0.98
WC	0.16	<0.0001	**0.11**	**<0.001**	0.21	<0.0001	0.20	**<0.0001**	0.13	<0.001	0.06	0.17
BMI	0.15	<0.0001	**0.12**	**<0.001**	0.20	<0.0001	0.20	**<0.0001**	0.11	<0.01	0.03	0.40
Total serum cholesterol	0.16	<0.0001	**0.11**	**<0.01**	0.13	<0.001	0.13	**<0.001**	0.20	<0.001	0.11	0.04
Serum triglycerides	0.13	<0.001	0.09	0.04	0.11	<0.01	0.10	0.02	0.20	0.001	0.12	0.07
Serum HDL cholesterol	0.00	0.98	0.00	0.85	−0.10	<0.001	−0.10	<0.001	0.05	0.09	0.04	0.11
Central obesity	0.32	<0.0001	**0.22**	**<0.001**	0.36	<0.0001	0.30	**<0.0001**	0.22	<0.01	0.05	0.58
Raised triglycerides	0.17	<0.01	0.01	0.90	0.09	0.17	−0.01	0.88	0.31	<0.01	0.13	0.20
Low HDL cholesterol	0.10	<0.01	0.04	0.12	0.14	0.02	0.10	0.08	0.02	0.69	−0.03	0.52
High blood pressure	0.31	<0.0001	0.08	0.16	0.32	<0.01	0.17	0.13	0.34	<0.001	0.02	0.83
Type 2 diabetes	0.30	<0.0001	0.04	0.55	0.24	0.02	0.00	0.98	0.33	0.001	0.07	0.47
Metabolic syndrome	0.32	<0.0001	0.16	0.05	0.29	0.01	0.19	0.11	0.29	0.06	0.09	0.62

*In this set, data on 2-hour glucose, 2-hour insulin and WHR were not available; †, adjusted for age, age^2, sex, age x sex interaction and age^2 x sex interaction; ††, adjusted for age and age^2; numbers in bold face indicate statistically significant associations after correcting for multiple testing.

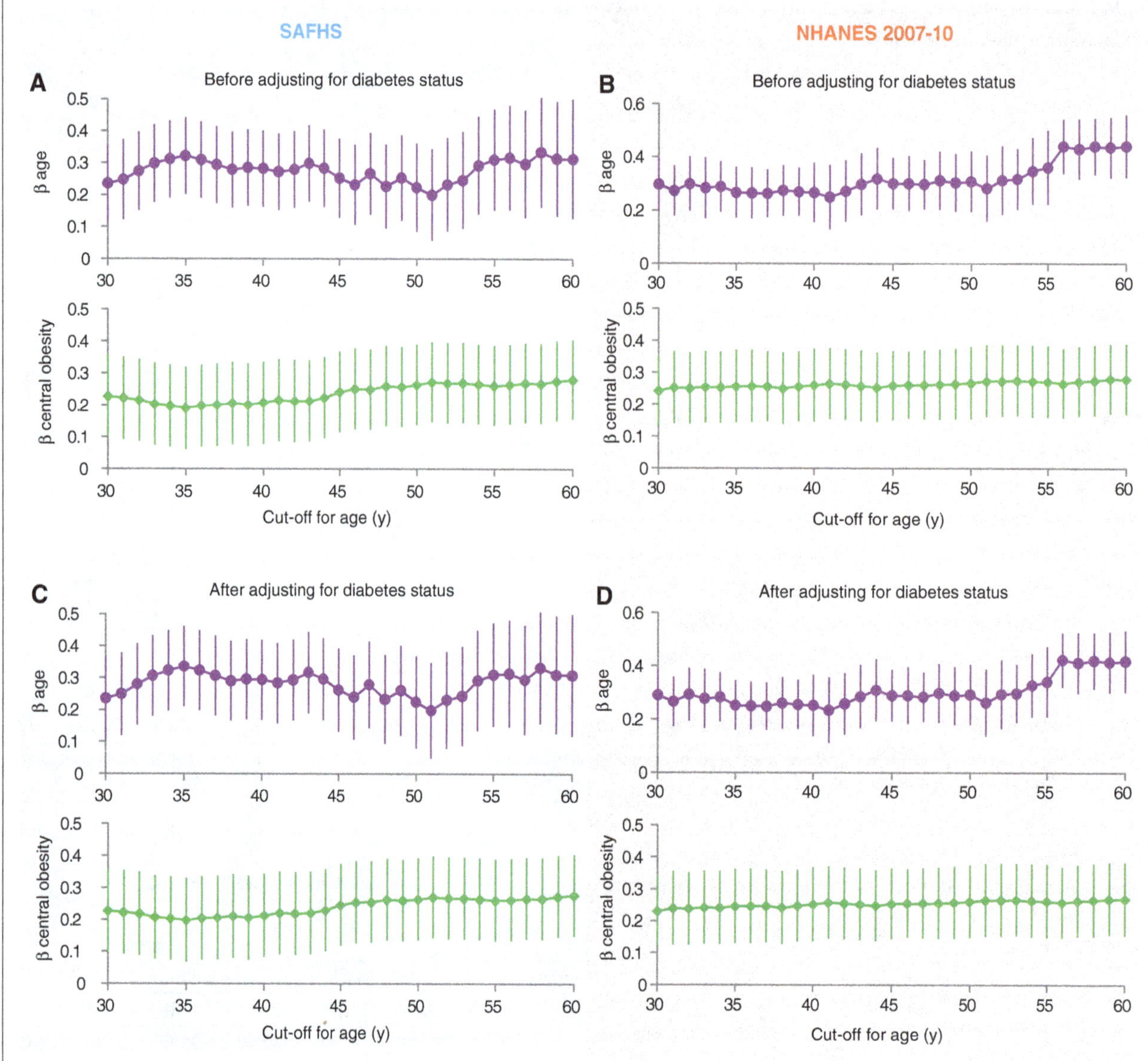

Figure 2 Association of central obesity with TFI is independent of age. Results for SAFHS participants are shown on the blue background on left while those for the NHANES 2007–10 participants are shown on pink background on right. **(A-B)** Estimated regression coefficients (β) for age (purple circles) and central obesity (green diamonds) in a single polygenic model for each cutoff of age. In these analyses age was dichotomized at the cutoffs shown on the abscissa and polygenic regression was run at each cutoff. Error bars represent 95% confidence intervals around the regression coefficient. **(C-D)** Analyses similar to those in **(A-B)** but additionally accounting for presence of type 2 diabetes.

expectedly the prevalence of hypothyroidism will be less than that reported here. We chose to use the cutoff of 3 μU/ml for the following three reasons: i) The main objective of this study was not to estimate prevalence of hypothyroidism but rather to compare the prevalence estimates across categories of predictor variables like waist circumference; ii) The criteria used for diagnosis of clinical thyroid states used in this study are based on clinical practice guidelines recommended by the American Association of Clinical Endocrinologists and the American Thyroid Association [34] and therefore follow the standards-of-care; and iii) Using these criteria, cross-ethnicity comparisons in American populations can be undertaken in future even if we have not included other ethnic groups in this study. In addition, we used TFI as a surrogate measure of thyroid function. This novel measure has the advantage that it combines the information content of TSH, FT3 and FT4 in the identification of hypothyroidism. However, we would like to point out that the clinical use of TFI has thus far not been validated in other populations and should be considered only illustrative rather than conclusive.

Biological plausibility in support of our findings is provided by a series of recent observations. First, thyroid

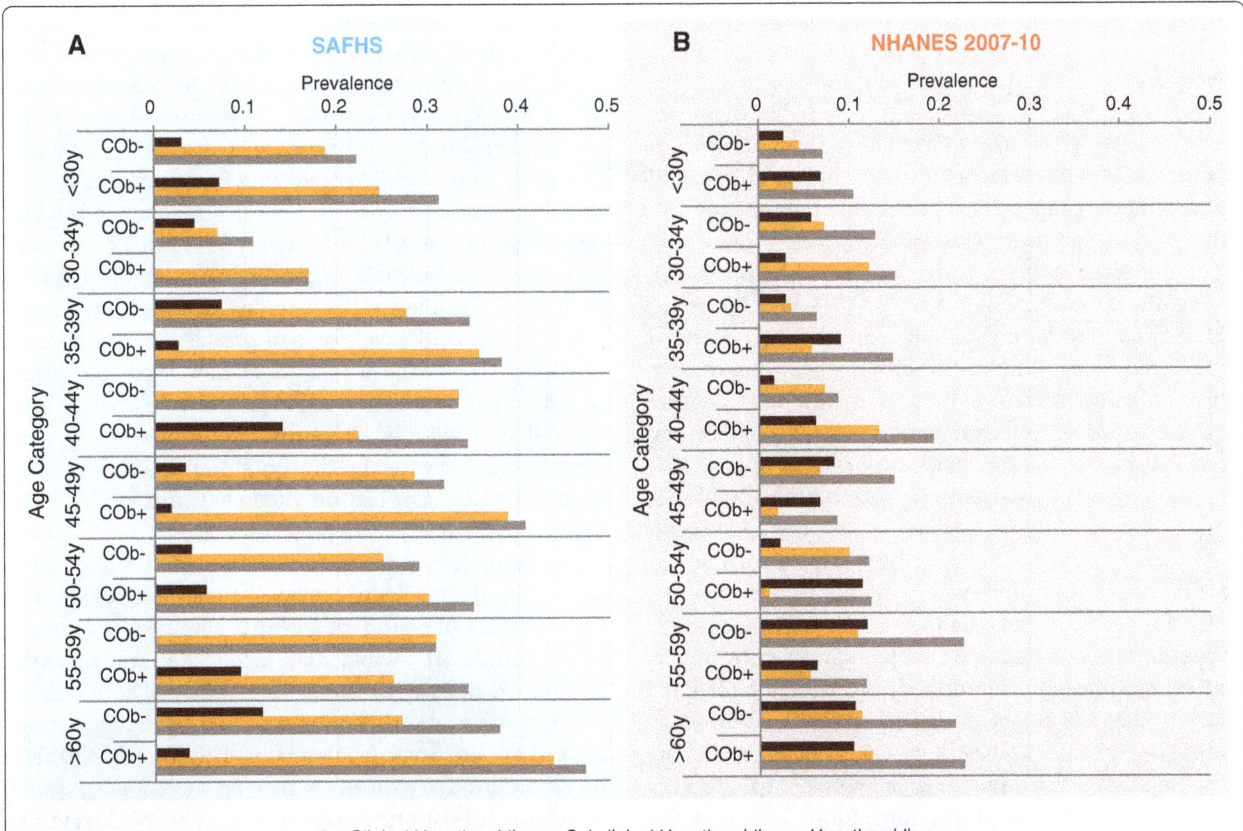

Figure 3 Utility of central obesity as an additional screening measure to detect thyroid dysfunction. Results for SAFHS participants are shown on the blue background in **(A)** while those for the NHANES 2007–10 participants are shown on pink background in **(B)**. Each panel shows color coded bars representing prevalence of the indicated clinical thyroid status within each age category. COb+, central obesity present; COb-, central obesity absent.

stimulating hormone receptors (TSHR) are present in tissues other than the thyroid, especially in differentiating adipocytes [35]. Whilst it is conceivable that increasing TSHR concentration in obesity may attract additional release of TSH through a positive feedback to the pituitary, direct data in this regard are currently unavailable. As explained by Skudlinski et al. [36] and Mueller et al. [37], however the interactions between TSH and TSHR are very complex and therefore expectation of a simple positive feedback loop conjectured here may be overly simplistic. Second, thyroid hormone has been shown [38] to regulate expression of the gene encoding apolipoprotein M by binding to a hormone response element in the promoter of this gene. It is noteworthy that apolipoprotein M plays an important role in MS and obesity [38-40]. Third, in the 3 T3-L1 adipocytes it was observed [41] that *in vitro* treatment with triiodothyronine and thyroxine increased the expression of the gene encoding Plasminogen activator inhibitor 1, a key contributor in the inflammatory and cardiovascular complications of obesity. Fourth, triiodothyronine regulates the expression of the apolipoprotein AV gene, another important contributor to the complex pathogenesis of obesity and its complications [42]. Considered in totality, these studies lend biological credibility to our observation that WC is associated with thyroid function although the exact mechanism of this association remains unknown.

Our results are conceptually in agreement with the observed association of WC-based indices with altered thyroid function in other populations like Chinese children [43], Turkish women [44], other US ethnic groups [4], Italian euthyroid subjects [45] and Korean adults [46]. It is interesting that these studies have addressed different aspects of metabolic syndrome but none of these studies has directly and simultaneously assessed associations of the components of MS with thyroid dysfunction. For example, the study by Kitahara et al. [4], demonstrated that in a predominantly non-Hispanic white population of US men and women, higher values of BMI and WC were associated with increased TSH levels. However, a direct comparison of WC and BMI was not done in that study. Similarly, two studies [44,45] have specifically evaluated the association with a focus on insulin sensitivity and resistance with thyroid dysfunction. The study by Jung et al., used WHR as the index of central obesity and found similar results as those of ours but they did not include all the components included in this study. As a consequence of these differences a direct comparison of our results with other studies is not possible but all these studies support the paradigm that obesity and thyroid dysfunction are associated with each other.

Some limitations need to be considered before generalizing these results. First, both SAFHS and NHANES 2007–10 studies did not permit a direct investigation of a predictive value of future hypothyroidism – an important requirement before central obesity can be considered as a marker of thyroid dysfunction. Also, it has been argued that hypothyroidism itself may lead to obesity [47]. The direction of causal pathways cannot be established from this study. Second, we did not use the age-specific diagnostic criteria for defining hypothyroidism that are now in vogue [48]. However, since our results were adjusted for age, age^2, sex and their interactions, we do not anticipate that our results would be influenced by any latent misclassification. Third, both SAFHS and NHANES 2007–10 datasets are, by design, cross-sectional in nature and follow-up data on these subjects is not available. Our reasoning that waist circumference might contribute to an increased risk of clinical hypothyroidism by predicting existing subclinical hypothyroidism is only a notional argument and can be affirmed only by longitudinal studies. Fourth, the reasons for some differences observed between males and females in the two SAFHS and NHANES 2007–10 datasets (for example, WC was significantly associated with TFI in females in SAFHS but in males in NHANES 2007–2010) are unclear and need to be investigated in future studies. It is possible that these significance values are primarily a result of the gender differential across the two datasets (SAFHS had 61% females while NHANES 2007–2010 had only 48% females). However, other reasons of biological of epidemiological dispositions cannot be overruled. Nevertheless, the fact that sex-adjusted results showed significant association of WC with TFI in both datasets demonstrates that the stratification due to sex may be minimal. Fifth, in our study we used the recommended [49] cutoffs for WC and BMI however there is now a growing opinion that "metabolically healthy obese" (MHO) subgroup [50] of MS is a special group with subclinical obesity or an overweight status that is associated with increased cardiovascular risks. Our study cannot directly comment on this but it is conceivable that this group may also be associated with altered thyroid disease risks. Future studies need to consider if central and general obesity are also associated with MHO status and therefore are able to identify individuals with increased likelihood of thyroid dysfunction.

Lastly, for dichotomizing the WC values we used cutoffs of ≥102 cm in men and ≥88 cm in women. While these cutoffs have been previously used for all US populations [49], lower cutoffs – especially those associated with increased likelihood of cardiovascular diseases – may provide even more sensitive prediction of thyroid dysfunction at the expense of specificity. The IDF recommends a cutoff of ≥90 cm and ≥80 cm for men and women of Mexican American and Hispanic origin [51]. As demonstrated by Ford et al. [52], these differences in the cutoffs can significantly influence the estimates of prevalence of abdominal obesity. At this time it is unclear how these definitions might impact the association of central obesity with thyroid dysfunction. Therefore, additional studies are required to investigate the potential effect of sliding cutoffs on the association of dichotomized WC with thyroid dysfunction.

Our study has an important indirect implication. Combined with the results of previous studies our results raise the possibility of considering central obesity as a screening adjunct to detect thyroid dysfunction. Recommendations for thyroid disease screening vary widely. The American Thyroid Association recommends [53] beginning screening at 35 y with 5-yearly follow-ups. The American College of Physicians recoomends screening in women over 50 who have at least one symptom suggestive of thyroid disease [54]. The American Academy of Family Physicians recommends [55] screening for high risk populations but the list of high-risk groups includes diabetes, autoimmune disorders, women with a history of thyroid disease, pregnant women and women over 35 years. The American Association of Clinical Endocrinologists recommends screening before childbearing age or pregnancy or during the first trimester [56]. Despite these varied recommendations the emerging common thread is that thyroid screening is likely to be beneficial in high-risk populations. In this vein, our observations raise the possibility that screening for thyroid dysfunction in Mexican Americans based on waist circumference, especially at younger ages, may yield additional benefits. Future studies need to carefully address this possibility.

Conclusions

In two disparate and large population based studies of Mexican Americans, we found that WC is an independent predictor of thyroid function. This association is independent of age, gender and BMI. These results implore that in high-risk, high-prevalence populations like Mexican Americans, consideration needs to be given to WC as a potential screening tool for thyroid dysfunction Future studies need to evaluate the screening benefits, harms and costs associated with prediction of incident thyroid dysfunction based on current evidence of central obesity.

Abbreviations

CDF: Cumulative density function; CO: Clinical hypothyroidism; CR: Clinical hyperthyroidism; FT3: Free triiodothyronine; FT4: Free thyroxine; HDL-C: High density lipoprotein cholesterol; MS: Metabolic syndrome; NHANES: National Health and Nutritiona Examination Survey; ROC: Receiver operating characteristic; RT3C: Reverse triiodothyronine; SAFHS: San Antonio Family Heart Study; SO: Subclinical hypothyroidism; SR: Subclinical hyperthyroidism; T2D: Type 2 diabetes; TBG: Thyroxine binding globulin; TFI: Thyroid function index; THG: Thyroglobulin; THRB: Thyroid hormone receptor beta; TSH: Thyroid stimulating hormone; TSHR: Thyroid stimulating hormone receptor; TT3: Total triiodothyronine; TT4: Total thyroxine; WC: Waist circumference; WHR: Waist-hip ratio.

Competing interests

The authors declare that they have no competing interests.

Authors' contributions

MM and HK conceptualized the study, conducted the analyses and drafted the manuscript. JEC and JB shared the data, helped in conceptualizing the study, reviewed and wrote parts of the manuscript. PBS, AGC, RD, JB and JEC collected the thyroid function data. TDD, LA and MCM reviewed and wrote parts of the manuscript. All authors read and approved the final manuscript.

Acknowledgements

This work was supported in part by NIH grants R01 DK082610, R01 DK079169 and R01 DK057003. Data collection for the San Antonio Family Heart Study was supported by NIH grant P01 HL045522. We are grateful to the participants of the San Antonio Family Heart Study for their continued involvement. The development of the analytical methods and software used in this study was supported by NIH grant R37 MH059490. The AT&T Genomics Computing Center supercomputing facilities used for this work were supported in part by a gift from the AT&T Foundation and with support from the National Center for Research Resources Grant Number S10 RR029392. This investigation was conducted in facilities constructed with support from Research Facilities Improvement Program grants C06 RR013556 and C06 RR017515 from the National Center for Research Resources of the National Institutes of Health.

Author details

[1]Department of Genetics, Texas Biomedical Research Institute, 7620 NW Loop 410, San Antonio, TX, USA. [2]Department of Veterinary Integrative Biosciences, College of Veterinary Medicine and Biomedical Sciences, Texas A&M University, College Station, TX, USA.

References

1. Gaitonde DY, Rowley KD, Sweeney LB: **Hypothyroidism: an update.** *Am Fam Physician* 2012, **86**(3):244–251.
2. Cooper DS, Biondi B: **Subclinical thyroid disease.** *Lancet* 2012, **379**(9821):1142–1154.
3. Hollowell JG, Staehling NW, Flanders WD, Hannon WH, Gunter EW, Spencer CA, Braverman LE: **Serum TSH, T(4), and thyroid antibodies in the United States population (1988 to 1994): National Health and Nutrition Examination Survey (NHANES III).** *J Clin Endocrinol Metab* 2002, **87**(2):489–499.
4. Kitahara CM, Platz EA, Ladenson PW, Mondul AM, Menke A, Berrington de Gonzalez A: **Body fatness and markers of thyroid function among U.S. men and women.** *PLoS One* 2012, **7**(4):e34979.
5. Perros P, McCrimmon RJ, Shaw G, Frier BM: **Frequency of thyroid dysfunction in diabetic patients: value of annual screening.** *Diabet Med* 1995, **12**(7):622–627.
6. Kadiyala R, Peter R, Okosieme OE: **Thyroid dysfunction in patients with diabetes: clinical implications and screening strategies.** *Int J Clin Pract* 2010, **64**(8):1130–1139.
7. Aoki Y, Belin RM, Clickner R, Jeffries R, Phillips L, Mahaffey KR: **Serum TSH and total T4 in the United States population and their association with participant characteristics: National Health and Nutrition Examination Survey (NHANES 1999–2002).** *Thyroid* 2007, **17**(12):1211–1223.
8. Vanderver GB, Engel A, Lamm S: **Cigarette smoking and iodine as hypothyroxinemic stressors in U.S. women of childbearing age: a NHANES III analysis.** *Thyroid* 2007, **17**(8):741–746.
9. Spencer CA, Hollowell JG, Kazarosyan M, Braverman LE: **National Health and Nutrition Examination Survey III thyroid-stimulating hormone (TSH)-thyroperoxidase antibody relationships demonstrate that TSH upper reference limits may be skewed by occult thyroid dysfunction.** *J Clin Endocrinol Metab* 2007, **92**(11):4236–4240.
10. Helfand M, Crapo LM: **Screening for thyroid disease.** *Ann Intern Med* 1990, **112**(11):840–849.
11. Ruhla S, Weickert MO, Arafat AM, Osterhoff M, Isken F, Spranger J, Schofl C, Pfeiffer AF, Mohlig M: **A high normal TSH is associated with the metabolic syndrome.** *Clin Endocrinol (Oxf)* 2010, **72**(5):696–701.
12. Waring AC, Rodondi N, Harrison S, Kanaya AM, Simonsick EM, Miljkovic I, Satterfield S, Newman AB, Bauer DC: **Thyroid function and prevalent and incident metabolic syndrome in older adults: the Health, Ageing and Body Composition Study.** *Clin Endocrinol (Oxf)* 2012, **76**(6):911–918.
13. Mitchell CS, Savage DB, Dufour S, Schoenmakers N, Murgatroyd P, Befroy D, Halsall D, Northcott S, Raymond-Barker P, Curran S, Henning E, Keogh J, Owen P, Lazarus J, Rothman DL, Farooqi IS, Shulman GI, Chatterjee K, Petersen KF: **Resistance to thyroid hormone is associated with raised energy expenditure, muscle mitochondrial uncoupling, and hyperphagia.** *J Clin Invest* 2010, **120**(4):1345–1354.
14. Kaur J: **A Comprehensive Review on Metabolic Syndrome.** *Cardiol Res Pract* 2014, **2014:**943162.
15. MacCluer JW, Stern MP, Almasy L, Atwood LA, Blangero J, Comuzzie AG, Dyke B, Haffner SM, Henkel RD, Hixson JE, Kammerer CM, Mahaney MC, Mitchell BD, Rainwater DL, Samollow PB, Sharp RM, VandeBerg JL, Williams JT: **Genetics of atherosclerosis risk factors in Mexican Americans.** *Nutr Rev* 1999, **57**(5 Pt 2):S59–S65.
16. Mitchell BD, Almasy LA, Rainwater DL, Schneider JL, Blangero J, Stern MP, MacCluer JW: **Diabetes and hypertension in Mexican American families: relation to cardiovascular risk.** *Am J Epidemiol* 1999, **149**(11):1047–1056.
17. Voruganti VS, Lopez-Alvarenga JC, Nath SD, Rainwater DL, Bauer R, Cole SA, Maccluer JW, Blangero J, Comuzzie AG: **Genetics of variation in HOMA-IR and cardiovascular risk factors in Mexican-Americans.** *J Mol Med (Berl)* 2008, **86**(3):303–311.
18. Samollow PB, Perez G, Kammerer CM, Finegold D, Zwartjes PW, Havill LM, Comuzzie AG, Mahaney MC, Göring HH, Blangero J, Foley TP, Barmada MM: **Genetic and environmental influences on thyroid hormone variation in Mexican Americans.** *J Clin Endocrinol Metab* 2004, **89**(7):3276–3284.
19. Dayan CM: **Interpretation of thyroid function tests.** *Lancet* 2001, **357**(9256):619–624.
20. Garber JR, Cobin RH, Gharib H, Hennessey JV, Klein I, Mechanick JI, Pessah-Pollack R, Singer PA, Woeber KA: **Clinical practice guidelines for hypothyroidism in adults: cosponsored by the American Association of Clinical Endocrinologists and the American Thyroid Association.** *Thyroid* 2012, **22**(12):1200–1235.
21. Rothwell CJ, Madans JH, Porter KS: **National Health and Nutrition Examination Survey: Estimation Procedures, 2007–2010.** *Vital and Health Stat* 2013, **2**(159):1–17.
22. Hanley JA, McNeil BJ: **The meaning and use of the area under a receiver operating characteristic (ROC) curve.** *Radiology* 1982, **143**(1):29–36.
23. Blangero J, Diego VP, Dyer TD, Almeida M, Peralta J, Kent JW Jr, Williams JT, Almasy L, Goring HH: **A kernel of truth: statistical advances in polygenic variance component models for complex human pedigrees.** *Adv Genet* 2013, **81:**1–31.
24. Blangero J: **Statistical genetic approaches to human adaptability.** *Hum Biol* 1993, **65**(6):941–966.
25. Almasy L, Blangero J: **Multipoint quantitative-trait linkage analysis in general pedigrees.** *Am J Hum Genet* 1998, **62**(5):1198–1211.
26. Li J, Ji L: **Adjusting multiple testing in multilocus analyses using the eigenvalues of a correlation matrix.** *Heredity (Edinb)* 2005, **95**(3):221–227.

27. Col NF, Surks MI, Daniels GH: **Subclinical thyroid disease: clinical applications.** *JAMA* 2004, **291**(2):239–243.
28. Tarcin O, Abanonu GB, Yazici D: **Association of metabolic syndrome parameters with TT3 and FT3/FT4 ratio in obese Turkish population.** *Metab Syndr Relat Disord* 2012, **10**(2):137–142.
29. Westerink J, van der Graaf Y, Faber DR, Visseren FL: **The relation between thyroid-stimulating hormone and measures of adiposity in patients with manifest vascular disease.** *Eur J Clin Invest* 2011, **41**(2):159–166.
30. Rotondi M, Leporati P, La Manna A, Pirali B, Mondello T, Fonte R, Magri F, Chiovato L: **Raised serum TSH levels in patients with morbid obesity: is it enough to diagnose subclinical hypothyroidism?** *Eur J Endocrinol* 2009, **160**(3):403–408.
31. Tagliaferri M, Berselli ME, Calo G, Minocci A, Savia G, Petroni ML, Viberti GC, Liuzzi A: **Subclinical hypothyroidism in obese patients: relation to resting energy expenditure, serum leptin, body composition, and lipid profile.** *Obes Res* 2001, **9**(3):196–201.
32. Dayan CM, Panicker V: **Novel insights into thyroid hormones from the study of common genetic variation.** *Nat Rev Endocrinol* 2009, **5**(4):211–218.
33. Dayan CM, Saravanan P, Bayly G: **Whose normal thyroid function is better–yours or mine?** *Lancet* 2002, **360**(9330):353.
34. Garber JR, Cobin RH, Gharib H, Hennessey JV, Klein I, Mechanick JI, Pessah-Pollack R, Singer PA, Woeber KA: **Clinical practice guidelines for hypothyroidism in adults: cosponsored by the American Association of Clinical Endocrinologists and the American Thyroid Association.** *Endocr Pract* 2012, **18**(6):988–1028.
35. Lu S, Guan Q, Liu Y, Wang H, Xu W, Li X, Fu Y, Gao L, Zhao J, Wang X: **Role of extrathyroidal TSHR expression in adipocyte differentiation and its association with obesity.** *Lipids Health Dis* 2012, **11**:17.
36. Szkudlinski MW, Fremont V, Ronin C, Weintraub BD: **Thyroid-stimulating hormone and thyroid-stimulating hormone receptor structure-function relationships.** *Physiol Rev* 2002, **82**(2):473–502.
37. Mueller S, Szkudlinski MW, Schaarschmidt J, Gunther R, Paschke R, Jaeschke H: **Identification of novel TSH interaction sites by systematic binding analysis of the TSHR hinge region.** *Endocrinology* 2011, **152**(8):3268–3278.
38. Mosialou I, Zannis VI, Kardassis D: **Regulation of human apolipoprotein m gene expression by orphan and ligand-dependent nuclear receptors.** *J Biol Chem* 2010, **285**(40):30719–30730.
39. Ooi EM, Watts GF, Chan DC, Nielsen LB, Plomgaard P, Dahlback B, Barrett PH: **Association of apolipoprotein M with high-density lipoprotein kinetics in overweight-obese men.** *Atherosclerosis* 2010, **210**(1):326–330.
40. Dullaart RP, Plomgaard P, de Vries R, Dahlback B, Nielsen LB: **Plasma apolipoprotein M is reduced in metabolic syndrome but does not predict intima media thickness.** *Clin Chim Acta* 2009, **406**(1–2):129–133.
41. Biz C, Oliveira C, Mattos AB, Oliveira J, Ribeiro EB, Oller do Nascimento CM: **The effect of thyroid hormones on the white adipose tissue gene expression of PAI-1 and its serum concentration.** *Braz J Med Biol Res* 2009, **42**(12):1163–1166.
42. Prieur X, Huby T, Coste H, Schaap FG, Chapman MJ, Rodriguez JC: **Thyroid hormone regulates the hypotriglyceridemic gene APOA5.** *J Biol Chem* 2005, **280**(30):27533–27543.
43. Chen H, Zhang H, Tang W, Xi Q, Liu X, Duan Y, Liu C: **Thyroid function and morphology in overweight and obese children and adolescents in a Chinese population.** *J Pediatr Endocrinol Metab* 2013, **26**(5–6):489–496.
44. Topsakal S, Yerlikaya E, Akin F, Kaptanoglu B, Erurker T: **Relation with HOMA-IR and thyroid hormones in obese Turkish women with metabolic syndrome.** *Eat Weight Disord* 2012, **17**(1):e57–e61.
45. Ambrosi B, Masserini B, Iorio L, Delnevo A, Malavazos AE, Morricone L, Sburlati LF, Orsi E: **Relationship of thyroid function with body mass index and insulin-resistance in euthyroid obese subjects.** *J Endocrinol Invest* 2010, **33**(9):640–643.
46. Jung CH, Sung KC, Shin HS, Rhee EJ, Lee WY, Kim BS, Kang JH, Kim H, Kim SW, Lee MH, Park JR, Kim SW: **Thyroid dysfunction and their relation to cardiovascular risk factors such as lipid profile, hsCRP, and waist hip ratio in Korea.** *Korean J Intern Med* 2003, **18**(3):146–153.
47. Weaver JU: **Classical endocrine diseases causing obesity.** *Front Horm Res* 2008, **36**:212–228.
48. Tabatabaie V, Surks MI: **The aging thyroid.** *Curr Opin Endocrinol Diabetes Obes* 2013, **20**(5):455–459.
49. Alberti KG, Eckel RH, Grundy SM, Zimmet PZ, Cleeman JI, Donato KA, Fruchart JC, James WP, Loria CM, Smith SC Jr: **Harmonizing the metabolic syndrome: a joint interim statement of the International Diabetes Federation Task Force on Epidemiology and Prevention; National Heart, Lung, and Blood Institute; American Heart Association; World Heart Federation; International Atherosclerosis Society; and International Association for the Study of Obesity.** *Circulation* 2009, **120**(16):1640–1645.
50. Roberson LL, Aneni EC, Maziak W, Agatston A, Feldman T, Rouseff M, Tran T, Blaha MJ, Santos RD, Sposito A, Al-Mallah MH, Blankstein R, Budoff MJ, Nasir K: **Beyond BMI: The "Metabolically healthy obese" phenotype & its association with clinical/subclinical cardiovascular disease and all-cause mortality – a systematic review.** *BMC Public Health* 2014, **14**:14.
51. Grundy SM, Brewer HB Jr, Cleeman JI, Smith SC Jr, Lenfant C: **Definition of metabolic syndrome: Report of the National Heart, Lung, and Blood Institute/American Heart Association conference on scientific issues related to definition.** *Circulation* 2004, **109**(3):433–438.
52. Ford ES, Li C, Zhao G: **Prevalence and correlates of metabolic syndrome based on a harmonious definition among adults in the US.** *J Diabetes* 2010, **2**(3):180–193.
53. Ladenson PW, Singer PA, Ain KB, Bagchi N, Bigos ST, Levy EG, Smith SA, Daniels GH, Cohen HD: **American Thyroid Association guidelines for detection of thyroid dysfunction.** *Arch Intern Med* 2000, **160**(11):1573–1575.
54. Helfand M, Redfern CC: **Clinical guideline, part 2. Screening for thyroid disease: an update. American College of Physicians.** *Ann Intern Med* 1998, **129**(2):144–158.
55. Surks MI, Ortiz E, Daniels GH, Sawin CT, Col NF, Cobin RH, Franklyn JA, Hershman JM, Burman KD, Denke MA, Gorman C, Cooper RS, Weissman NJ: **Subclinical thyroid disease: scientific review and guidelines for diagnosis and management.** *JAMA* 2004, **291**(2):228–238.
56. Wier FA, Farley CL: **Clinical controversies in screening women for thyroid disorders during pregnancy.** *J Midwifery Womens Health* 2006, **51**(3):152–158.

16

Differences and associations of metabolic and vitamin D status among patients with and without sub-clinical hypothyroid dysfunction

Naji J Aljohani[1,3], Nasser M Al-Daghri[2,3*], Omar S Al-Attas[2,3,4], Majed S Alokail[2,3], Khalid M Alkhrafy[2,3,5], Abdulaziz Al-Othman[2,6], Sobhy Yakout[2,3], Abdulaziz F Alkabba[1], Ahmed S Al-Ghamdi[1], Mussa Almalki[1], Badurudeen Mahmood Buhary[1] and Shaun Sabico[2,3]

Abstract

Background: Sub-clinical hypothyroid dysfunction, a relatively understudied disorder in the Kingdom of Saudi Arabia (KSA), has significant clinical implications if not properly monitored. Also from KSA, more than 50% of the population suffer from hypovitaminosis D (<50 nmol/l). In this cross-sectional case-control study, we described the differences and associations in the metabolic patterns of adult Saudis with and without hypothyroid dysfunction in relation to their vitamin D status, PTH, calcium and lipid profile.

Methods: A total of 94 consenting adult Saudis [52 controls (without subclinical hypothyroidism), 42 cases (previously diagnosed subjects)] were included in this cross-sectional study. Anthropometrics were obtained and fasting blood samples were taken for ascertaining lipid and thyroid profile, as well as measuring PTH, 25(OH) vitamin D and calcium.

Results: Cases had a significantly higher body mass index than the controls ($p < 0.001$). Circulating triglycerides was also significantly higher in cases than the controls ($p = 0.001$). A significant positive association between HDL-cholesterol and PTH ($R = 0.56$; $p = 0.001$), as well as a negative and modestly significant negative association between LDL-cholesterol and PTH ($R = - 20.0$; $p = 0.04$) were observed. FT3 was inversely associated with circulating 25 (OH) vitamin D ($R = -0.25$; $p = 0.01$).

Conclusions: Patients with hypothyroid dysfunction possess several cardiometabolic risk factors that include obesity and dyslipidemia. The association between PTH and cholesterol levels as well as the inverse association between vitamin D status and FT3 needs to be reassessed prospectively on a larger scale to confirm these findings.

Keywords: Thyroid dysfunction, Obesity, Dyslipidemia, Saudi

Background

Thyroid diseases are one of the more commonly encountered endocrine disorders in the Kingdom of Saudi Arabia (KSA), next to diabetes mellitus (DM) [1]. While current demographics point to less alarming prevalence of thyroid dysfunction, certain populations such as children with Down syndrome appear to manifest conditions related to thyroid dysfunction [2]. In the Middle East in general, thyroid dysfunction, specifically subclinical hypothyroid dysfunction, is a relatively understudied field as compared to other metabolic disorders such as obesity and insulin resistance. In a recent study, Bahammam and colleagues observed that subclinical hypothyroid dysfunction was prevalent among Saudi patients suffering from obstructive sleep apnea (OSA), with an estimated 1 out of 10 OSA patients harboring the condition [3]. Granted that hypothyroid dysfunction is not as endemic as the previously mentioned disorders, it nevertheless deserves attention as it can lead to serious repercussions if left ignored. Several studies point to an association between thyroid diseases, particularly Grave's disease and vitamin D status

* Correspondence: aldaghri2011@gmail.com
[2]Biochemistry Department, Biomarkers Research Program, College of Science, King Saud University, Riyadh, Saudi Arabia
[3]Prince Mutaib Chair for Biomarkers of Osteoporosis, King Saud University, Riyadh, Saudi Arabia

in several ethnic groups, but none if not limited in the Middle East [4-6]. In this cross-sectional case-control study, we describe the differences and associations in the metabolic patterns of adult Saudis with and without subclinical hypothyroid dysfunction in relation to lipid and calcium metabolism in an attempt to stimulate further clinical investigations with respect to this understudied disorder.

Methods

Subjects

A total of 94 consenting adult Saudis [52 control (6 males; 46 females), 42 cases (3 males, 39 females)] were included in this cross-sectional study. All subjects were recruited at the Endocrinology Unit of King Fahad Medical City, Riyadh Saudi Arabia. Adult Saudis aged 20-50, who are known cases of subclinical hypothyroid dysfunction based on previous clinical assessment (elevated TSH with normal FT4 levels), medications taken and laboratory tests with no complications were included. Control subjects were those who tested negative for subclinical hypothyroid dysfunction with no history of thyroid medications. Non-Saudis and pregnant women as well as children were excluded. Written and informed consent were secured prior to inclusion. Ethical approval was obtained from the Institutional Review Board of King Fahad Medical City, Riyadh, KSA.

Anthropometrics

Anthropometric parameters were obtained while the subject was standing erect and barefoot. Height and weight were determined using standardized conventional methods. Body mass index (BMI) was calculated using the formula: weight in kilograms (kg) divided by height in squared meters (m^2).

Blood measurements

Blood (≈ 10cc) was withdrawn after an overnight fast (> 10 hours). Serum calcium was measured using standard analytical techniques (Konelab, Finland). Fasting blood lipids which included triglycerides, total, HDL- and LDL-cholesterol as well as calcium were measured routinely using a chemical analyzer (Konelab, Finland). Serum TSH, FT3, and FT4 were estimated using commercially available kits by Roche Elecsys Modular Analytics Cobas e411 utilizing electrochemiluminescence immunoassay (Roche Diagnostics, Mannheim, Germany). TSH upper normal limit for males is 3.69 μIU/ml and 3.94 μIU/ml for females. Intact PTH and 25(OH)D were measured by specific ELISAs in accordance with the instructions provided by the manufacturer (IDS, Tyne & Wear, UK). 25(OH) vitamin D has been the preferred metabolite for the measurement of vitamin D status instead of 1, 25(OH)D, and remains the basis for the diagnosis of vitamin D deficiency [7]. The inter- and intra-assay variabilities were 5.8% and 3.4% respectively for the intact PTH ELISA, 5.3% and 4.6% respectively for the 25(OH)D ELISA. Anti-thyroid peroxidase (TPO) antibodies (Ab) were also measured using commercially available ELISA kits (Bio-Line S.A, Brussels, Belgium) with a sensitivity of 1.4 U/ml (intra-assay variability 6.9%; inter-assay variability 13.4%).

Data analysis

Data was analyzed using the Statistical Package for the Social Sciences (SPSS) version 16.5 (Chicago, IL, USA). Frequencies were presented as N and continuous variables if normal were presented as mean ± standard deviation and median (inter-quartile range) for variables with non-normal distribution. For group comparisons (controls versus cases), independent T-test if normally distributed continuous variables, and Mann-Whitney U-test for variables with non-Gaussian distribution were utilized. Significance set at $p < 0.05$.

Results

Table 1 shows the general characteristics of both cases and controls. There was no significant difference in the mean age of both groups. Subjects with thyroid dysfunction had a significantly higher body mass index than controls ($p < 0.001$). Circulating triglycerides were also

Table 1 Differences in metabolic characteristics of controls versus cases

	Controls	Cases	P value
N	52	42	
Age (years)	36.1 ± 8.1	35.5 ± 10.1	0.75
Gender (M/F)	6/46	3/39	
Body Mass Index (kg/m^2)	27.8 ± 3.9	32.3 ± 6.8	<0.001
Triglycerides (mmol/l)	1.2 ± 0.26	1.9 ± 0.46	0.001
Total Cholesterol (mmol/l)	5.1 ± 0.80	5.2 ± 1.0	0.56
LDL-Cholesterol (mmol/l)	3.9 ± 0.88	3.9 ± 0.87	0.99
HDL-Cholesterol (mmol/l)	0.90 ± 0.37	0.88 ± 0.30	0.78
Iodine (μg/l)	119.5 ± 35.9	97.6 ± 38.5	0.009
TSH (mIU/l)#	2.4 (1.6, 3.3)	3.7 (1.5, 7.6)	0.04
FT3 (pmol/l)	6.0 ± 1.3	4.8 ± 1.2	<0.001
FT4 (pmol/l)	17.2 ± 1.3	17.5 ± 1.2	0.80
TPOAb (U/ml) #	17.7 (14.1, 25.0)	164.9 (15.8, 582.9)	0.001
PTH (pg/ml)	5.3 ± 1.5	8.0 ± 1.2	0.15
Albumin (g/l)	33.8 ± 5.4	36.5 ± 6.8	0.03
Corrected Ca (mmol/l)	2.4 ± 0.23	2.1 ± 0.18	< 0.001
Ca (mmol/l)	2.5 ± 0.19	2.1 ± 0.45	0.002
25 (OH) Vitamin D (nmol/l)	18.3 ± 1.5	37.3 ± 1.9	< 0.001

Note: # denotes non-Gaussian distribution and presented as median (interquartile range); *p*-value significant at < 0.05.

Table 2 Correlation coefficients (R) of Lipids to thyroid function tests, PTH and vitamin D adjusted for age and BMI

	TSH	FT3	FT4	PTH	Iodine	TPO Ab	Vitamin D
Total Cholesterol (mmol/l)	-0.05	-0.02	-0.06	-0.04	0.05	0.03	-0.02
HDL-Cholesterol (mmol/l)	-0.12	-0.13	-0.13	**0.56****	-0.04	0.08	-0.04
Triglycerides (mmol/l)	0.12	0.04	-0.10	-0.16	-0.09	0.01	-0.19
LDL-Cholesterol (mmol/l)	-0.04	0.02	0.003	**-0.20***	0.08	0.001	0.04

Note: * denotes significance at < 0.05; ** denotes significance at < 0.01; *p*-value significant at < 0.05.

significantly higher among the cases than the controls ($p = 0.001$). The rest of the lipid parameters (Total, LDL- and HDL-cholesterol) were not significant. Among the thyroid tests, median TSH and median TPO Ab were significantly higher in the cases (consistent with Hashimoto's Thyroiditis) who also had a significantly lower mean FT3 and iodine than the controls (p values 0.03, 0.001, 0.009 and < 0.001, respectively). Only 2 subjects had TPOAb levels below 1.7 U/ml (cases). Mean FT4 was similar in both cases and controls. Lastly, mean serum calcium as well as corrected calcium were significantly lower in cases than controls ($p = 0.002$ and $p \leq 0.001$, respectively). Cases also had a significantly higher 25 (OH) vitamin D levels than the controls ($p < 0.001$), although both groups fall below sufficiency levels. Intact PTH was not significantly different between groups. Table 2 shows the regression coefficients of the lipid parameters versus the different thyroid tests, as well as 25(OH) vitamin D and PTH. A significant positive association between HDL-cholesterol and PTH ($R = 0.56$; $p = 0.001$) as well as a negative and modestly significant association between LDL-cholesterol and PTH were detected ($R = - 20.0$; $p = 0.04$). The rest of the associations were not significant. Finally, Figure 1 shows the inverse and significant association between FT3 and circulating 25 (OH) vitamin D ($R = -0.25$; $p = 0.01$). TSH was not significantly associated with 25(OH) vitamin D.

Discussion

The main finding of this study is that aside from the conventional and expected differences in the expression of thyroid tests, including iodine and TPOab, patients with hypothyroid dysfunction also exhibited obesity and elevated levels of triglycerides as compared to controls. How subclinical hypothyroid dysfunction influences weight gain can be explained via the peripheral effects of thyroid hormones and their local regulation of central nervous system (CNS) in the physiologic regulation of appetite that is independent of their conventional role in basal energy expenditure as well as regulation of resting energy expenditure [8,9]. With respect to obesity per se, it has been found out that visceral adipose tissue has a direct effect in TSH levels among obese, and this is independent of insulin resistance [10]. Regarding triglycerides, our results were in accordance with the study of Wanjia and colleagues, who also observed elevated TSH levels among patients with hypertriglyceridemia [11]. The exact mechanisms accountable for the effects of thyroid function with respect to lipid profile are unclear. Nevertheless it is almost established that TSH receptors are present in tissues other than the thyroid gland which include kidneys, bone marrow and adipose tissue, and that variations ion TSH levels among euthyroid patients are partially explained by lipid components and hypercholesterolemia which are independent of thyroid hormones [12,13]. Furthermore, there are several factors not accounted for in this study that may influence thyroid function and lipid profile, including smoking and insulin resistance [14], as well as obesity and abnormalities in glucose tolerance.

One striking and unexpected finding in this study is the significantly higher mean 25(OH) vitamin D levels among patients with subclinical hypothyroid dysfunction

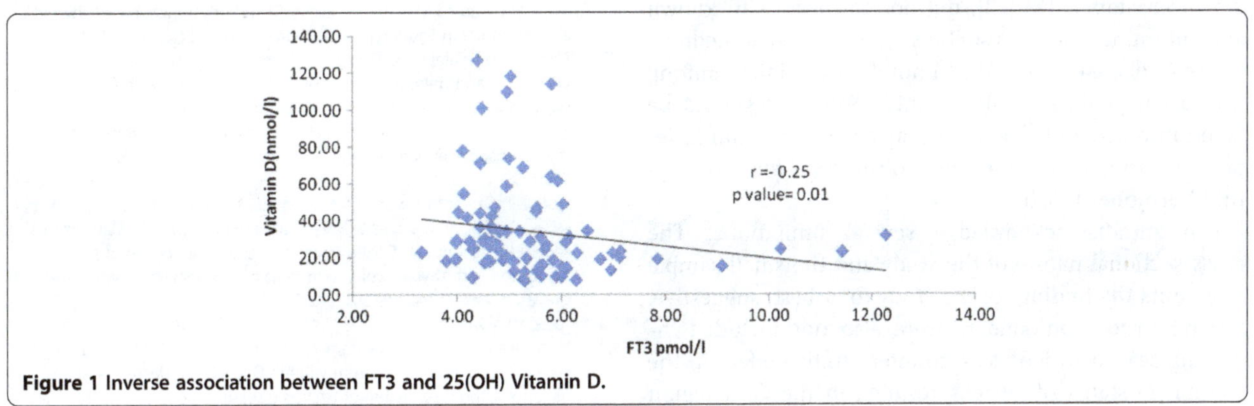

Figure 1 Inverse association between FT3 and 25(OH) Vitamin D.

than controls despite the presence of established risk factors for vitamin D deficiency including obesity and hypetriglyceridemia [15-17]. Calcium levels while also significantly different, still fall within normal range, although the possibility of other causes such as malabsorption or decreased dietary calcium intake in some subjects cannot be ruled out. Furthermore, PTH levels were higher, although not significant in the case group than controls. These differences this can be attributed to several confounders unaccounted for in the study which include differences in dietary calcium and vitamin D intake, undocumented comorbidities such as malabsorption and existing renal disorders which were not evident at the time of selection, as well as sun exposure, and needs further investigation. Nevertheless, while the vitamin D status of cases was significantly higher as compared to controls, both mean levels were still far below sufficiency levels and the corresponding PTH levels were not significantly different from one another, and as such the interpretation is comparable. Furthermore we recently observed that PTH levels do not correlate with 25(OH) vitamin D levels in Saudis despite severely low levels [18].

The association of PTH with lipid concentrations, specifically the cholesterol levels was demonstrated earlier and we suggest that this is mainly due to the positive association of PTH to body composition and adiposity, rather than the cholesterol itself [19,20]. Also, the inverse association of FT3 to circulating levels of 25(OH) D should be interpreted with caution. It was previously reported that higher vitamin D status was associated with low TSH only among younger individuals and not in adults [21]. Furthermore, while vitamin D deficiency has been implicated in several autoimmune thyroid diseases, no association was elicited between the antibodies measured in the present study and vitamin D, confirming a recent study among Dutch natives about the lack of correlation of low vitamin D levels and the early stages of thyroid auto-immunity [22]. Similarly, polymorphisms of vitamin D alpha-hydroxylase (CYP)1alpha, a key enzyme for regulating both systemic and tissue levels of 1, 25-dihydroxyvitamin D3 [23], did not correlate with known auto-immune disorders such as type 1 diabetes mellitus, Grave's disease and Hashimoto's thyroidits among Caucasian pedigrees [24]. In this context, it should be taken into account that TSH may have direct and independent effects on bone metabolism regardless of thyroid hormones [25,26].

The authors acknowledge several limitations. The cross-sectional nature of the study and the small sample size limits the findings of the study to at best, suggestive. Several major confounders were also not included including season which has a counterintuitive effect in the vitamin D status of citizens residing in the Gulf region [27]. Gender difference could not be elicited due to the big discrepancy in the numbers between male and female subjects. Nevertheless, the study has its own strength as being the first to document several metabolic differences among Saudi patients with and without hypothyroid dysfunction and the first to associate vitamin D status in relation to thyroid function profile.

Conclusions

In summary, adult Saudi patients with subclinical hypothyroid dysfunction harbor several cardiometabolic abnormalities, including obesity and dyslipidemia, the latter being associated positively with PTH levels. Higher vitamin D levels were associated with lower FT3 in the patents. Further prospective studies are needed to determine whether the associations elicited are causal to one another.

Competing interests

The authors declare that they have no competing interest.

Authors' contributions

NJA and NMA conceived the study. OSA, MSA, KMA and AA carried out data acquisition and interpretation. SY, AFA, ASA, MA and BMB analyzed the data and prepared the manuscript. NJA and SS drafted the revised and final version of the manuscript. All authors provided intellectual contributions to the manuscript and has read and approved the final version.

Acknowledgments

The author would like to thank the nursing staff of KFMC for the recruitment, data and sample collection of patients. The authors also thank Mr. Benjamin Vinodson for the statistical analysis of the data.

Author details

[1]Faculty of Medicine, King Saud bin Abdulaziz University for Health Sciences, King Fahad Medical City, Riyadh, Saudi Arabia. [2]Biochemistry Department, Biomarkers Research Program, College of Science, King Saud University, Riyadh, Saudi Arabia. [3]Prince Mutaib Chair for Biomarkers of Osteoporosis, King Saud University, Riyadh, Saudi Arabia. [4]Center of Excellence in Biotechnology Research Center, King Saud University, Riyadh, Saudi Arabia. [5]Clinical Pharmacy Department, College of Pharmacy, King Saud University, Riyadh, Saudi Arabia. [6]College of Applied Medical Sciences, King Saud University, Riyadh, KSA, Saudi Arabia.

References

1. Akbar DH, Ahmed MM, Al-Mughales J: **Thyroid dysfunction and thyroid autoimmunity in Saudi type 2 diabetics.** *Acta Diabetol* 2006, **43**:14–18.
2. Abdullah MA, Salman H, Al-Habib S, Ghareeb A, Abanamy A: **Antithyroid antibodies and thyroid dysfunction in Saudi children with Down syndrome.** *Ann Saudi Med* 1994, **14**:283–285.
3. Bahammam SA, Sharif MM, Jammah AA, Bahammam AS: **Prevalence of thyroid disease in patients with obstructive sleep apnea.** *Respir Med* 2011, **105**:1755–1760.
4. Yasuda T, Okamoto Y, Hamada N, Miyashita K, Takahara M, Sakamoto F, Miyatsuka T, Kitamura T, Katakami N, Kawamori D, Otuski M, Matsuoka TA, Kaneto H, Shinomura I: **Serum vitamin D levels are decreased and associated with thyroid volume in female patients with newly onset Grave's disease.** *Endocrine* 2012, **42**:739–741.
5. Yasuda T, Okamoto Y, Hamada N, Miyashita K, Takahara M, Sakamoto F, Miyatsuka T, Kitamura T, Katakami N, Kawamori D, Otsuki M, Matsuoka TA, Kaneto TH, Shimomura I: **Serum vitamin D levels are decreased in patients without remission of Grave's disease.** *Endocrine* 2013, **43**:230–232.

6. Rotondi M, Chiovato L: **Vitamin D deficiency in patients with Grave's disease: probably something more than a casual association.** *Endocrine* 2013, **43**:3–5.
7. Rizzoli R, Boonen S, Brandi ML, Bruyere O, Cooper C, Kanis JA, Kaufman JM, Ringe JD, Weryha G, Reginster JY: **Vitamin D supplementation in elderly or postmenopausal women: a 2013 update of the 2008 recommendations from the European Society for Clinical and Economic Aspects of Osteoporosis and Osteoarthritis (ESCEO).** *Curr Med Res Opin* 2013, **29**:305–313.
8. Amin A, Dhillo WS, Murphy KG: **The central effects of thyroid hormones on appetite.** *J Thyroid Res* 2011, **2011**:306510.
9. Al-Adsani H, Hoffer LJ, Silva JE: **Resting energy expenditure is sensitive to small dose changes in patients on chronic thyroid hormone replacement.** *J Clin Endocrinol Metab* 1997, **82**:1118–1125.
10. Muscogiuri G, Sorice GP, Mezza T: **High normal TSH values in obesity: is it insulin resistance or adipose tissue's guilt?** *Obesity (Silver Spring)* 2013, **21**:101–106.
11. Wanjia X, Chenggang W, Aihong W, Xiaomei Y, Jiajun Z, Chunxiao Y, Jin X, Yinglong H, Ling G: **A high normal TSH levels is associated with an atherogenic lipid profile in euthyroid non-smokers with newly diagnosed asymptomatic coronary heart disease.** *Lipids Health Dis* 2012, **11**:44.
12. Williams GR: **Extrathyroidal expression of TSH receptor.** *Ann Endocrinol (Paris)* 2011, **72**:68–73.
13. Wang F, Tan Y, Wang C, Zhang X, Zhao Y, Song X, Zhang B, Guan Q, Xu J, Zhang J, Zhang D, Lin H, Yu C, Zhao J: **Thyroid-stimulating hormone levels within the reference range are associated with serum lipid profiles independent of thyroid hormones.** *J Clin Endocrinol Metab* 2012, **97**:2724–2731.
14. Palmieri EA, Fazio S, Lombardi G, Biondi B: **Subclinical hypothyroidism and cardiovascular risk: a reason to treat?** *Treat Endocrinol* 2004, **3**:233–244.
15. Al-Daghri NM, Al-Attas OS, Al-Okail MS, Alkharfy KM, Al-Yousef MA, Nadhrah HM, Sabico SB, Chrousos GP: **Severe hypovitaminosis D is widespread in Saudi adults and is more common in non-diabetics than diabetics.** *Saudi Med J* 2010, **31**:775–780.
16. Al-Daghri NM, Al-Attas OS, Alokail MS, Alkharfy KMK, Yousef M, Nadhrah HM, Al-Othman A, Al-Saleh Y, Sabico S, Chrousos GP: **Hypovitaminosis D and cardiometabolic risk factors among non-obese youth.** *Cent Eur J Med* 2010, **5**:752–757.
17. Tamer G, Mesci B, Tamer I, Kilic D, Arik S: **Is vitamin D deficiency an independent risk factor for obesity and abdominal obesity in women?** *Endokrynol Pol* 2012, **63**:196–201.
18. Al-Saleh Y, Al-Daghri NM, Alkharfy KM, Al-Attas OS, Alokail MS, Al-Othman A, Sabico S, Chrousos GP: **Normal circulating PTH in Saudi healthy individuals with hypovitaminosis D.** *Horm Metab Res* 2013, **45**:43–46.
19. Williams DM, Fraser A, Lawlor DA: **Association of vitamin D, parathyroid hormone and calcium with cardiovascular risk factors in US adolescents.** *Heart* 2011, **97**:315–320.
20. Kayaniyil S, Vieth R, Harris SB, Retnakaran R, Knight JA, Gerstein HC, Perkins BA, Zinman B, Hanley AJ: **Association of 25(OH)D and PTH with metabolic syndrome and its traditional and nontraditional components.** *J Clin Endocrinol Metab* 2011, **96**:168–175.
21. Chailurkit LO, Aekplakorn W, Ongphiphadhanakul B: **High vitamin D status in younger individuals is associated with low circulating thyrotropin.** *Thyroid* 2013, **23**:25–30.
22. Effraimidis G, Badenhoop K, Tijssen JG, Wiersinga WM: **Vitamin D deficiency is not associated with early stages of thyroid autoimmunity.** *Eur J Endocrinol* 2012, **167**:43–48.
23. Kozai M, Yamamoto H, Ishiguro M, Harada N, Masuda M, Kagawa T, Takei Y, Otani A, Nakahashi O, Ikeda S, Taketani Y, Takeyama K, Kato S, Takeda E: **Thyroid hormones decrease plasma 1α,25-dihydroxyvitamin D levels through transcriptional repression of the renal 25-hydroxyvitamin D3 1α-hydroxylase gene (CYP27B1).** *Endocrinology* 2013, **154**:609–622.
24. Pani MA, Regulla K, Segni M, Krause M, Hofmann S, Hufner M, Herwig J, Pasquino AM, Usadel KH, Badenhoop K: **Vitamin D1alpha-hydroxylase (CYP1alpha) polymorphism in Grave's disease, Hashimoto's thyroidits and type 1 diabetes mellitus.** *Eur J Endocrinol* 2002, **146**:777–781.
25. Mazziotti G, Porcelli T, Patelli I, Vescovi PP, Giustina A: **Serum TSH values and risk of vertebral fractures in euthyroid post-menopausal women with low bone mineral density.** *Bone* 2010, **46**:747–751.
26. Maziotti G, Sorvillo F, Piscopo M, Cioffi M, Pilla P, Biondi B, Iorio S, Giustina A, Amato G, Carella C: **Recombinant human TSH modulates in vivo C-telopeptides of type-1 collagen and bone alakaline phosphatase, but not osteoprotegerin production in postmenopausal women monitored for differentiated thyroid carcinoma.** *J Bone Miner Res* 2005, **20**:480–486.
27. Al-Daghri NM, Al-Attas OS, Alokail MS, Alkharfy KM, El-Kholie E, Yousef M, Al-Othman A, Al-Saleh Y, Sabico S, Kumar S, Chrousos GP: **Increased vitamin D supplementation recommended during summer season in the gulf region: a counterintuitive seasonal effect in vitamin D levels in adult, overweight and obese Middle Eastern residents.** *Clin Endcrinol (Oxf)* 2012, **76**:346–350.

17

Coexistence of Graves' disease and unilateral functioning Struma ovarii

Tullaya Sitasuwan[1], Suchanan Hanamornroongruang[2], Thavatchai Peerapatdit[1] and Nuntakorn Thongtang[1*]

Abstract

Background: Coexisting of Graves' disease and functioning struma ovarii is a rare condition. Although the histology of struma ovarii predominantly composed of thyrocytes, the majority of the patients did not have thyrotoxicosis. The mechanism underlying the functioning status of the tumor is still unclear but the presence of thyroid stimulating hormone receptor (TSHR) is thought to play a role. Here we describe the patient presentation and report the TSHR expression of the tumor.

Case presentation: A 56-year old Asian woman presented with long standing thyrotoxicosis for 23 years. She was diagnosed with Graves' disease and thyroid nodules. She had bilateral exophthalmos and had high titer of plasma TSHR antibody. Total thyroidectomy was performed and the histologic findings confirmed the clinical diagnosis. The patient had persistent thyrotoxicosis postoperatively. Thyroid uptake demonstrated the adequacy of the thyroid surgery and the whole body scan confirmed the presence of functioning thyroid tissue at pelvic area. The surgery was scheduled and the patient had hypothyroidism after the surgery. The pathological diagnosis was struma ovarii at right ovary. We performed TSHR staining in both the patient's struma ovarii and in 3 cases of non-functioning struma ovarii. The staining results were all positive and the intensity of the TSHR staining of functioning struma ovarii was the same as that in other cases of non-functioning tumors, suggesting that the determinant of functioning struma ovarii might be the presence of TSHR stimuli rather than the intensity of the TSHR in the ovarian tissue.

Conclusion: In patients with Graves' disease with persistent or recurrent thyrotoxicosis after adequate ablative treatment, the possibility of ectopic thyroid hormone production should be considered. TSHR expression is found in patients with functioning and non-functioning struma ovarii and cannot solely be used to determine the functioning status of the tumor.

Keywords: Graves' disease, Functioning struma ovarii

Background

Coexisting of Graves' disease and functioning struma ovarii is a rare condition. Struma ovarii is a rare ovarian tumor. Most affected patients are asymptomatic; however thyrotoxicosis from struma ovarii has been reported in 5 % to 15 % of the confirmed cases [1, 2]. Although the histology of struma ovarii predominantly composed of thyrocytes, the majority of the patients do not have thyrotoxicosis. The mechanism underlying the functioning status of the tumor is still unclear. The expression of thyroid-stimulating hormone receptor (TSHR) is thought to play a role [3, 4]. The diagnosis of functioning struma ovarii is challenging especially when the patient had functioning thyroid gland. Here we report an usual case of coexisting Graves' disease with functioning struma ovarii and the TSHR staining result, including the TSHR staining of the patient with non-functioning struma ovarii.

Case presentation

A 56-year-old woman presented with persistent thyrotoxicosis. She was first diagnosed with thyrotoxicosis 23 years previously and had been periodically treated with antithyroid drugs for several years at a time. On examination, she had bilateral exophthalmos. Her thyroid gland was enlarged

* Correspondence: nuntakorn@hotmail.com
[1]Division of Endocrinology and Metabolism, Faculty of Medicine Siriraj Hospital, Mahidol University, Bangkok 10700, Thailand
Full list of author information is available at the end of the article

with palpable thyroid nodules. Her serum TSHR antibody level was elevated at 3.86 IU/L (reference range, <1.00 IU/L), thus confirming the diagnosis of Graves' disease with thyroid nodules.

A thyroid scan with $Tc^{99}m$ showed generalized increased uptake in the thyroid gland with visualized activity in the pyramidal lobe. One hyperfunctioning nodule at the upper pole of the right lobe and another hypofunctioning nodule in the middle aspect of the right lobe were demonstrated (Fig. 1). The provisional diagnosis at that time was Graves' disease with thyroid nodules, and ablative treatment was planned. Ultrasound-guided fine-needle aspiration yielded an area of undetermined significance. Total thyroidectomy was performed without perioperative complications. The surgical specimen contained 57.7 g of thyroid tissue. The histological findings supported the clinical diagnosis of Graves' disease and benign thyroid nodules.

Two weeks after total thyroidectomy, the patient's symptoms of thyrotoxicosis recurred. The differential diagnosis included inadequate thyroidectomy or a source of extrathyroidal thyrotoxicosis such as functioning struma ovarii. A thyroid function test confirmed the presence of post-thyroidectomy thyrotoxicosis (Table 1). The radioactive iodine uptake was evaluated to check the adequacy of the thyroid surgery, and very low uptake of 0.2 % was found in the thyroid bed (reference range, 15 %–45 %). A radioactive iodine (I^{131}) whole-body scan demonstrated intense radiotracer uptake with a star artifact in the pelvic region. Single-photon emission computed tomography/computed tomography of the pelvis confirmed the presence of inhomogeneous increased radiotracer uptake by an 8.5- × 7.2-cm mixed multicystic-solid mass with internal calcification in the right adnexal region (Fig. 2). The plasma level of cancer antigen 125 was elevated at 48.55 U/ml (reference range, 0–35 U/ml). Therefore the patient was diagnosed with coexisting Graves' disease and functioning struma ovarii and surgery is scheduled. Preoperative control of thyrotoxicosis is required to prevent thyroid storm during the surgery. In the present case, therefore, the patient's methimazole was restarted, and a euthyroid state was achieved before scheduling total abdominal hysterectomy with bilateral salpingo-oophorectomy (TAH with BSO).

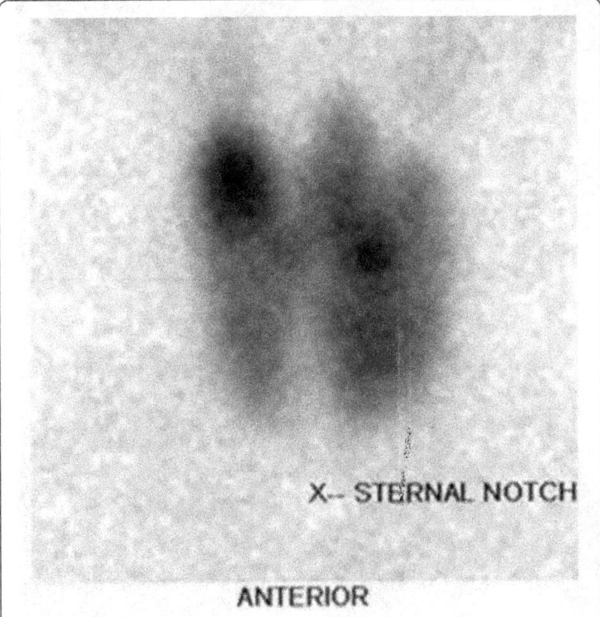

Fig. 1 $Tc^{99}m$ thyroid scan showed diffusely increased uptake by the thyroid tissue with thyroid nodules

The patient's perioperative course was uneventful. An 8.0- × 5.5- × 5.0-cm right ovarian mass with minimal ascites was found, the cut surfaces of the ovary showed solid-cystic appearance. The solid component showed soft red-brown and yellowish semitranslucent tissue resembling thyroid tissue. The cystic spaces contained clear yellow fluid.

The histological diagnosis was struma ovarii of the right ovary, without evidence of malignancy. Immunohistochemical staining for thyroglobulin (clone 2H11 + 6E1; Cell Marque) was positive; this result confirmed the thyroid epithelial nature of the lesion (Fig. 3b). Moreover, immunohistochemical staining for TSHR (clone 4C1/E1/G8; Abcam) was performed with normal thyroid tissue as a positive control and normal ovarian tissue as a negative control. Immunohistochemical staining was performed by autostainer (Ventana Benchmark XT). The result showed that the struma ovarii tissue in our patient was positive for TSHR, indicating the presence of TSHR expression in the struma ovarii tissue (Fig. 3c). Two weeks postoperatively, the patient's thyroid hormone levels were in the hypothyroid range. Replacement therapy with levothyroxine was initiated, and euthyroidism was achieved.

Discussion

Struma ovarii is a rare ovarian germ cell tumor which is entirely or predominantly composed of thyroid tissue [5]. Struma ovarii has been reported in 0.3 % to 1.0 % of all ovarian tumors and 2.0 % to 4.0 % of all ovarian teratomas [1]. It commonly occurs in the fourth to sixth decades of life, and it is usually benign and unilateral. Most affected patients are asymptomatic. However, patients may seek medical attention because of compressive symptoms involving a nearby organ, ascites, or even thyrotoxicosis. Thyrotoxicosis from struma ovarii has been reported in 5 % to 15 % of the confirmed cases [1–3, 6], but it is noted to be rare for tumors of <3 cm [7]. However, the actual incidence remains unclear owing to a lack of precise data on thyroid function in affected patients. Thyrotoxicosis in patients with struma ovarii has three potential causes: a hyperfunctioning struma ovarii alone, both a

Table 1 Thyroid hormone levels and management at baseline and during follow-up

	At first presentation	Before total thyroidectomy	2 weeks after total thyroidectomy	Before TAH with BSO	2 weeks after TAH with BSO
Free T_4 (0.93–1.70 ng/dl)	–	1.14	4.8	1.43	0.11
Total T_4 (4.50–11.70 μg/dl)	17.27	–	–	–	–
Total T_3 (80–200 ng/dl)	233	167.5	380.7	153.2	–
TSH (0.27-4.20 mIU/ml)	<0.005	0.01	<0.005	0.16	>100
Treatment	Start propylthiouracil 300 mg/day	Methimazole 7.5 mg/day	Stop methimazole for 2 weeks	Methimazole 2.5 mg/day	Start levothyroxine 100 mcg/day

hyperfunctioning thyroid gland and a struma ovarii, or a hyperfunctioning thyroid gland with an incidental non-functioning struma ovarii [7]. The diagnosis of a functioning struma ovarii is challenging, especially in a patient with a hyperfunctioning thyroid gland. The evidence for the presence of a hyperfunctioning struma ovarii is based on increased radioiodine uptake by the ovary on an I^{131} whole-body scan [6]. Cervical goiter is quite common in patients with struma ovarii (16 %–40 %) [1, 2]. Because Graves' disease is the most common cause of hyperthyroidism with diffuse thyroid gland enlargement, a number of previous cases of thyrotoxicosis due to struma ovarii were incorrectly treated by thyroidectomy [6, 7]. The coexistence of Graves' disease and a hyperfunctioning struma ovarii is extremely rare. The characteristic of the prior case reports were summarized in Table 2. In most cases, the diagnosis was based on persistent postoperative thyrotoxicosis. In only two cases were both coexisting diseases simultaneously diagnosed [1, 8]. The optimal preoperative method for diagnosis of hyperfunctioning struma ovarii is either confirmation of the presence of thyrotoxicosis despite the absence of hyperfunctioning thyroid tissue or low radioiodine uptake at the neck along with high ovarian uptake of radioiodine tracer. Increased uptake of radioiodine by an ovarian tumor on a whole-body scan alone is insufficient for diagnosis of hyperfunctioning struma ovarii because it reportedly yields both false-positive and false-negative results [9–14]. The main differential diagnosis for increased uptake of radiotracer in the abdomen is ovarian metastasis from primary thyroid cancer.

Similar to most cases, the hyperthyroidism in our patient was thought to have arisen only from Graves' disease based on typical signs of diffuse thyroid gland enlargement, bilateral exophthalmos, diffuse thyroid uptake with visualized activity in the pyramidal lobe, and an elevated level of plasma TSHR antibody. However, persistent post-thyroidectomy thyrotoxicosis with low I^{131} uptake at the

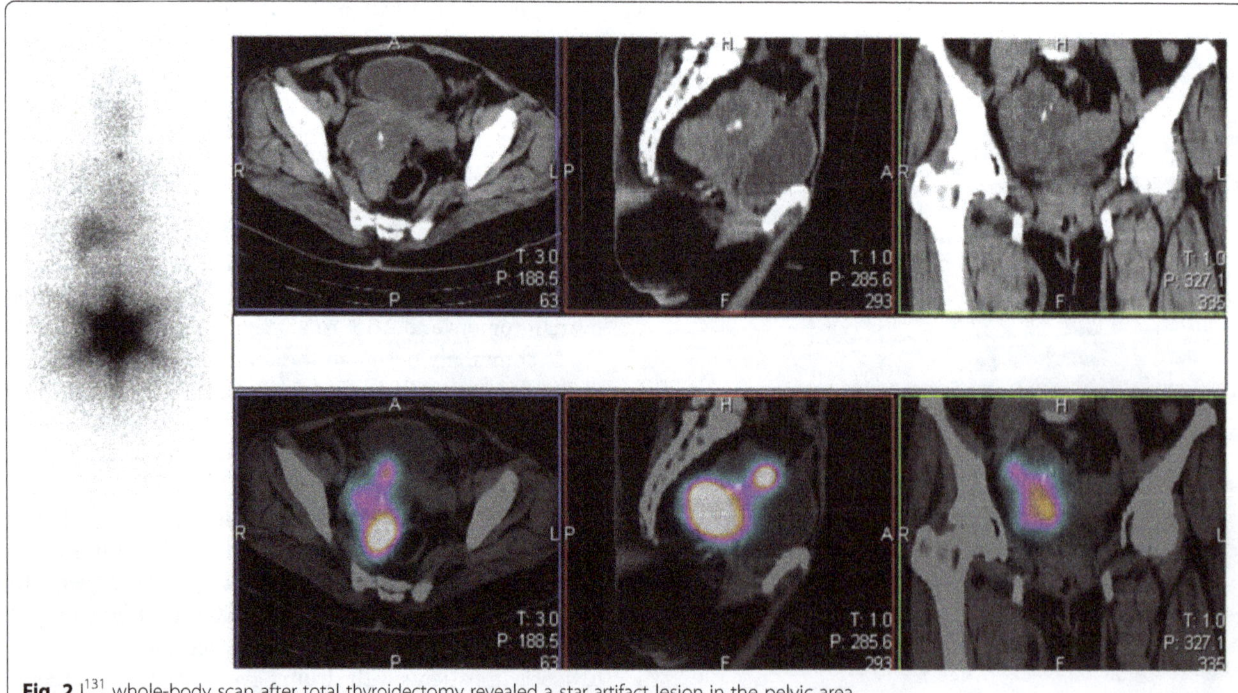

Fig. 2 I^{131} whole-body scan after total thyroidectomy revealed a star artifact lesion in the pelvic area

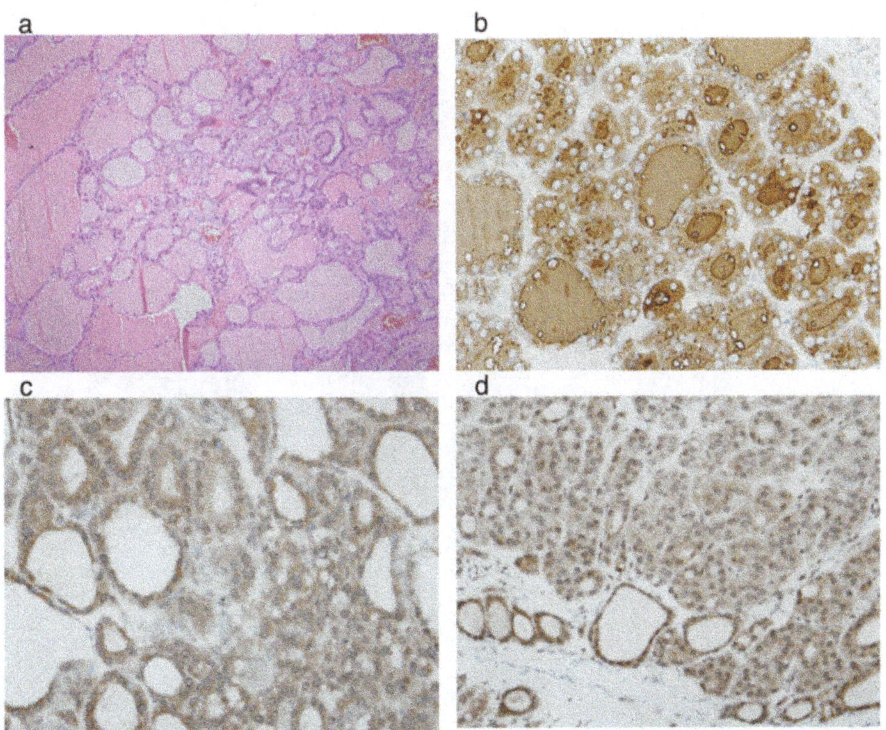

Fig. 3 a H&E staining of our patient's ovarian section revealed typical thyroid follicles. **b** The thyroid tissue in our patient's ovarian tumor was highlighted by thyroglobulin antibody. **c** Immunostaining for TSH receptor showed positive staining in our patient's struma ovarii. **d** TSH receptor also expressed on the tumor cells from other patient with non-functioning struma ovarii

thyroid bed and biochemical hypothyroidism after removal of the struma ovarii confirmed the diagnosis of a functioning struma ovarii.

The pathophysiology of thyrotoxicosis from struma ovarii remains unclear. The finding of tall thyroidal epithelium with scattered papillary infoldings, which is frequently found in struma ovarii, has a poor correlation with the presence of clinical thyrotoxicosis [7]. There are two proposed mechanisms underlying the pathophysiology of functioning struma ovarii. First, the ovarian tumor may have autonomous function, as in toxic multinodular goiter [7]. Second, in patients with coexisting Graves' disease, TSHR antibodies stimulate the struma ovarii in the same way that they stimulate the thyroid tissue to cause Graves' disease. Our patient's ovarian section revealed typical thyroid follicles without features of malignancy. Immunohistochemical staining for the TSHR in the struma ovarii tissue was positive (Fig. 3c), thus supporting the second hypothesis [3, 4]. We performed TSHR staining in the struma ovarii of another patient with normal thyroid function test preoperatively and two other patients without confirm thyroid function test but was clinically euthyroid preoperatively. The staining results were all positive and the intensity of the TSHR staining of functioning strum ovarii was the same as that in other cases of nonfunctioning struma ovarii (Fig. 3d), suggesting that the determinant of functioning struma ovarii might be the presence of TSHR stimuli rather than the intensity of the TSHR in the ovarian tissue. In prior case reports of coexisting Graves' disease and struma ovarii, the diagnosis of functioning struma ovarii almost always follows the diagnosis of Graves' disease by several years. The circulating TSHR antibody in Graves' disease presumably has a stimulatory effect on the thyroid tissue in the ovary, resulting in gradual growth and increased thyroid hormone production [3, 15].

Approximately 5 % of struma ovarii are malignant, regardless of whether they are functional, and tissue sampling for malignancy testing is very difficult. Therefore, struma ovarii should be surgically removed in all cases. Meanwhile, the coexisting Graves' disease can be managed medically, surgically, or by radioactive iodine ablation.

Conclusions

In patients with Graves' disease with persistent or recurrent thyrotoxicosis after adequate ablative treatment, the possibility of ectopic thyroid hormone production such as that from struma ovarii or a metastatic differentiated thyroid cancer should be considered. TSHR expression is found in patients with functioning and non-functioning

Table 2 Cases of Coexisting Graves' disease and Functioning Struma Ovarii

Author, year	Age at diagnosis	Presentation					TSH receptor antibody	Cervical thyroidectomy before diagnosis struma ovarii	Prior pelvic exam that result negative	Ovarian scan before abdominal surgery	Ovarian findings			Years after Graves' disease diagnosis
		Exoph-thalmos	Thyroid bruit	Pelvic pressure symptoms	Pleural effusion	Ascites					Side	Maximum diameter (cm)	Malignancy	
Kampers, 1970 [7]	64	Yes	NA	NA	NA	NA	NA	Yes	NA	NA	NA	NA	No	18
Lefort, 1981 [9]	38	Yes	NA	NA	No	No	Positive	NA	NA	Positive	Right	7	No	12
Lazarus, 1987 [15]	48	Yes	NA	NA	NA	Few	Positive	Yes	14 years	Positive	Left	9	No	24
Kung, 1990 [10]	40	No	NA	No	NA	No	Positive	No	23 weeks	NA	Right	5	No	4
Banyot, 1995 [1]	30	No	No	Yes	NA	NA	Negative	No	NA	Positive	Right	7	NA	0
Grandet, 2000 [16]	78	NA	NA	NA	NA	Few	NA	Yes	NA	Positive	Bilateral	10	No	4
Kano, 2000 [8]	50	NA	NA	NA	NA	Yes	Positive	No	NA	NA	Left	7	Yes	0
Mimura, 2001 [6]	26	No	No	NA	NA	NA	Positive	No	NA	Positive	Left	16	No	4
Sussman, 2002 [17]	53	No	NA	No	NA	NA	NA	No	NA	NA	Right	7.5	Yes	5
Bartel, 2005 [18]	54	NA	NA	NA	NA	NA	Positive	Yes	NA	Positive	Left	NA	No	23
Guida, 2005 [11]	42	Yes	NA	NA	No	Marked	NA	Yes	NA	Negative	Right	12	No	1
Teale, 2006 [4]	36	Yes	NA	NA	NA	NA	Positive	Yes	NA	NA	Left	13.5	No	8
Chiofalo, 2007 [19]	42	No	NA	Yes	NA	Yes	Positive	Yes	NA	Positive	Right	12	No	0.5
Wong, 2009 [2]	44	Yes	Yes	Yes	NA	NA	Positive	Yes	NA	NA	Left	NA	Yes	1
Anastasilakis, 2013 [3]	49	No	NA	NA	Yes	Moderate	Positive	No	NA	NA	Right	18	No	2
Our case, 2015	56	Yes	No	No	No	Minimal	Positive	Yes	Not done	Positive	Right	8	No	23

struma ovarii and cannot solely be used to determine the functioning status of the tumor.

Consent

Written informed consent was obtained from the patient for publication of this case report and any accompanying images. A copy of the written consent is available for review by the editor of this journal.

Abbreviations

TSHR: Thyroid-stimulating hormone receptor; I^{131}: Radioactive iodine; TAH with BSO: Total abdominal hysterectomy with bilateral salpingo-oophorectomy; NA: Not available.

Completing interests

The authors declare that they have no competing interests.

Authors' contributions

TS treated the patient, gathered data and drafted the manuscript. SH prepared, analysed, and interpreted the histopathological samples, and critically reviewed the manuscript. TP critically reviewed the manuscript. NT treated the patient, conceptualized the case report, gathered data, and critically reviewed the manuscript. All authors approved the final version of the manuscript.

Acknowledgements

Language editing by Edanz.

Author details

[1]Division of Endocrinology and Metabolism, Faculty of Medicine Siriraj Hospital, Mahidol University, Bangkok 10700, Thailand. [2]Department of Pathology, Faculty of Medicine Siriraj Hospital, Mahidol University, Bangkok 10700, Thailand.

References

1. Bayot MR, Chopra IJ. Coexistence of struma ovarii and Graves' disease. Thyroid. 1995;5(6):469–71.
2. Wong LY, Diamond TH. Severe ophthalmopathy developing after treatment of coexisting malignant struma ovarii and Graves' disease. Thyroid. 2009;19(10):1125–7. doi:10.1089/thy.2008.0422.
3. Anastasilakis AD, Ruggeri RM, Polyzos SA, Makras P, Molyva D, Campenni A, et al. Coexistence of Graves' disease, papillary thyroid carcinoma and unilateral benign struma ovarii: case report and review of the literature. Metabolism. 2013;62(10):1350–6. doi:10.1016/j.metabol.2013.05.013.
4. Teale E, Gouldesbrough DR, Peacey SR. Graves' disease and coexisting struma ovarii: struma expression of thyrotropin receptors and the presence of thyrotropin receptor stimulating antibodies. Thyroid. 2006;16(8):791–3. doi:10.1089/thy.2006.16.791.
5. Devaney K, Snyder R, Norris HJ, Tavassoli FA. Proliferative and histologically malignant struma ovarii: a clinicopathologic study of 54 cases. Int J Gynecol Pathol. 1993;12(4):333–43.
6. Mimura Y, Kishida M, Masuyama H, Suwaki N, Kodama J, Otsuka F, et al. Coexistence of Graves' disease and struma ovarii: case report and literature review. Endocr J. 2001;48(2):255–60.
7. Kempers RD, Dockerty MB, Hoffman DL, Bartholomew LG. Struma ovarii–ascitic, hyperthyroid, and asymptomatic syndromes. Ann Intern Med. 1970;72(6):883–93.
8. Kano H, Inoue M, Nishino T, Yoshimoto Y, Arima R. Malignant struma ovarii with Graves' disease. Gynecol Oncol. 2000;79(3):508–10. doi:10.1006/gyno.2000.5966.
9. Lefort G, Commenges-Ducos M, Denechaud M, Rivel J, Latapie JL. Ovarian goiter in Basedow's disease. Role of thyroid-stimulating immunoglobulins? Nouv Presse Med. 1981;10(26):2209–10.
10. Kung AW, Ma JT, Wang C, Young RT. Hyperthyroidism during pregnancy due to coexistence of struma ovarii and Graves' disease. Postgrad Med J. 1990;66(772):132–3.
11. Guida M, Mandato VD, Di Spiezio SA, Di Carlo C, Giordano E, Nappi C. Coexistence of Graves' disease and benign struma ovarii in a patient with marked ascites and elevated CA-125 levels. J Endocrinol Invest. 2005;28(9):827–30.
12. Ghander C, Lussato D, Conte Devolx B, Mundler O, Taieb D. Incidental diagnosis of struma ovarii after thyroidectomy for thyroid cancer: functional imaging studies and follow-up. Gynecol Oncol. 2006;102(2):378–80. doi:10.1016/j.ygyno.2006.01.047.
13. Joja I, Asakawa T, Mitsumori A, Nakagawa T, Akaki S, Yamamoto M, et al. I-123 uptake in nonfunctional struma ovarii. Clin Nucl Med. 1998;23(1):10–2.
14. Nodine JH, Maldia G. Pseudostruma ovarii. Obstet Gynecol. 1961;17:460–3.
15. Lazarus JH, Richards AR, MacPherson MJ, Dinnen JS, Williams ED, Owen GM, et al. Struma ovarii: a case report. Clin Endocrinol (Oxf). 1987;27(6):715–20.
16. Grandet PJ, Remi MH. Struma ovarii with hyperthyroidism. Clin Nucl Med. 2000;25(10):763–5.
17. Sussman SK, Kho SA, Cersosimo E, Heimann A. Coexistence of malignant struma ovarii and Graves' disease. Endocr Pract. 2002;8(5):378–80. doi:10.4158/EP.8.5.378.
18. Bartel TB, Juweid ME, O'Dorisio T, Sivitz W, Kirby P. Scintigraphic detection of benign struma ovarii in a hyperthyroid patient. J Clin Endocrinol Metab. 2005;90(6):3771–2. doi:10.1210/jc.2005-0147.
19. Chiofalo MG, Misso C, Insabato L, Lastoria S, Pezzullo L. Hyperthyroidism due to coexistence of Graves' disease and Struma ovarii. Endocr Pract. 2007;13(3):274–6. doi:10.4158/EP.13.3.274.

Papillary thyroid carcinoma with pleomorphic tumor giant cells in a pregnant woman

Johan O. Paulsson[1], Jan Zedenius[2,3] and C. Christofer Juhlin[1,4*]

Abstract

Background: Papillary thyroid carcinoma with pleomorphic tumor giant cells (PTC-PC) is characterized by the occurrence of bizarre, pleomorphic cells within a small area of a conventional PTC. The histologic distinction between PTC-PC and PTC's with a focal anaplastic thyroid cancer (ATC) component (denoted in the 2004 WHO classification as "papillary thyroid carcinoma with spindle and giant cell carcinoma", PTC-SGC) is debated, however the prognosis is thought to be different (excellent for PTC-PC, poor for PTC-SGC). Therefore, this diagnostic challenge is significant for any endocrine pathologist to recognize. Herein, we report the histological and clinical workup of a PTC-PC case, with particular focus on the molecular analyses that facilitated the establishment of the final diagnosis.

Case presentation: The patient was a pregnant, 28-year-old female presenting with a 30 mm conventional PTC, with focal areas with undifferentiated cells exhibiting exaggerated nuclear pleomorphism. No foci of extrathyroidal extension, angioinvasion or lymph node engagement were seen. Immunohistochemical analyses revealed the pleomorphic cells exhibiting retained differentiation. Molecular genetic analyses demonstrated a codon V600 missense mutation of the *BRAF* gene, but no *TP53* or *TERT* promoter mutations. The absence of an aggressive phenotype in addition to the lack of mutations in two major ATC-related genes led to the diagnosis of a PTC-PC. Postoperative MRI showed no evidence of metastatic disease. Radioiodine ablation was performed seven months post-operatively, and a SPECT-CT imaging did not show signs of residual tissue. She is well and without signs of disease 16 months post-operatively.

Conclusions: PTC-PC is a differential diagnosis to PTC-SGC that mandates careful considerations. Taken together with previous publications, PTC-PC seems to be histologically similar to PTC-SGC, but clinically distinct. Even so, the distinction is not easily made given the different therapeutic consequences for each individual patient. This is the first report that includes molecular genetics to aid in finalizing the diagnosis. Exclusion of mutations in *TP53* and the *TERT* promoter could be considered as an adjunct tool when assessing papillary thyroid cancer with focal pleomorphism.

Keywords: Papillary thyroid cancer, Pleomorphism, Pathology, Anaplastic thyroid cancer, Molecular testing

* Correspondence: christofer.juhlin@ki.se
[1]Department of Oncology-Pathology, Karolinska Institutet, Stockholm, Sweden
[4]Department of Pathology and Cytology, Karolinska University Hospital, Stockholm, Sweden
Full list of author information is available at the end of the article

Background

When evaluating thyroid tumors in the microscope, exaggerated pleomorphic cells and elevated Ki67-labeling index constitute two alarming histological features. These factors are almost always present in anaplastic (undifferentiated) thyroid cancer (ATC), but very seldom in papillary thyroid cancer (PTC) [1]. No clear guidelines in how to interpret focal areas with dedifferentiation have been established, as these tumors are so rarely encountered in clinical practice. Two different histological entities associated to pleomorphism (with great disparities in overall prognosis and outcomes) exist; namely papillary thyroid carcinoma with pleomorphic tumor giant cells (PTC-PC) and PTC's with a focal anaplastic thyroid cancer (ATC) component (entitled "papillary thyroid carcinoma with spindle and giant cell carcinoma", PTC-SGC) [1]. While PTC-PC cases generally display excellent prognosis, the survival rates for PTC-SGC are much poorer and often coupled to the extension of the anaplastic component. Therefore, the pleomorphic features in PTC-PC are not thought to be a result from a dedifferentiation to anaplastic carcinoma, as opposed to PTC-SGC, in which the focal pleomorphism constitute a bona fide ATC component [1].

In this case report, we depict a case of PTC with a focal pleomorphic component and how different clinical, histological and immunhistochemical analyses were used in the workup of this patient. We also describe for the first time how molecular testing steered the final histopathological diagnosis towards PTC-PC.

Case presentation

The patient was a pregnant, 28-year-old female of Swedish ethnicity with no previous medical conditions or familial history, who experienced a lump in the neck during the summer of 2016. Physical examination was normal apart from the neck tumor. She did not exhibit any signs of dysphagia, hoarseness or discomfort. A 30 mm nodule was visible on neck ultrasound, and a first round of cytology was inconclusive (Bethesda I). A second round of cytology was performed, and a diagnosis of papillary thyroid cancer (Bethesda VI) was put forward based on the findings of follicular epithelium with nuclear atypia, nuclear inclusions and nuclear grooves. The tumor cells were positive for CK19 and HBME1, and the cytological Ki-67-index was estimated as 3–5%. Pleomorphic giant cells were not reported. Subsequent ultrasonographical mapping revealed no evident lateral lymph node engagements, and a total thyroidectomy with an associated lymph node dissection of regio VI was performed. The operation was carried out during the 2nd trimester and was uneventful without any postoperative complications.

The thyroid specimen exhibited a weight of 33,1 g. In the right lobe, a 30 × 30 × 25 mm well-defined nodule with firm, white to gray cut surface was visualized during macroscopic grossing. No macroscopic evidence of additional nodules were found in the isthmus or left thyroid lobe. Microscopy revealed a partly encapsulated, infiltrating tumor with a predominant papillary growth pattern, in addition to areas with follicular and solid growth patterns. Within most of the tumor area, the tumor cell nuclei were medium-sized, oval and exhibited a light chromatin, in addition to nuclear pseudo-inclusions and nuclear grooves (Fig. 1a). A few psammoma bodies were also seen scattered across the tumor area. This histological phenotype is consistent with a conventional papillary thyroid carcinoma (PTC) [1]. No extrathyroidal extension or foci with angioinvasion were seen. In the solid areas (constituting less than 10% of the tumor), PTC-like nuclear changes were more infrequent, but still present in small subsets of nuclei. Multifocally, areas with tumor necrosis (Fig. 1b) and elevated mitosis counts (5 mitoses/10 high power fields, but no atypical mitoses) were observed – but since the vast majority of the nuclei carried PTC-associated features (inclusions, grooves) in addition to the fact that the predominant growth pattern was papillary and no blood vessel infiltration was seen, no clear-cut diagnosis of poorly differentiated thyroid carcinoma (PDTC) could be made either by the older 2004 WHO criteria [1] or the proposed Turin criteria [2] supported by the novel 2017 WHO classification of tumors of endocrine organs [3]. The observed necrosis was believed to be tumor-related, as it was multifocal and without other degenerative changes usually associated to previous cytology aspiration.

In several foci near the tumor capsule, pleomorphic tumor cells with bizarre features were observed, including scattered giant cells (Fig. 1c and d). Strikingly, many of these giant nuclei exhibited prominent pseudo-inclusions, and a few had smudged chromatin. These cells were intermingled with more normal-sized tumor nuclei. The single, largest area with pleomorphic cells was 6 mm. The mitotic count was 5 mitoses/10 high power fields.

A tumor-free lymph node was found near the thyroid capsule, and an additional six tumor-free lymph nodes were visualized from the central compartment. As of this, no local metastatic disease could be found.

Immunhistochemical analyses were performed, and the tumor cells were uniformly positive for TTF1 (Fig. 1e), CK19 and Bcl-2. The cells were negative for chromogranin A and calcitonin, thereby excluding medullary thyroid cancer. Approximately 25% of all tumor cells expressed thyroglobulin. The p53 staining was weak and not diffuse, arguing against an underlying *TP53* mutation. A positive signal was obtained using the V600E mutation-specific BRAF antibody, arguing in favor for

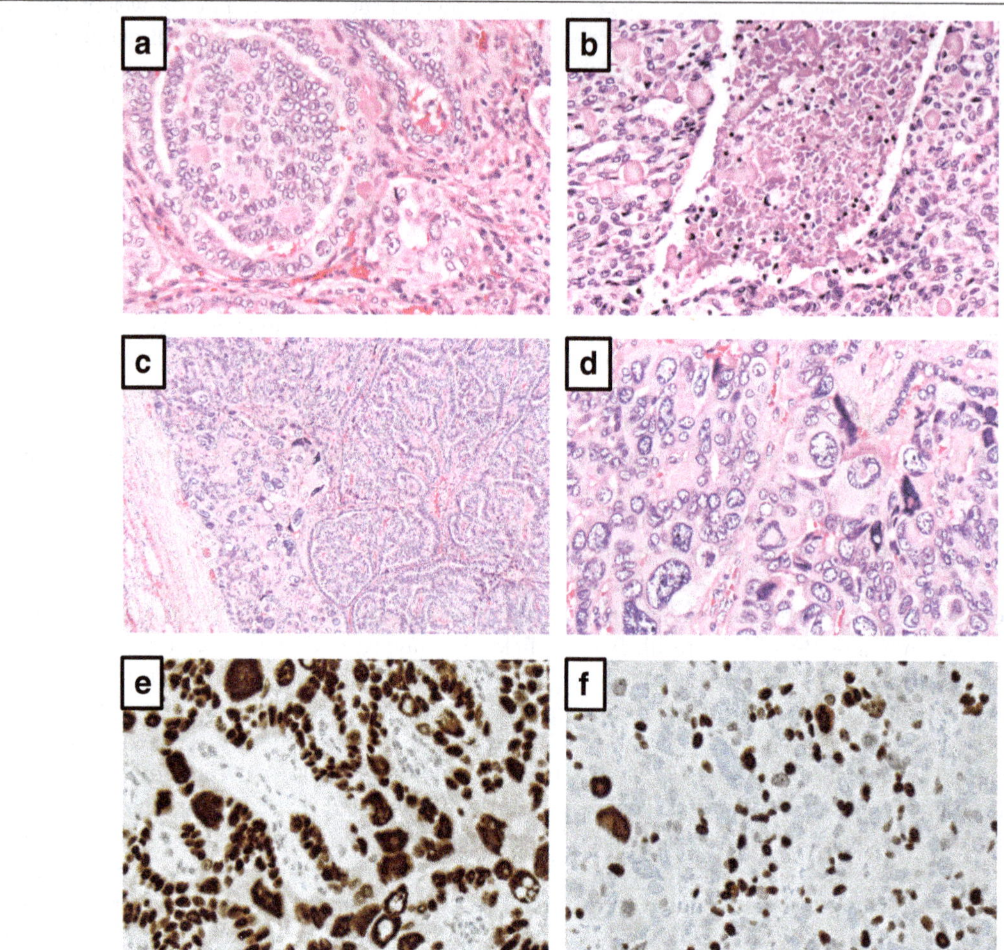

Fig. 1 Photomicrographs of the PTC-PC case. **a** Routine sections of the conventional PTC area demonstrate clear-cut PTC-related nuclear features. **b** Focal tumor necrosis (central) within the conventional PTC area (left and right). **c-d** Focal areas with exaggerated pleomorphism and bizarre giant cells at 100× and 400× magnifications respectively. **e** Retained TTF1 immunoreactivity within the pleomorphic areas. **f** Markedly increased Ki67-labeling index within the same area (30% positive nuclei using immunohistochemistry with an anti-Ki-67 antibody)

an underlying *BRAF* V600E missense mutation. There were no differences in the immunohistochemical profile when comparing the pleomorphic areas to the more conventional PTC areas, except for the Ki-67 proliferation labeling index, which was 10% in the conventional areas and up to 30% in the pleomorphic areas (Fig. 1f).

Although the immunohistochemical profile suggested retained differentiation (TTF1 positivity) and thus supported the diagnosis of PTC-PC [4], the focally observed high-proliferative areas with aggravated pleomorphism and bizarre nuclei led to the suspicion of tumor dedifferentiation into a local ATC component, consistent with PTC-SGC [1]. To better try to distinguish the two entities, a microdissection of formalin-fixated paraffin-embedded material representing the largest pleomorphic areas was performed. Tumor cell content was appreciated as 80%. Tissue was then deparaffinized and genomic DNA was extracted by established methods used in the clinical routine (Maxwell 16 FFPE Plus LEV DNA Purification Kit, Promega, WI, USA). Quality and quantity of genomic DNA was established using Nanodrop technology (NanoDrop Technologies). After DNA extraction, a control section was obtained and showed adequate representation of tumor tissue.

Three different genes were then assayed; *BRAF* (codon 600), *TP53* (exons 4–8) and *TERT* (promoter hotspot mutations C228T and C250T).

A 116 bp sequence of *BRAF* including codon 600 (part of exon 15) was amplified and analyzed using a real time PCR technique (Cobas 4800 *BRAF* V600 Mutation Test Kit, Roche Molecular Systems, NJ, USA). An activating mutation was found at codon V600. The test does not discriminate between V600E, V600 K and V600D.

For *TP53* and *TERT*, bi-directional Sanger sequencing was performed using conventional protocols (Genetic Analyzer 3500, Applied Biosystems, CA, USA). No *TP53* mutation in exons 4–8 was found, however, a known *TP53* single nucleotide polymorphism (SNP) in exon 4 was observed (c.215 C > G, p. P72R, rs1042522). This SNP has a reported minor allele frequency of 25,5% in the European American population according to the Exome Variant Server (http://evs.gs.washington.edu/EVS). Moreover, no C228T or C250T *TERT* promoter mutations were detected.

The case was presented at a multidisciplinary tumor board meeting held weekly at the Karolinska University Hospital. If the conclusive diagnosis would have been PTC-SGC, the patient would have continued with a much more aggressive and urgent treatment which would have required to abort the fetus, however with regards to the histopathology and the molecular profile of the tumor, a diagnosis of PTC-PC was argued for. But given the uncertainty of the histology as well as the high Ki67-labeling index, the patient was referred for magnetic resonance imaging (MRI) of the neck and chest, which was negative for pulmonary involvement, however displayed enlarged left-sided cervical lymph nodes in regio 2. Using ultrasonographic mapping, a fine needle biopsy was performed. The subsequent cytological examination however, could not detect any malignant cells.

Postoperative radioiodine ablation using 5400 MBq was performed six weeks after childbirth, seven months post-operatively. Whole body scintigraphy showed uptake in the neck, but a subsequent SPECT-CT did not show any sign of residual tissue. Serum thyroglobulin during stimulation by recombinant TSH was 2.1 micrograms/L. Basal thyroglobulin was 0.2 micrograms/L, without detectable thyroglobulin antibodies. Today, 16 months after surgery, the woman is well with no biochemical signs of disease.

Discussion and conclusions

In the final pathology report, two different possibilities are discussed. Either the tumor represents a papillary thyroid carcinoma with pleomorphic tumor giant cells (PTC-PC), or the local finding of high-proliferative bizarre cells represents dedifferentiation into a focal anaplastic component (PTC-SGC). The WHO classification from 2004 [1] "rule-in" criteria for PTC-SGC is a focal undifferentiated component in minority compared to the PTC component, and hence this tumor could in theory be classified as such based on the focal findings of exaggerated pleomorphism. Indeed, the disturbingly high Ki67-labeling index within this area (30%) supports the notion of this minor component as highly aggressive. On the other hand, many factors argue in favor of the alterative diagnosis of PTC-PC. For example, the age of the patient and the clinical presentation is not typical for a focal ATC component. Moreover, the pleomorphic cells exhibited strong TTF1 and CK19 expression, which is often lost in ATCs [1]. Moreover, no histological signs of aggressive behavior existed, as the current case lacked extrathyroidal extension, an angio-invasive component and lymph node involvement [1, 4].

The molecular genetics in this case could pinpoint a codon V600 missense mutation in the *BRAF* gene, thereby proving the tumor as PTC-related [5]. However, since a large subset of ATCs de-differentiate from pre-existing PTCs, this marker does not exclude the occurrence of a synchronous ATC [6]. *TP53* mutations are seen in 50–80% of ATC cases but are rare in PTCs [7], and *TERT* promoter mutations are detected in 50–95% of ATC cases, but only in 10% of PTCs [8]. Interestingly, when co-occurring in the same patient, PTC and ATC cases display very high frequencies of *TERT* promoter mutations; 91 and 95% respectively [9]. The lack of *TP53* and *TERT* promoter mutations in our case could not entirely rule out ATC, but certainly not rule in ATC either. Therefore, the molecular genetics could not pinpoint the diagnosis, however speaks in favor of a PTC-PC diagnosis. Additional candidate genes arguing for dedifferentiation exist but were not tested as a part of the clinical workup as they are not established in our clinical pathology laboratory from a methodological standpoint. It is also worth mentioning that *TERT* promoter mutations in well-differentiated forms of thyroid cancer (such as PTC) are heavily coupled to older patient age [8]. Therefore, the young age of our patient could in theory affect the result of the *TERT* promoter mutational screening – which should be considered when screening adolescents for these aberrations. However, as the reason for conducting this molecular analysis was to exclude an overt ATC component, we believe a positive outcome (i.e. finding of a *TERT* promoter mutation) in such a young patient would strongly point towards a more aggressive form of the disease and support a focal ATC component.

ATCs arise either de novo or from a preexisting well or poorly differentiated thyroid carcinoma [1]. Nevertheless, the ATC component could be in minority, with the clear majority of the tumor constituting a well or poorly differentiated thyroid carcinoma. When the well differentiated tumor is a PTC, this focal ATC variant is denoted PTC-SGC [1]. However, the distinction between this tumor entity and a clear-cut ATC diagnosis is not easily established, and the prognosis of patients diagnosed with PTC-SGC is not entirely characterized. In a few series, patients with PTC-SGC have prolonged survival rates as compared to classical ATC cases, in other publications however, the prognosis was equally grim for PTC-SGC as for ATC [10, 11].

In a previous study, the authors describe four cases of PTC-PC, in which the pleomorphic areas constituted 5 to 25% of the tumor [4]. These four patients (three females and one male with a mean age of 36 years) remained alive without disease following thyroidectomy and ^{131}I ablation therapy (with a mean follow-up time of 52 months), which is in strong contrast to the course of disease in patients with ATC or PTC-SGC. The authors therefore conclude that, based on the clinical and prognostic features of these cases, the bizarre cells found within these four tumors do not represent dedifferentiation and progression to ATC, and also argues against the diagnosis of PTC-SGC. Our patient mirrors the four previously published cases in regards to that no recurrences have been reported postoperatively, and no signs of extrathyroidal extension or lymph node metastasis have been found.

Moreover, there might be histological differences separating PTC-PC from PTC-SGC tumors as well, in that no areas of necrosis or inflammation was seen within the pleomorphic areas within our case (as well as in the previous four reported cases). Usually, the ATC component of a PTC-SGC is usually seen with tumor necrosis, a prominent inflammatory response as well as areas of fibrosis and hemorrhage [1]. Moreover, the bizarre pleomorphism in our case could in theory occur as a degenerative phenomenon rather than a feature associated to an aggressive malignant behavior. Indeed, the 2017 WHO classification of tumors of endocrine organs now lists "follicular adenoma with bizarre nuclei" as an acknowledged entity, thereby recognizing that well-differentiated thyroid tumors might exhibit highly atypical cell nuclei, similarly as PTC-PC cases.

We conclude that PTC-PC could constitute a separate histopathological variant of PTC, separate from PTC-SGC. PTC-PC should be considered as a differential diagnosis in younger patients when assessing PTCs with focal pleomorphism but retained differentiation (TTF1+, CK19+), no visible necrosis or inflammation and no obvious signs of extrathyroidal extension or lymph node involvement. As our final diagnosis relied heavily on the molecular testing, exclusion of mutations in *TP53* and the *TERT* promoter could be considered helpful when evaluating papillary thyroid cancer with focal pleomorphism.

Abbreviations

ATC: Anaplastic thyroid cancer; bp: Base pairs; BRAF: B-Raf proto-oncogene, serine/threonine kinase; CK19: Cytokeratin 19; MBq: Megabecquerel; MRI: Magnetic resonance imaging; PCR: Polymerase chain reaction; PDTC: Poorly differentiated thyroid cancer; PTC: Papillary thyroid cancer; PTC-PC: Papillary thyroid carcinoma with pleomorphic tumor giant cells; PTC-SGC: Papillary thyroid carcinoma with spindle and giant cell carcinoma; SPECT-CT: Single-photon emission computed tomography; TERT: Telomerase reverse transcriptase; TSH: Thyroid stimulating hormone; TTF1: Thyroid transcription factor 1

Funding

This study was supported by grants provided from the Swedish Cancer Society and the Swedish Society for Medical Research.

Authors' contributions

JOP and CCJ reviewed the case histologically and analyzed the tumor immunohistochemically and by molecular genetics. JOP prepared the figure JZ reviewed the clinical course of the patient and performed follow-up. All authors drafted, read and approved the final manuscript.

Competing interests

The authors declare that they have no competing interests.

Author details

[1]Department of Oncology-Pathology, Karolinska Institutet, Stockholm, Sweden. [2]Department of Molecular Medicine and Surgery, Karolinska Institutet, Stockholm, Sweden. [3]Department of Breast and Endocrine Surgery, Karolinska University Hospital, Stockholm, Sweden. [4]Department of Pathology and Cytology, Karolinska University Hospital, Stockholm, Sweden.

References

1. RA DL, Lloyd RV, Heitz PU, Eng C. International Agency for Research on Cancer, World Health Organization. Pathology and genetics of tumours of endocrine organs, World Health Organization classification of tumours. 3rd ed. Lyon: IARC Press; 2004.
2. Volante M, Collini P, Nikiforov YE, Sakamoto A, Kakudo K, Katoh R, Lloyd RV, LiVolsi VA, Papotti M, Sobrinho-Simoes M, Bussolati G, Rosai J. Poorly differentiated thyroid carcinoma: the Turin proposal for the use of uniform diagnostic criteria and an algorithmic diagnostic approach. Am J Surg Pathol. 2007;31:1256–64.
3. Lloyd RV, Osamura RY, Klöppel G, Rosai J. International Agency for Research on Cancer, World Health Organization. WHO classification of tumours of endocrine organs. World Health Organization classification of tumours. 4th ed. Lyon: IARC Press; 2017.
4. Hommell-Fontaine J, Borda A, Ragage F, Berger N, Decaussin-Petrucci M. Nonconventional papillary thyroid carcinomas with pleomorphic tumor giant cells: a diagnostic pitfall with anaplastic carcinoma. Virchows Arch. 2010;456:661–70.
5. Adeniran AJ, Zhu Z, Gandhi M, Steward DL, Fidler JP, Giordano TJ, Biddinger PW, Nikiforov YE. Correlation between genetic alterations and microscopic features, clinical manifestations, and prognostic characteristics of thyroid papillary carcinomas. Am J Surg Pathol. 2006;30:216–22.
6. Kunstman JW, Juhlin CC, Goh G, Brown TC, Stenman A, Healy JM, Rubinstein JC, Choi M, Kiss N, Nelson-Williams C, Mane S, Rimm DL, Prasad ML, Höög A, Zedenius J, Larsson C, Korah R, Lifton RP, Carling T. Characterization of the mutational landscape of anaplastic thyroid cancer via whole-exome sequencing. Hum Mol Genet. 2015;24:2318–29.
7. Nikiforov YE. Nikiforova MN (2011) molecular genetics and diagnosis of thyroid cancer. Nat Rev Endocrinol. 2011;7:569–80.
8. Landa I, Ganly I, Chan TA, Mitsutake N, Matsuse M, Ibrahimpasic T, Ghossein RA, Fagin JA. Frequent somatic TERT promoter mutations in thyroid cancer: higher prevalence in advanced forms of the disease. J Clin Endocrinol Metab. 2013;98:E1562–6.
9. Oishi N, Kondo T, Ebina A, Sato Y, Akaishi J, Hino R, Yamamoto N, Mochizuki K, Nakazawa T, Yokomichi H, Ito K, Ishikawa Y, Katoh R. Molecular alterations of coexisting thyroid papillary carcinoma and anaplastic carcinoma: identification of TERT mutation as an independent risk factor for transformation. Mod Pathol. 2017; https://doi.org/10.1038/modpathol.2017.75.
10. Aldinger KA, Samaan NA, Ibanez M, Hill CS. Anaplastic carcinoma of the thyroid: a review of 84 cases of spindle and giant cell carcinoma of the thyroid. Cancer. 1978;41:2267–75.
11. Voutilainen PE, Multanen M, Haapiainen RK, Leppäniemi AK, Sivula AH. Anaplastic thyroid carcinoma survival. World J Surg. 1999;23:975–8. discussion 978-979

19

Utility of repeat cytological assessment of thyroid nodules initially classified as benign: clinical insights from multidisciplinary care in an Irish tertiary referral centre

Nigel Glynn[1], Mark J. Hannon[1], Sarah Lewis[1], Patrick Hillery[1], Mohammed Al-Mousa[1], Arnold D. K. Hill[2], Frank Keeling[3], Martina Morrin[3], Christopher J. Thompson[1], Diarmuid Smith[1], Derval Royston[4], Mary Leader[4] and Amar Agha[1*]

Abstract

Background: Fine needle aspiration biopsy (FNAB) is the tool of choice for evaluating thyroid nodules with the majority classified as benign following initial assessment. However, concern remains about false negative results and some guidelines have recommended routine repeat aspirates. We aimed to assess the utility of routine repeat FNAB for nodules classified as benign on initial biopsy and to examine the impact of establishing a multidisciplinary team for the care of these patients.

Methods: We performed a retrospective review of 400 consecutive patients (413 nodules) who underwent FNAB of a thyroid nodule at our hospital between July 2008 and July 2011. Data recorded included demographic, clinical, histological and radiological variables.

Results: Three hundred and fifty seven patients (89 %) were female. Median follow-up was 5.5 years. Two hundred and fifty eight (63 %) nodules were diagnosed as benign. The rate of routine repeat biopsy increased significantly over the time course of the study (p for trend = 0.012). Nine Thy 2 nodules were classified differently on the basis of routine repeat biopsy; one patient was classified as malignant on repeat biopsy and was diagnosed with papillary thyroid carcinoma. Eight were classified as a follicular lesions on repeat biopsy—six diagnosed as benign following lobectomy; two declined lobectomy and were followed radiologically with no nodule size increase.

Conclusions: The false negative rate of an initial benign cytology result, from a thyroid nodule aspirate, is low. In the setting of an experienced multidisciplinary thyroid team, routine repeat aspiration is not justified.

Keywords: Thyroid nodule, Fine needle aspiration, Thyroid cytology

* Correspondence: amaragha@beaumont.ie
[1]Department of Endocrinology, Beaumont Hospital and RCSI Medical School, Dublin 9, Ireland
Full list of author information is available at the end of the article

Background

Thyroid nodules are palpable in 5 % of the population in iodine sufficient regions and in a much higher percentage in iodine deficient countries [1, 2]. However, neck ultrasound (US) identifies nodules in almost 40 % of the population [3]. The majority of nodules are benign with malignancy diagnosed in approximately 5–12 % of ultrasound detected nodules [4, 5].

An increasing number of thyroid nodules are incidentally detected by various modalities of imaging of the neck and thorax and contribute to an increased workload for endocrinologists, pathologists and radiologists. Several international societies have produced multidisciplinary guidelines for the assessment and management of thyroid nodules [6–9]. The overall objective of clinicians is to diagnose malignancy pre-operatively in patients with thyroid carcinoma and to limit unnecessary surgery in the vast majority with benign nodules. Neck ultrasound and fine-needle aspiration biopsy (FNAB) are promoted as the tools of choice for diagnosis.

Nodules classified as "benign" on cytology, following FNAB, account for the greatest proportion of cases seen in routine clinical practice [10]. However, cytological assessment of samples is somewhat subjective with several factors influencing the diagnostic outcome including the experience of the cytopathologist, as well as the adequacy of the sample [11, 12]. The negative predictive value of a "benign" cytology result is difficult to define and concern exists over false negative (falsely reassuring) results typically ranging from 1–11 %, potentially resulting in missed cancer diagnosis [13–18]. All guidelines recommend clinical follow-up for this group of patients. However, debate exists regarding the need for repeat cytological aspiration for nodules initially classified as benign [6].

Methods

The primary aim of the study was to evaluate the utility of routine repeat FNAB for nodules initially classified as benign. Secondary aims were to determine the distribution of cytological diagnostic categories among a large cohort of unselected patients with thyroid nodules and to examine the effect of a multidisciplinary team on the assessment and care pathway of patients with thyroid nodules.

We performed a retrospective review of 400 consecutive patients (413 nodules) who underwent FNAB of a thyroid nodule at our hospital between July 2008 and July 2011. Thirteen patients had assessment of more than one nodule.

Patients were identified from the Department of Pathology database (WINPATH). All FNA biopsy results were reported according to the Royal College of Pathologists Thy Classification System (Table 1) [19]. Nodules were aspirated routinely if they were greater than 1.5 cm in diameter with any solid component or if they were less than 1.5 cm in diameter with suspicious clinical or sonographic features. Data recorded include demographic, clinical, cytological and radiological variables.

Table 1 Cytological classification following first FNAB [19]

Thy category	Description	No. of biopsies (%)
Thy 1	Inadequate/non-diagnostic	63 (15)
Thy 2	Benign	258 (63)
Thy 3	Follicular lesion	75 (18)
Thy 4	Suspicious for malignancy	8 (2)
Thy 5	Malignant	9 (2)

Data were collected by retrospective chart review of patients receiving routine clinical care and follow-up. All patients gave informed consent for FNAB in the context their standard clinical care. No further measures were taken beyond those of routine clinical practice. Data collection was undertaken via clinical audit by physicians caring for the patients; formal review and approval by the Research Ethics Committee was not required.

The first year of the study (July 2008–June 2009 inclusive) preceded the establishment of a formal multidisciplinary team for the management of thyroid nodules. During this period, thyroid aspirates were reported in a descriptive fashion rather than being stratified according to a cytological classification system. For all nodules evaluated during this period, the original slides were reviewed by a single cytopathologist and a Thy grade was assigned. Prospective reporting of thyroid aspirates according to the Thy classification system was implemented after June 2009.

A multidisciplinary team (MDT) for the management of thyroid nodules and thyroid cancer was established in July 2009 including specialists from thyroidology, endocrine surgery, histocytopathology, radiology, chemical pathology and radiation oncology. In addition to the routine reporting of Thy grade on cytology samples, the MDT developed an agreed protocol for the assessment of thyroid nodules based on the guidelines of the British Thyroid Association: 2007 Update (5).

The initial cytology category assigned to each nodule informed the management and surveillance as follows:

- Thy 1 (insufficient sample)—cases were discussed by the MDT and follow up involved repeat biopsy, surgical resection or clinical/radiological follow-up based on the risk profile and patient preference.
- Thy 2 (benign)—Routine repeat FNAB, after 6 months, was recommended to exclude a false negative result.
- Thy 3 (atypia or follicular lesion)—A lobectomy was offered for formal histological diagnosis

- Thy 4 (suspicious for malignancy)—Thyroidectomy was recommended due to the high risk of malignancy.
- Thy 5 (malignant)—Thyroidectomy was recommended due to the very high risk of malignancy.

Eighty nine percent of aspirates were performed under US guidance. The MDT met twice monthly during the study period to discuss both routine and complex cases.

Statistics

Mean and standard error of the mean (SEM) were determined for normally distributed continuous data and median (standard deviation or range) was used for data not normally distributed.

The study period was divided into quartiles. MDT performance indicators were assessed in each quarter and trend analysis was performed using Chi square test. Statistical analysis was performed using GraphPad Prism 5 software (GraphPad Inc., La Jolla, CA, 2010).

Results

Three hundred and fifty seven patients (89 %) were female. Median age was 54 years (range 16–89). Median nodule size (measured on ultrasound in 217 cases) was 25 mm in maximum transverse diameter. Only seven nodules were less than 10 mm in size. Median follow-up was 5.5 years (range 4.4–7.9).

Two hundred and thirty nine (58 %) nodules underwent a single biopsy; 156 (38 %) had a second biopsy. 14(3 %) and 4(1 %) underwent a third and fourth biopsy respectively. The distribution of initial Thy category is outlined in Table 1.

Nodules with benign cytology (Thy2)

Overall, 258 nodules (63 %) were initially classified as Thy 2 (benign). Management of patients with a nodule initially classified as Thy 2 (benign) is outlined in Fig. 1. Twenty three patients (9 %) elected, subsequently, to have surgery rather than conservative follow-up (lobectomy or thyroidectomy), principally due to local compressive symptoms (subjective or objective) or for cosmetic reasons—all were diagnosed as benign nodules. Among the remainder of this patient group, 126/235 (54 %) underwent routine repeat biopsy. The rate of routine repeat biopsy increased significantly over the time course of the study; p for trend = 0.012 (Fig. 2).

Nine Thy 2 nodules were classified differently following routine repeat biopsy (Fig. 1, Table 2). One patient was classified as Thy 5 (malignant) on repeat FNAB and was diagnosed with a solitary 3 cm papillary thyroid carcinoma (PTC) following a thyroidectomy—the entire nodule was malignant; the lesion had classical PTC morphology in some areas and in others demonstrated a Warthin-like tumour appearance. Two level VI cervical lymph nodes contained metastatic PTC - (Stage 1, pT2N1aM0). Eight were classified as Thy 3 after repeat aspiration; six underwent thyroid lobectomy and were diagnosed as benign; two declined lobectomy—they were followed with surveillance ultrasound and the nodules remained stable in size during 3 year follow up.

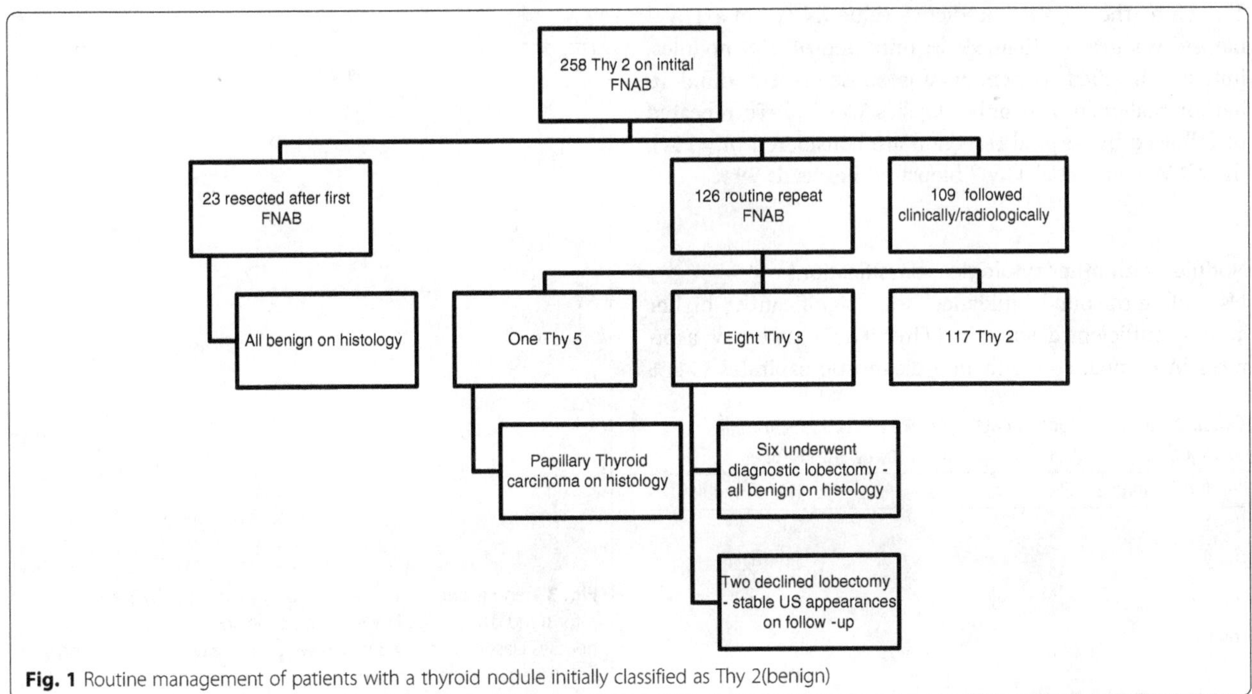

Fig. 1 Routine management of patients with a thyroid nodule initially classified as Thy 2(benign)

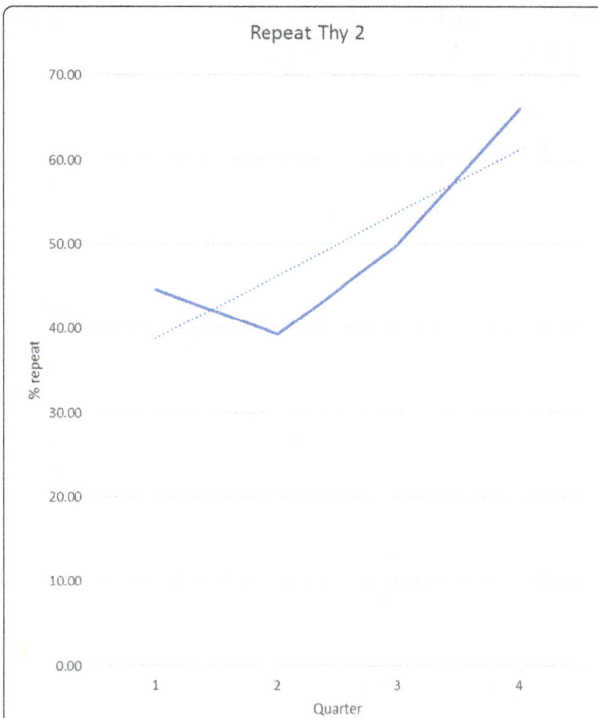

Fig. 2 Trend (dotted line) for repeat FNA after initial aspirate classified as Thy 2 (benign); p for trend = 0.012. Solid line represents the absolute percentage of aspirates, initially classified as Thy 2, which were repeated in each quarter of the study period

The majority of patients with a nodule initially classified as Thy 2, who did not have surgery or a repeat biopsy, were followed for between 4–8 years without clinical or sonographic evidence of significant nodule enlargement. Therefore, the negative predictive value (NPV) of a Thy 2 biopsy was greater than 99 %; only one of 258 nodules, initially classified as benign, was subsequently found to harbor malignancy. If only biopsies which were repeated or followed by surgical resection are considered ($n = 149$), the NPV of an initial Thy 2 biopsy still exceeds 99 %.

Nodules with other cytological classifications

Use of ultrasound guidance was significantly higher among sufficient/diagnostic (Thy2-Thy5) category aspirates in comparison with non-diagnostic aspirates (94 % versus 76 % of aspirates respectively). Therefore, lack of ultrasound guidance was strongly associated with insufficient biopsy material (p value < 0.0001).

Table 2 Final cytological category of 126 nodules, initially classified as Thy2 (benign) after routine repeat FNAB

Result of routine 2nd FNAB	No. of nodules (%)
Thy 1	0 (0)
Thy 2	117 (92.8)
Thy 3	8 (6.4)
Thy 4	0 (0)
Thy 5	1 (0.8)

Sixty three nodules (15 %) were initially classified as Thy 1 (insufficient). Twenty seven (43 %), of the nodules initially classified as Thy1, were predominantly or partially cystic in nature. Nineteen percent (12/63) of those initially classified as Thy 1 underwent surgical resection while 52 % (33/63) were re-biopsied. In the former group (surgically resected nodules), 4/12 patients were diagnosed with a malignant lesion. Repeat biopsy of a nodule originally classified as Thy 1 yielded a diagnostic sample in 57 %. Among those patients with two consecutive biopsies classified as Thy 1 ($n = 12$), four underwent surgery and 1 of the 4 had a malignant lesion diagnosed –2.7 cm locally invasive papillary thyroid carcinoma. The remaining patients, with either one or two insufficient cytology samples ($n = 28$), were followed clinically and/or radiologically and did not develop any concerning features to warrant resection.

Seventy five (18 %) of nodules were assigned to the Thy 3 category (atypia, follicular lesion or follicular neoplasm). The majority of Thy 3 nodules (55/75) were surgically excised; 29 % (16 nodules) were ultimately diagnosed as malignant. The rate of lobectomy for Thy 3 nodules increased significantly over the course of the study—p for trend 0.026 (Fig. 3). The remaining 20 patients have been followed with serial ultrasound—no nodule has increased significantly in size or developed any new suspicious radiological features.

Eight (2 %) nodules were initially classified as Thy 4 (suspicious for malignancy)—all proceeded to surgical resection. One patient was diagnosed with medullary thyroid carcinoma. Among the remainder, one patient

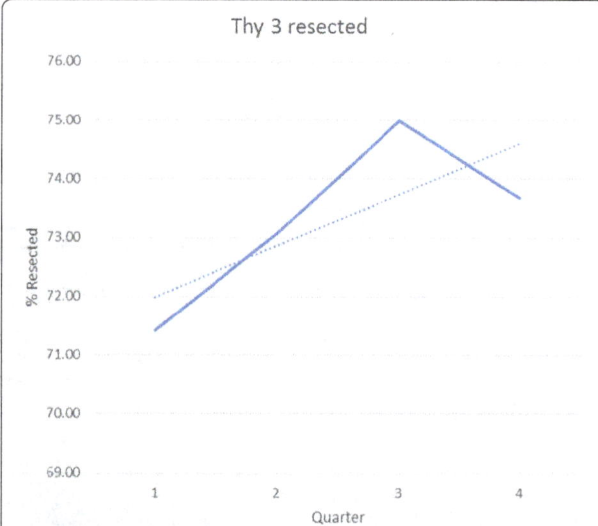

Fig. 3 Trend (dotted line) for lobectomy following Thy 3 aspirate; p for trend 0.026. Solid line represents the absolute percentage of nodules classified as Thy 3 which were surgically resected during each quarter of the study period

was diagnosed with stage IV papillary thyroid carcinoma (PTC) while all others had stage I PTC. Thy 5 (malignant) nodules accounted for 2 % of cases (9 nodules). All had malignancy diagnosed following thyroidectomy—all patients had stage I differentiated thyroid cancer.

Discussion

We describe the cytological findings and outcome in a large, consecutive series of patients who underwent diagnostic evaluation of thyroid nodules. The gender distribution and nodule size in our cohort are comparable to other large case series. However, length of follow up in our cohort is considerably longer than many studies in this field.

In keeping with previous research, most nodules in our cohort were classified as benign (Thy 2) after cytological assessment [10]. There is on-going debate, internationally, about the appropriate follow up of such cases. Guidance varies between repeat clinical, ultrasound and/or cytological assessment [6–9]. During the time course of this study, we adopted the contemporary recommendations of The British Thyroid Association to perform a routine repeat aspiration of lesions initially classified as benign (Thy 2) to rule out a false negative result [6].

Among the Thy 2 nodules in our cohort, 7 % had a different classification on repeat biopsy. However, amongst 126 patients who had a repeat FNAB, only one patient (0.8 %) initially classified Thy 2 was ultimately diagnosed with differentiated papillary carcinoma. Considering all nodules initially categorised as Thy 2 or only those who underwent repeat biopsy or surgery, the negative predictive value (NPV) of an initial benign cytology assessment exceeded 99 %. The majority of patients with benign cytology findings do not proceed to thyroidectomy and, given the indolent nature of many differentiated thyroid malignancies, there are concerns that a short follow up interval may lead to a verification bias and consequent overestimate of the NPV. In our study, only 23 (9 %) patients with initial benign cytology underwent surgical resection; however the long follow up (range 4–8 years) gives more credence to our conclusions.

Advocates of routine repeat FNAB of benign thyroid nodules on initial cytology voice concerns about false negative results and missed diagnoses of thyroid cancer. False negative rates, following a benign biopsy result, have been reported to be as high as 11 % in some historical series [17]. This led some authors to conclude that repeat aspiration is useful to reduce the rate of false negative results [17, 20, 21]. However, much of this data precede the widespread use of ultrasound-guided FNA resulting in a better cytological yield. In addition, cytology results were, previously, often not reported according to a validated classification system. Furthermore, repeat biopsies were not undertaken on a routine basis but, rather, were performed on the basis of clinical suspicion in many cases, leading to a somewhat biased study cohort.

Hamburger et al., in one of the few studies to perform routine repeat aspiration of benign thyroid nodules (not guided by ultrasound), reported that 9 % were assigned a different classification on repeat biopsy; 3 % were diagnosed with malignancy following thyroidectomy [13]. More recent research by *Singh Ospina* et al. reported that 1.2 % of nodules were classified as malignant when the FNAB was repeated after an initial benign cytological assessment-334 nodules, initially classified as benign, underwent repeat aspiration over a 10 year period; however, the authors do not report what proportion of initially benign biopsies were repeated [14]. Higher false negative biopsy rates-approximately 2.5 %—have been described in other recent retrospective studies [15, 22]. However, re-biopsy was undertaken on a selective basis, based on clinical or radiological concern during follow up, as opposed to the routine policy favoured in our study. Recent research has more accurately defined the natural history of nodules initially classified as benign; in a study of over 2000 such nodules, followed for over 8 years, there were no deaths due to thyroid cancer; thyroidectomy was undertaken in 24 % and the false negative rate was estimated at 1.3 % [18].

Enhanced resolution of ultrasound scanners has improved risk stratification of thyroid nodules. Several ultrasound features (e.g. irregular border, intranodular vascularity, hypoechoic echotexture, microcalcifications) have been shown to be more common in malignant thyroid lesions [23]. Ultrasound characteristics, combined with clinical features and specific risk factors can be used to risk stratify patients and inform the decision about the need for repeat biopsy [24, 25]. This approach is now advocated by many international experts and professional societies, who have suggested that routine repeat biopsy of nodules classified as Thy 2 (benign) may not be necessary in all cases [7]. Alternatively, nodules could be risk assessed according to the patient's history as well as clinical and ultrasound features. Low risk lesions may not require biopsy. Furthermore, the size of the lesion is now recognised as a less important independent determinant of risk, unless the lesion has increased in size [26].

Multidisciplinary care is advocated for all patients with thyroid nodules and cancer [7]. However, there is a paucity of clinical data evaluating this approach to the care of this subgroup of patients [10]. Our local MDT was established towards the beginning of the study period and the temporal trends allow some assessment of its impact on patient care.

There was a high rate of Thy 1 (non-diagnostic/inadequate) aspirates in our series. Previous research has shown the value of US guidance in attaining a diagnostic sample [27]. Lack of US guidance in our study was strongly associated a non-diagnostic aspirate. Our rate of routine repeat biopsy increased significantly throughout the duration of the study (Fig. 1). This temporal trend supports the notion of increased integration of the MDT over time with improved implementation of a shared-care protocol.

Cytology has been shown to be inaccurate in distinquishing benign and malignant follicular lesions—ie Thy 3 lesions. International guidelines advise diagnostic lobectomy in such cases with predominantly follicular features (as opposed to those with only atypical cellular features) [7]. Our rate of lobectomy for Thy 3 lesions increased significantly throughout the study period—Fig. 2. We believe this may due to the establishment of the MDT which promoted a protocolisedapproach to care in line with international guidelines. The malignancy rate in Thy3 nodules in our study is somewhat higher than other series. However, only 75 % of our Thy 3 nodules were excised and this sample may be biased due to clinical and/or radiological concern about patients sent for surgery. Long-term clinical follow-up of non-operated Thy 3 nodules has not raised any concern or led to a recommendation for surgery.

Thy 4 category (suspicious for malignancy) only accounted for 2 % of nodules. However, all cases were diagnosed with malignancy after thyroidectomy. This may represent an over-reliance on this category as similar studies report malignancy rates between 60–80 % for this cytological category [10, 28, 29]. However, the number of Thy 5 (malignant) lesions is in keeping with international literature with no false positive cases. This emphasises the positive predictive value of fine-needle aspiration in the preoperative diagnosis of thyroid cancer.

This study supports and extends the findings of similar studies in this field. Very few previous studies have examined the impact of a routine repeat FNAB in patients with a thyroid nodule initially classified as benign, regardless of the clinical or radiological features. Our data support a very high accuracy of an initial, well-targeted FNAB with only 7 % of nodules receiving a different classification on re-biopsy and <1 % diagnosed with malignancy. The long follow up of our cohort adds further weight to our findings.

This study is limited mainly by the retrospective design. There may be a selection bias in the patients that had repeat biopsy, influenced by clinician and patient opinion at the time of evaluation but this is unlikely to have resulted in an underestimation of false negative results, as one would expect that if selection bias was a factor, it would have resulted in more diagnoses of thyroid carcinoma on repeat FNAB. In addition, greater detail of the ultrasound characteristics of nodules would have permitted analysis of these features for risk stratification of nodules. Finally, the study reports routine practice in a tertiary referral centre and the results may be challenging to reproduce in centres with a smaller case load, less complex case mix and where a similar, broad-based multidisciplinary team is not available.

Conclusion

We conclude that the risk of malignancy in thyroid nodules initially classified as Thy 2 (benign), by an experienced cytopathologist, is very low when the FNAB is well-targeted and cases are managed by a MDT. Repeat biopsy is not necessary in all patients but could be reserved for selected cases with high risk clinical and/or radiological features.

In addition, the establishment of a multidisciplinary team, for the care of patients with thyroid nodules, is associated with improved implementation of international guidelines.

Abbreviations

FNAB, fine needle aspiration biopsy; MDT, multidisciplinary team; US, ultrasound; NPV, negative predictive value; SEM, standard error of mean; SD, standard deviation

Acknowledgements

We gratefully acknowledge the work of the technical and clinical staff of the Department of Histopathology, Beaumont Hospital.

Funding

No funding was received for this project.

Authors' contributions

NG, ML & AA conceived of and designed the study. NG, MJH, SL, PH & MAM assembled the data. FK, MM & ML contributed to analysis and interpretation of the data. NG performed the statistical analysis. ADKH, DS, CJT & DR contributed to clinical care of the patients, interpretation of the data and review of the manuscript. NG & AA drafted the manuscript. All authors read and approved the manuscript.

Competing interests

The authors declare that they have no competing interests.

Author details

[1]Department of Endocrinology, Beaumont Hospital and RCSI Medical School, Dublin 9, Ireland. [2]Department of Surgery, Beaumont Hospital and RCSI Medical School, Dublin 9, Ireland. [3]Department Radiology, Beaumont Hospital and RCSI Medical School, Dublin 9, Ireland. [4]Department of Pathology, Beaumont Hospital and RCSI Medical School, Dublin 9, Ireland.

References

1. Wiest PW, Hartshorne MF, Inskip PD, Crooks LA, Vela BS, Telepak RJ, et al. Thyroid palpation versus high-resolution thyroid ultrasonography in the detection of nodules. J Ultrasound Med. 1998;17(8):487–96.
2. Tomimori E, Pedrinola F, Cavaliere H, Knobel M, Medeiros-Neto G. Prevalence of incidental thyroid disease in a relatively low iodine intake area. Thyroid. 1995;5(4):273–6.
3. Frates MC, Benson CB, Charboneau JW, Cibas ES, Clark OH, Coleman BG, et al. Management of thyroid nodules detected at US: Society of Radiologists in Ultrasound consensus conference statement. Radiology. 2005;237(3):794–800.
4. Hegedüs L. Clinical practice. The thyroid nodule. N Engl J Med. 2004;351(17): 1764–71.
5. Nam-Goong IS, Kim HY, Gong G, Lee HK, Hong SJ, Kim WB, et al. Ultrasonography-guided fine-needle aspiration of thyroid incidentaloma: correlation with pathological findings. Clin Endocrinol (Oxf). 2004;60(1):21–8.
6. British Thyroid Association, Royal College of Physicians Guidelines for the Management of Thyroid Cancer. Second edition. Royal College of Physicians, London. 2007.
7. Perros P, Boelaert K, Colley S, Evans C, Evans RM, Gerrard Ba G, et al. Guidelines for the management of thyroid cancer. Clin Endocrinol (Oxf). 2014;81 Suppl 1:1–122.
8. Haugen BR, Alexander EK, Bible KC, Doherty GM, Mandel SJ, Nikiforov YE, Pacini F, Randolph GW, Sawka AM, Schlumberger M, Schuff KG. 2015 American Thyroid Association management guidelines for adult patients with thyroid nodules and differentiated thyroid cancer: the American Thyroid Association guidelines task force on thyroid nodules and differentiated thyroid cancer. Thyroid. 2016;26(1):1-33.
9. Gharib H, Papini E, Paschke R, Duick DS, Valcavi R, Hegedüs L, et al. American Association of Clinical Endocrinologists, Associazione Medici Endocrinologi, and EuropeanThyroid Association Medical Guidelines for Clinical Practice for the Diagnosis and Management of Thyroid Nodules. Endocr Pract. 2010;16 Suppl 1:1–43.
10. Yassa L, Cibas ES, Benson CB, Frates MC, Doubilet PM, Gawande AA, et al. Long-term assessment of a multidisciplinary approach to thyroid nodule diagnostic evaluation. Cancer. 2007;111(6):508–16.
11. Giles WH, Maclellan RA, Gawande AA, Ruan DT, Alexander EK, Moore FD, et al. False negative cytology in large thyroid nodules. Ann Surg Oncol. 2015;22(1):152–7.
12. Cibas ES, Baloch ZW, Fellegara G, Livolsi VA, Raab SS, Rosai J, et al. A prospective assessment defining the limitations of thyroid nodule pathologic evaluation. Ann Intern Med. 2013;159(5):325–32.
13. Hamburger JI. Consistency of sequential needle biopsy findings for thyroid nodules. Mang implications Arch Intern Med. 1987;147(1):97–9.
14. Singh Ospina N, Sebo TJ, Morris JC, Castro MR. The Value of Repeat Thyroid Fine-Needle Aspiration Biopsy in Patients with a Previously Benign Result: How Often Does It Alter Management? Thyroid. 2015;25(10):1121–6.
15. Gabalec F, Cáp J, Ryska A, Vasátko T, Ceeová V. Benign fine-needle aspiration cytology of thyroid nodule: to repeat or not to repeat? Eur J Endocrinol. 2009;161(6):933–7.
16. Lewis CM, Chang KP, Pitman M, Faquin WC, Randolph GW. Thyroid fine-needle aspiration biopsy: variability in reporting. Thyroid. 2009;19(7):717–23.
17. Oertel YC, Miyahara-Felipe L, Mendoza MG, Yu K. Value of repeated fine needle aspirations of the thyroid: an analysis of over ten thousand FNAs. Thyroid. 2007;17(11):1061–6.
18. Nou E, Kwong N, Alexander LK, Cibas ES, Marqusee E, Alexander EK. Determination of the optimal time interval for repeat evaluation after a benign thyroid nodule aspiration. J Clin Endocrinol Metab. 2014;99(2):510–6.
19. Cross P, Chandra A, Giles T, Johnson S, Kocjan G, Poller D, Stephenson T: Guidance on the reporting of thyroid cytology specimens. *Royal College of Pathologists* 2009.
20. Furlan JC, Bedard YC, Rosen IB. Single versus sequential fine-needle aspiration biopsy in the management of thyroid nodular disease. Can J Surg. 2005;48(1):12–8.
21. Flanagan MB, Ohori NP, Carty SE, Hunt JL. Repeat thyroid nodule fine-needle aspiration in patients with initial benign cytologic results. Am J Clin Pathol. 2006;125(5):698–702.
22. Illouz F, Rodien P, Saint-André JP, Triau S, Laboureau-Soares S, Dubois S, et al. Usefulness of repeated fine-needle cytology in the follow-up of non-operated thyroid nodules. Eur J Endocrinol. 2007;156(3):303–8.
23. Brito JP, Gionfriddo MR, Al Nofal A, Boehmer KR, Leppin AL, Reading C, et al. The accuracy of thyroid nodule ultrasound to predict thyroid cancer: systematic review and meta-analysis. J Clin Endocrinol Metab. 2014;99(4): 1253–63.
24. Kwak JY, Koo H, Youk JH, Kim MJ, Moon HJ, Son EJ, et al. Value of US correlation of a thyroid nodule with initially benign cytologic results. Radiology. 2010;254(1):292–300.
25. Kwak JY, Kim EK, Kim HJ, Kim MJ, Son EJ, Moon HJ. How to combine ultrasound and cytological information in decision making about thyroid nodules. Eur Radiol. 2009;19(8):1923–31.
26. Kamran SC, Marqusee E, Kim MI, Frates MC, Ritner J, Peters H, et al. Thyroid nodule size and prediction of cancer. J Clin Endocrinol Metab. 2013;98(2): 564–70.
27. Cesur M, Corapcioglu D, Bulut S, Gursoy A, Yilmaz AE, Erdogan N, et al. Comparison of palpation-guided fine-needle aspiration biopsy to ultrasound-guided fine-needle aspiration biopsy in the evaluation of thyroid nodules. Thyroid. 2006;16(6):555–61.
28. Wang CC, Friedman L, Kennedy GC, Wang H, Kebebew E, Steward DL, et al. A large multicenter correlation study of thyroid nodule cytopathology and histopathology. Thyroid. 2011;21(3):243–51.
29. Wu HH, Jones JN, Osman J. Fine-needle aspiration cytology of the thyroid: 10 years experience in a community teaching hospital. Diagn Cytopathol. 2006;34(2):93–6.

Acute airway compromise due to parathyroid tumour apoplexy: an exceptionally rare and potentially life-threatening presentation

Aoife Garrahy[1*], David Hogan[2], James Paul O'Neill[2] and Amar Agha[1]

Abstract

Background: Spontaneous haemorrhage into a parathyroid adenoma is a rare and potentially life-threatening presentation.

Case presentation: We report the case of a 45 year old female recently diagnosed with primary hyperparathyroidism who presented with chest discomfort and acute airway compromise due to spontaneous extracapsular haemorrhage into a parathyroid adenoma. Computed tomography (CT) imaging showed a hypopharyngeal haematoma extending 10 cm into the superior mediastinum. Surgical decompression of the cyst followed by enbloc resection of the parathyroid tumour was performed after elective intubation. Calcium and parathyroid hormone (PTH) levels had fallen prior to surgery and remain normal post-operatively.

Conclusion: Spontaneous parathyroid haemorrhage should be considered in any patient with unexplained spontaneous cervical haemorrhage, particularly if there is a history of hyperparathyroidism. Initial evaluation of such patients should include serum calcium and PTH as well as imaging.

Keywords: Parathyroid haemorrhage, Parathyroid tumour apoplexy, Primary hyperparathyroidism

Background

Spontaneous parathyroid haemorrhage is an exceptionally rare but potentially life-threatening presentation. Haemorrhage may be contained within the gland, but often presents as extracapsular haemorrhage extending into the neck or mediastinum, manifesting as acute painful neck swelling, discomfort and cervical ecchymosis. Tracheal compression may lead to airway compromise while compression of the recurrent laryngeal nerve and oesophagus may lead to hoarseness and dysphagia respectively. We describe a case of spontaneous haemorrhage into a parathyroid adenoma presenting with acute airway compromise requiring surgical evacuation.

* Correspondence: aoife.garrahy@gmail.com
[1]Department of Endocrinology, Beaumont Hospital, Dublin, Ireland

Case Presentation

A 45 year old female presented to the emergency department (ED) with a 3 days history of progressive dyspnoea, cough, throat and chest discomfort and palpitations.

Eight weeks prior to her ED visit, she was diagnosed with primary hyperparathyroidism (adjusted calcium 3.33 mmol/L (13.3 mg/dl) (normal range 2.2–2.6 mmol/L), PTH 367 (normal range 15–65) pg/ml) and 24 h urinary calcium 5.4 mmol/24 h (normal range 2.5–7.5 mmol/24 h). At her initial assessment she had no symptoms of hypercalcaemia apart from mild constipation. Family history was unremarkable. She received intravenous zolendronic acid and serum calcium fell to a nadir of 2.9 mmol/l. Neck ultrasound reported to show a 6 mm probable parathyroid lesion intimately related to the inferior pole of the right lobe of thyroid. One day prior to her acute presentation, and 6 weeks on from the ultrasound scan, a Sestamibi/SPECT CT revealed a 3.7 cm mass in

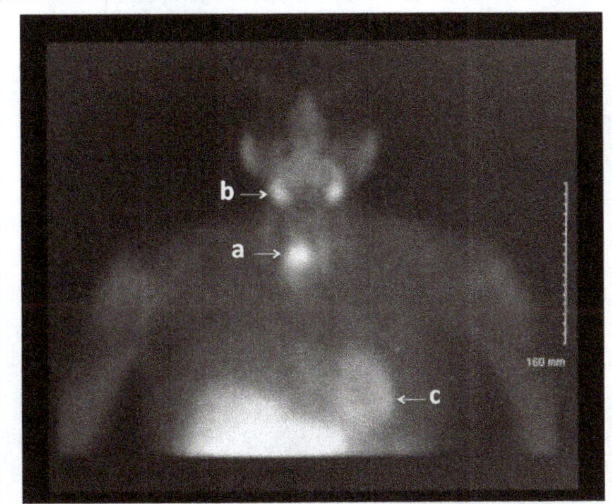

Fig. 1 Technetium 99 m sestamibi scan showing intense tracer uptake relative to the right lower pole of thyroid (**a**), and physiological uptake in the salivary glands (**b**) and myocardium (**c**)

the right tracheoesophageal groove extending to the posterior upper mediastinum at T1-T2 level (Figs. 1 & 2).

On arrival to ED, she was dyspnoeic and tachycardic. A biphasic stridor was noted. Flexible nasendoscopy identified no supraglottic or glottic cause for her stridor. The admitting medical team arranged a CT pulmonary angiogram to outrule a pulmonary embolism. CT thorax and subsequent emergency CT neck revealed significant increase in size of the mass since the scan 2 days prior, measuring 5.2 × 4.2 × 10.7 cm, with a hypodense fluid level, beginning at the level of the hypopharynx and extending into the superior mediastinum to the level of the aortic arch (Fig. 3). The trachea was narrowed with the smallest antero-posterior (AP) diameter measuring 0.4 cm at the level of the sternoclavicular joints.

She was admitted to the intensive care unit, electively intubated and brought to theatre the following morning. Preoperatively calcium levels had normalised and PTH had fallen to 77 pg/ml from a peak value of 496 pg/ml suggesting infarction of the gland (Fig. 4). There was no tracheal invasion on bronchoscopy. The cystic mass was identified in level 6 posterior and inferior to the right hemi-thyroid with evidence of recent haemorrhage into the surrounding tissues. The right recurrent laryngeal nerve (RLN) lay over the tumour (Fig. 5). The close proximity of the tumour to the adjacent thyroid necessitated that a right hemi-thyroidectomy was performed with preservation of the RLN. Decompression of the cyst revealed old blood products and allowed complete dissection and removal of the tumour en-bloc (Fig. 6). Intra-operative PTH monitoring was not used.

She was extubated without complication on the first post-operative day. There was no stridor and vocal cord examination was normal. Histology confirmed a

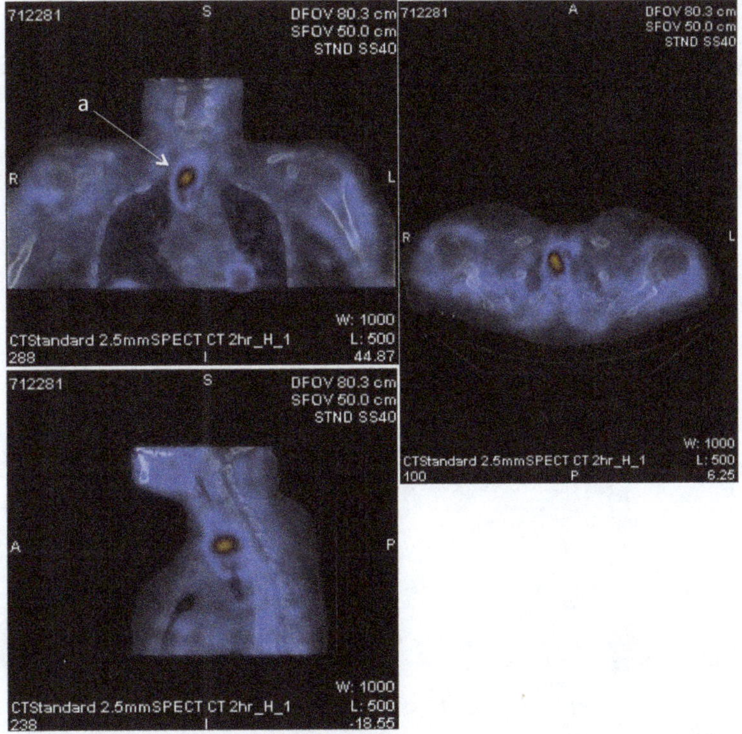

Fig. 2 SPECT CT showing 3.7 cm soft tissue mass (**a**) in the right tracheoesophageal groove extending into the posterior upper mediastinum. There is some associated compression of the upper oesophagus which is slightly deviated to the left

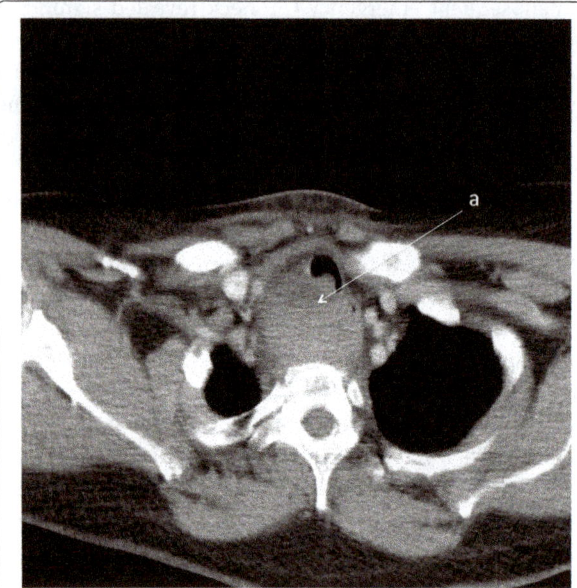

Fig. 3 CT Neck showing large mass with a hypodense fluid level (**a**)

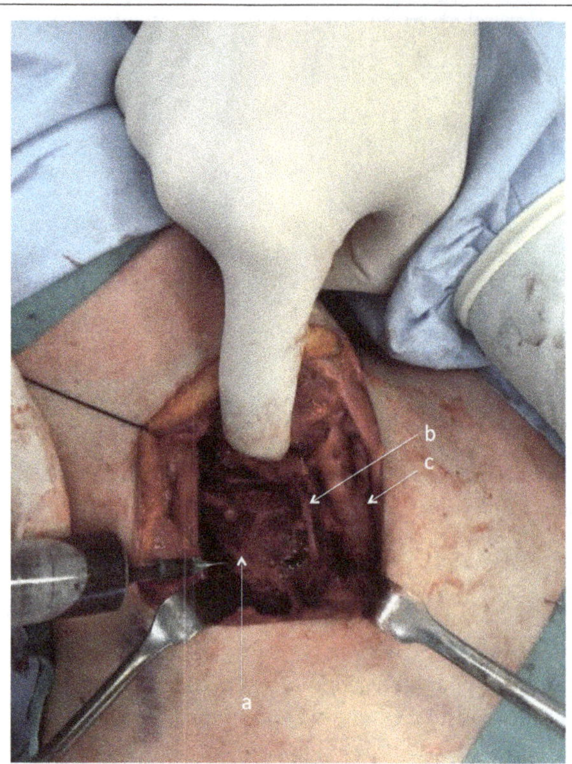

Fig. 5 Aspiration of blood from parathyroid cyst prior to enbloc excision of the tumour. (**a**) parathyroid cyst, (**b**) recurrent laryngeal nerve, (**c**) tracheal rings

parathyroid neoplasm with extensive haemorrhage and necrosis; MIB-1 index <5% (Figs. 7 & 8). Serum calcium level remains normal 5 months post-operatively.

Discussion

Spontaneous parathyroid haemorrhage is a rare but potentially life-threatening complication of parathyroid disease. *Capps* first reported a case of fatal haemorrhage due to rupture of a parathyroid adenoma in 1934. Since then, over 80 cases have been described in the English literature; ten of these associated with acute airway compromise requiring emergency intervention, and more than half of cases presenting with compressive symptoms due to haemorrhage.

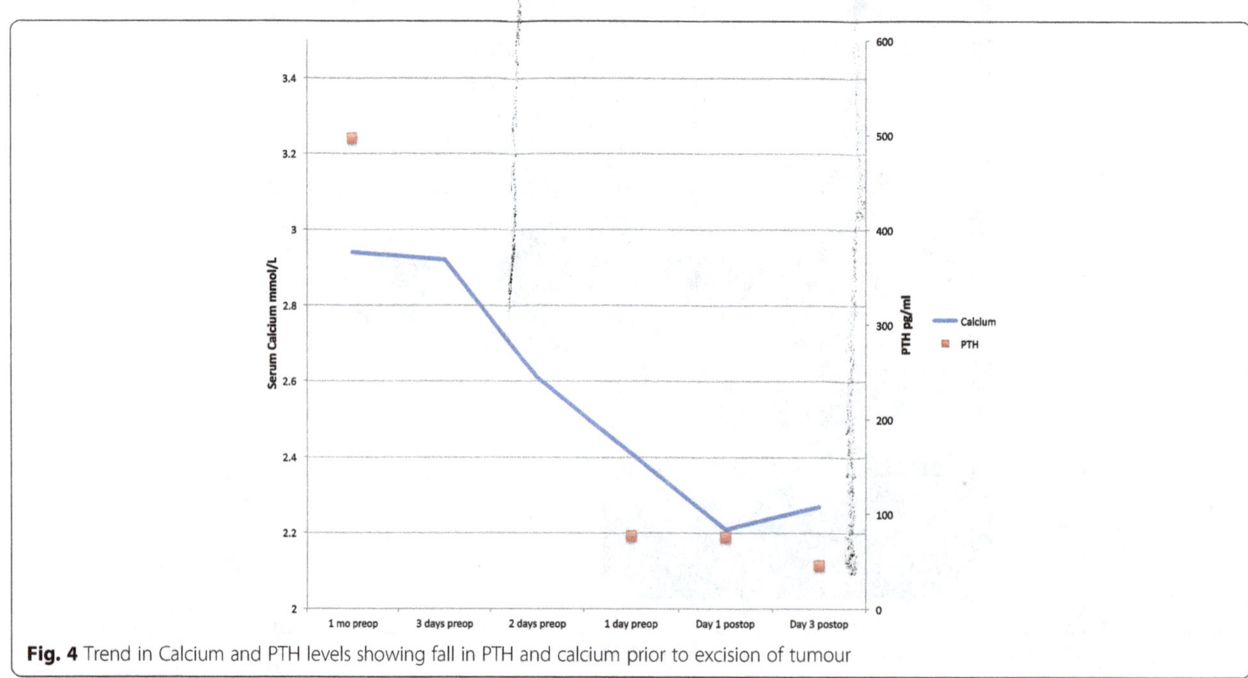

Fig. 4 Trend in Calcium and PTH levels showing fall in PTH and calcium prior to excision of tumour

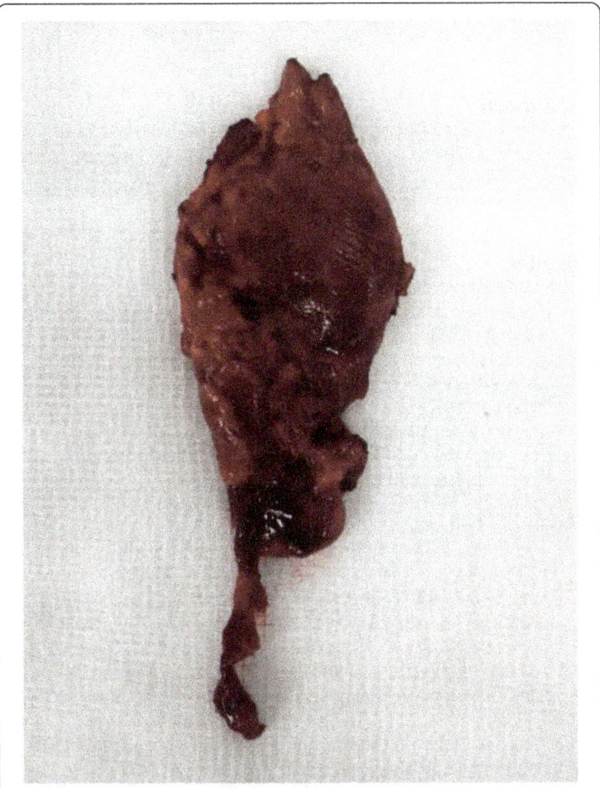

Fig. 6 Gross specimen: Haemorrhagic parathyroid tumour

Haemorrhage may occur into a parathyroid adenoma (cervical or ectopic), parathyroid hyperplasia or a parathyroid cyst and is thought to occur due to a lack of balance between cell growth and blood supply, somewhat similar to apoplexy seen in other endocrine neoplasia. It may be contained within the parathyroid gland, but often presents as extracapsular haemorrhage extending into the neck and/or mediastinum due to rupture of the haemorrhage through the relatively thin parathyroid tumour wall [1].

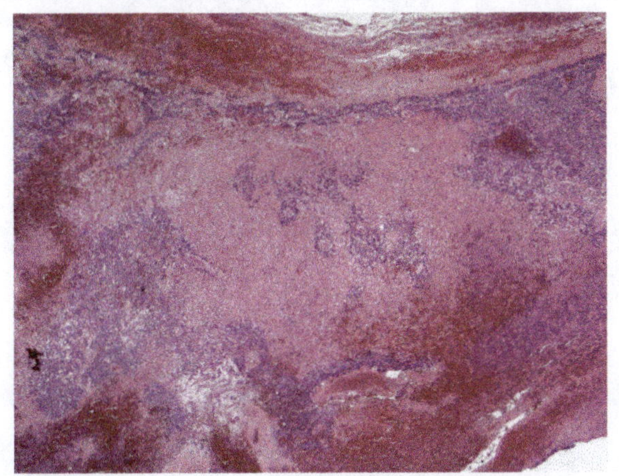

Fig. 7 *X2*: H&E, objective lens *X2*. Periphery of gland showing marked haemorrhage within residual parathyroid tissue

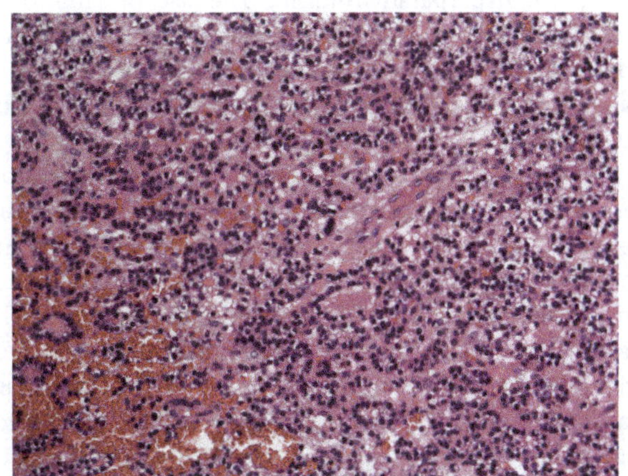

Fig. 8 X20: H&E, objective lens X20. High power of parathyroid tissue showing bland nuclear features and lack of mitoses. There was no evidence of perineural or vascular invasion

Clinical features are determined by the extent of the haemorrhage and degree of hyperparathyroidism. Spontaneous extracapsular parathyroid haemorrhage into the neck may present with acute painful neck swelling, discomfort and cervical ecchymosis [2]. External compression of the trachea can lead to airway compromise necessitating emergency intervention. Hoarseness and dysphagia may be presenting symptoms due to compression of the RLN and oesophagus respectively. Haemorrhage extending inferiorly into the mediastinum can manifest as cough, chest pain, dyspnoea, respiratory distress and may mimic aortic dissection. Haemorrhage has also been reported into hyperplastic parathyroid glandular tissue in secondary hyperparathyroidism in patients undergoing haemodialysis [3] and in one patient after suppression of PTH with cinacalcet [4]. The parathyroid gland may be functional or non-functional, and the serum calcium can range from high to low depending on the occurrence of gland infarction. Cases of parathyroid haemorrhage presenting as hypercalcemic crisis have been described [5]. Rarely, the underlying lesion may represent a parathyroid carcinoma [6].

Initial evaluation of an intracervical haematoma should include serum calcium levels; however patients may be normocalcemic. Imaging with CT, magnetic resonance imagine (MRI) and nuclear medicine is essential to delineate the anatomy of the haemorrhage and, if possible, identify the source of the haemorrhage [7]. In our case, although the ultrasound radiologist was experienced in neck ultrasound, it is likely that the adenoma was low down in the neck and was not seen on ultrasound hence the value of SPECT CT. The possibility of parathyroid haemorrhage should be considered in anyone presenting with retropharyngeal or mediastinal haemorrhage, particularly if there is a documented history of hyperparathyroidism. The use of anticoagulants should be avoided if possible, as the empiric administration of low molecular weight heparin in our case may have resulted in enlargement of the haematoma.

Surgical exploration is the treatment of choice and offers definitive management of the hyperparathyroidism aswell as addressing local haemorrhage; however timing remains controversial. Airway compromise necessitates emergency surgical exploration and evacuation of the haemorrhage, as in our case. Some suggest a watch-and-wait approach with surgery deferred to 3 months [8], particularly as many cases of primary hyperparathyroidism can be cured as a result of apoplexy of the gland [1]. Indeed, in our case the excised parathyroid gland was necrotic and the patient's calcium had normalized before surgical intervention suggesting haemorrhagic infarction of the gland had led to autoparathyroidectomy. Recurrence of primary hyperparthyroidism following initial spontaneous remission has been described, suggestive that in some cases remission may be due to impaired perfusion of the tumour due to local pressure effects rather than gland necrosis[9], therefore careful biochemical monitoring is required.

Conclusion

Spontaneous parathyroid haemorrhage is a rare but potentially life-threatening complication. The diagnosis should be considered in any patient presenting with a spontaneous cervical haemorrhage of unknown aetiology, particularly if there is evidence of hypercalcemia, history of hyperparathyroidism or ecchymosis of the neck or chest wall. Initial evaluation should include a calcium and PTH level although these may have fallen if significant glandular haemorrhage has led to infarction of the gland. While some propose conservative management, surgery is the preferred option, particularly in the presence of acute airway compromise.

Abbreviations

AP: Antero-posterior; CT: Computed tomography; ED: Emergency department; MRI: Magnetic resonance imaging; PTH: Parathyroid hormone; RLN: Recurrent laryngeal nerve; SPECT: Single-photon emission computed tomography

Acknowledgements

Not applicable.

Funding

Not applicable.

Authors' Contributions

AG drafted the manuscript and treated the patient. DH and JPON performed the surgery, provided perioperative care of the patient and helped draft the manuscript. AA treated the patient and supervised drafting of the manuscript. All authors read and approved the final manuscript.

Competing interests

The authors declare that they have no competing interests.

Author details

[1]Department of Endocrinology, Beaumont Hospital, Dublin, Ireland.
[2]Department of Otolaryngology, Head and Neck Surgery, Beaumont Hospital, Dublin, Ireland.

References

1. Nylen E, Shah A, Hall J. Spontaneous remission of primary hyperparathyroidism from parathyroid apoplexy. J Clin Endocrinol Metab. 1996;81(4):1326–8.
2. Simcic KJ, McDermott MT, Crawford GJ, Marx WH, Ownbey JL, Kidd GS. Massive extracapsular hemorrhage from a parathyroid cyst. Arch Surg (Chicago, Ill : 1960). 1989;124(11):1347–50.
3. Akimoto T, Saito O, Muto S, Hasegawa T, Nokubi M, Numata A, et al. A case of thoracic hemorrhage due to ectopic parathyroid hyperplasia with chronic renal failure. Am J Kidney Dis. 2005;45(6):e109–14.
4. Nagasawa M, Ubara Y, Suwabe T, Yamanouchi M, Hayami N, Sumida K, et al. Parathyroid hemorrhage occurring after administration of cinacalcet in a patient with secondary hyperparathyroidism. Intern Med (Tokyo, Japan). 2012;51(24):3401–4.
5. Chodack P, Attie JN, Groder MG. Hypercalcemic crisis coincidental with hemorrhage in parathyroid adenoma. Arch Intern Med. 1965;116:416–23.
6. Erdas E, Licheri S, Lai ML, Pisano G, Pomata M, Daniele GM. Cervico-mediastinal hematoma secondary to extracapsular hemorrhage of parathyroid carcinoma. Clinical case and review of the literature. Chir Ital. 2003;55(3):425–34.
7. Koulouris G, Pianta M, Stuckey S. The 'sentinel clot' sign in spontaneous retropharyngeal hematoma secondary to parathyroid apoplexy. Ear Nose Throat J. 2006;85(9):606–8.
8. Chaffanjon PC, Chavanis N, Chabre O, Brichon PY. Extracapsular hematoma of the parathyroid glands. World J Surg. 2003;27(1):14–7.
9. Kataoka K, Taguchi M, Takeshita A, Miyakawa M, Takeuchi Y. Recurrence of primary hyperparathyroidism following spontaneous remission with intracapsular hemorrhage of a parathyroid adenoma. J Bone Miner Metab. 2008;26(3):295–7.

21

Orbital radiotherapy plus three-wall orbital decompression in a patient with rare ocular manifestations of thyroid eye disease

Shuo Zhang, Yang Wang, Sisi Zhong, Xingtong Liu, Yazhuo Huang, Sijie Fang, Ai Zhuang, Yinwei Li, Jing Sun, Huifang Zhou* and Xianqun Fan*

Abstract

Background: Thyroid eye disease (TED) is a debilitating autoimmune orbital disease that is often a result of Graves' disease. Dysthyroid optic neuropathy (DON) is a rare but sight-threatening manifestation of TED with therapeutic challenges that can potentially lead to visual loss.

Case presentation: A 74-year-old man experienced active TED with extremely severe redness and swelling of the conjunctiva, loss of visual acuity and exacerbation of disfiguring proptosis. Computed tomography revealed the involvement of extraocular muscles resulting in optic nerve compression. He was in poor general condition and was intolerant to steroids. To achieve the optimal operating conditions for orbital decompression surgery, the patient was initially treated with orbital radiotherapy. The patient responded well, with improvements in clinical activity score and visual acuity.

Conclusion: This case demonstrates a rare and severe case of DON with therapeutic challenges. To date, no cases has been reported of a patient with such severe and unusual ocular manifestations. Early awareness of the occurrence of optic nerve compression and prompt treatment are important to prevent irreversible outcomes. Orbital radiotherapy should be considered as a useful surgery-delaying alternative for DON, especially in patients who have contraindications to steroids.

Keywords: Thyroid eye disease, Dysthyroid optic neuropathy, Orbital radiotherapy, Three-wall decompression

Background

Thyroid eye disease (TED) is an autoimmune orbital disease characterized by inflammation and edema of the periorbital connective tissues that results in expansion of the extraocular muscles and fat in the orbit [1]. It typically affects patients with hyperthyroidism due to Graves' disease.

Dysthyroid optic neuropathy (DON) is a rare but potentially sight-threatening complication that occurs in patients with TED. Only 3–5% of patients with TED suffer from DON [2]. High doses of intravenous methylprednisolone (iv-MP) therapy are usually the first-line treatment. Orbital decompression surgery should be performed for patients who fail to adequately respond to iv-MP [3]. The management of patients with DON with contraindications to steroids and urgent surgery remains uncertain. Orbital radiation is administered to patients without DON in most cases [3]. However, limited reports have described the efficacy of orbital radiotherapy and subsequent decompression surgery in DON patients.

Herein, we present a rare and severe case of active DON treated with orbital radiotherapy followed by three-wall orbital decompression in a poor surgical candidate previously intolerant to steroids. To the best of our knowledge, a case of active DON with

* Correspondence: fangzzfang@163.com; fanxq@sh163.net
Department of Ophthalmology, Ninth People's Hospital, Shanghai Jiao Tong University School of Medicine, No. 639 ZhiZaoJu Road, Shanghai 200011, China

such severe and unusual ocular manifestations has not been previously reported. This case has major clinical significance because it highlights the potential severe presentation of DON and suggests that orbital radiotherapy can be an optimal surgery-delaying treatment for patients who have contraindications to steroids.

Case presentation

A 74-year-old man presented to the Department of Ophthalmology, Shanghai Ninth People's Hospital, for extremely severe redness and swelling of the conjunctiva, loss of visual acuity and exacerbation of disfiguring proptosis. The patient had a history of Graves' disease and underwent a bilateral subtotal thyroidectomy in 1978. He experienced relapse of Graves' disease three months after surgery and was treated with methimazole with limited response. Due to uncontrolled hyperthyroidism, the patient underwent a left total thyroidectomy in 1985 and radioiodine treatment in 2002. He exhibited proptosis 20 years ago and the proptosis had gradually worsened over the previous years. He underwent iv-MP therapy with doses of 0.84 g (consecutive daily infusions of 0.12 g for 3 days and 0.08 g for 6 days) in 2014 and with doses of 1.8 g (consecutive daily infusions of 0.48 g for 3 days, 0.24 g for 1 day and 0.12 g for 1 day) twice in 2015 with limited response. The patient also suffered from intolerable side effects of steroids, such as dizziness and headache, had profound muscle weakness and was unable to walk. He also experienced iv-MP-related hepatotoxicity with elevated alanine aminotransferase (ALT) levels. The patient had a history of myocardial infarction, atrial fibrillation and multiple lacunar infarctions. He denied any other comorbid conditions such as hypertension and diabetes mellitus.

An ophthalmic examination showed reduction of best corrected visual acuity to hand movement in the right eye and 0.3 in the left eye, eyelids edema, swelling and hyperemia of the caruncle and plica, redness of the conjunctiva, remarkable chemosis and severe conjunctival prolapse (Fig. 1a and b). He was found to have severe restrictions in ocular movement in all directions with pain on attempted upward and downward gaze and spontaneous retrobulbar pain. He suffered from lagophthalmos and severe corneal exposure with diffuse punctate keratopathy and ulcers. Color vision, pupillary function and optic discs were normal in both eyes. His clinical activity score (CAS) was 6 points. Exophthalmometry showed proptosis of 32 mm of the right eye and 30 mm of the left eye. His intraocular pressures were 11 mmHg and 12 mmHg for the right and left eyes, respectively. He exhibited a free triiodothyronine (FT3) level of 3.43 pg/mL, low free thyroxin (FT4) level of 0.54 ng/dL, low thyroid-stimulating hormone (TSH) level of 0.06 μIU/mL, thyroid stimulating hormone receptor antibody (TRAb) level greater than 40.00 IU/L, an extremely high thyroid peroxidase antibody (TPOAb) level of 511.50 IU/mL, an elevated thyroglobulin antibody (TgAb) level of 433.10 IU/mL, high C-reactive protein (CRP) level of 2.06 mg/dL,

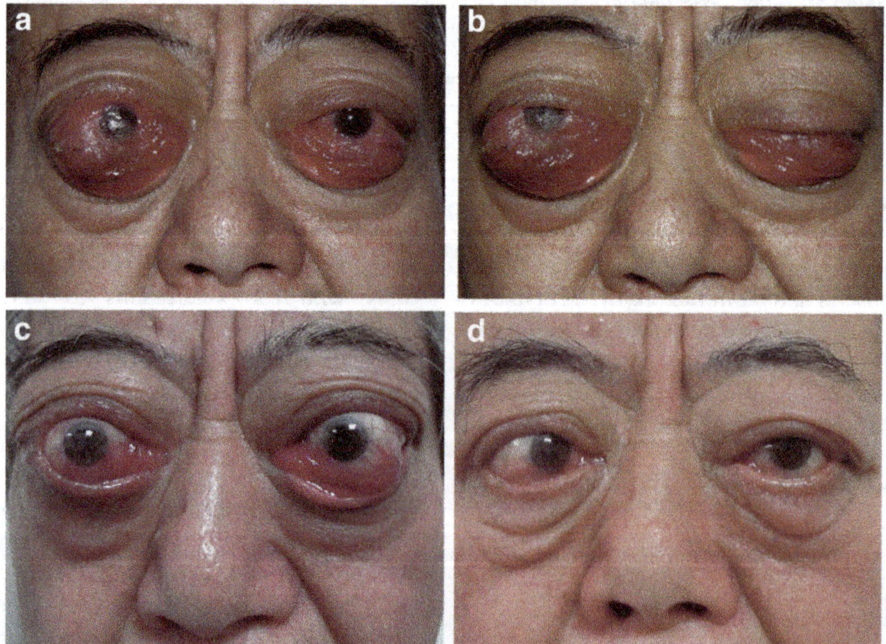

Fig. 1 Ophthalmologic symptoms of the patient. A 74-year-old man developed highly active TED with DON. An ophthalmic examination showed eyelids edema, redness of the conjunctiva, chemosis and severe conjunctival prolapse (**a** and **b**). One month after orbital radiotherapy (**c**). Six months after bilateral orbital decompression (**d**)

high interleukin-6 (IL-6) level of 127.58 pg/mL, high tumor necrosis factor-α (TNF-α) level of 259.42 pg/mL, normal immunoglobulin (Ig) G, IgA, IgM and IgG4 levels and an elevated IgE level of 465 IU/mL (Table 1). The patient received 7.5 mg of methimazole per day and 12.5 μg of levothyroxine sodium per day. An orbital computed tomography (CT) scan showed enlargement of the extraocular muscles bilaterally with marked enlargement of the medial rectus and inferior rectus muscles resulting in apical crowding and optic nerve compression (Fig. 2a–c). A diagnosis of active TED with DON and exposure keratitis was made [3].

The patient was evaluated as an urgent case and required prompt intervention (Fig. 3). Bilateral tarsorrhaphy and local therapy were performed to prevent worsening of chemosis and development of corneal ulcers. The patient was suggested to start 500 mg iv-MP for 3 consecutive days, but he had strong concerns about the use of glucocorticoids. At that time, the severe and terrible ocular signs including remarkable chemosis and severe conjunctival prolapse prevented immediate decompression surgery due to high intraorbital pressure and inaccessibility to the small surgical field. Therefore, decompression surgery was deemed high risk for optic nerve impairment. His poor general status due to multiple comorbidities and increased risk under anesthesia also interfered with urgent decompression surgery. Therefore, orbital radiotherapy with 20 Gy per orbit divided into 10 doses was given over a two-week period. Concomitant low-dose oral glucocorticoids were administered. The chemosis, conjunctival prolapse and corneal lesions significantly improved within 1 month (Fig. 1c). Spontaneous retrobulbar pain and pain on attempted eye movement were also significantly decreased. His CAS was also reduced by 2 points. Thus, an additional 10 Gy per orbit divided into in 5 doses was given. However, the impairment in best corrected visual acuity remained. Orbital radiotherapy significantly improved the ocular signs and offered the possibility of decompression surgery.

Table 1 Laboratory data before and after radiotherapy

	Before radiotherapy	Two months after radiotherapy	Normal range
FT3	3.43	3.48	2.5–3.9 pg/mL
FT4	0.54	0.45	0.58–1.64 ng/dL
TSH	0.06	1.99	0.34–5.6 μIU/mL
TPOAb	511.5	603.6	0–9 IU/mL
TRAb	> 40.00	> 40	0–1.75 IU/L
TgAb	433.1	122.9	0–115 IU/mL
CRP	2.06	0.60	0–0.80 mg/dL
IL-6	127.58	42.40	< 3.4 pg/mL
TNF-α	259.42	86.33	< 8.1 pg/mL
IgG	9.56	11.20	7–16 g/L
IgA	2.23	2.23	0.7–4 g/L
IgM	0.54	0.55	0.4–2.3 g/L
IgE	465.0	312.0	0–100 IU/mL
IgG4	0.555	0.637	0.03–2.01 g/L

Abbreviations: *FT3* free triiodothyronine, *FT4* free thyroxin, *TSH* thyroid-stimulating hormone, *TRAb* thyroid stimulating hormone receptor antibody, *TPOAb* thyroid peroxidase antibody, *TgAb* thyroglobulin antibody, *Ig* immunoglobulin, *CRP* C-reactive protein, *IL-6* interleukin-6, *TNF-α* tumor necrosis factor-α

Two months later, after extensive discussion of the risks and benefits of surgery, such as haemorrhage, cerebrospinal fluid (CSF) leakage, postoperative diplopia, postoperative lateral orbit depression and scarring, the patient agreed to proceed with right three-wall orbital decompression surgery under general anesthesia. A horizontal skin incision along with the double eyelid fold and lateral to the lateral canthus was made for lateral wall decompression. The deep lateral wall into the trigone of the greater wing of the sphenoid was removed, and the lateral orbital rim was removed en bloc. Transconjunctival and transcaruncular incisions were made for medial and inferior wall decompression. The patient subsequently underwent left three-wall orbital decompression using the same surgical techniques (Fig. 1d).

Following bilateral orbital decompression, the patient's best corrected visual acuity gradually improved. Six months following surgery, the final best corrected visual acuity improved to 0.5 in both the right and left eyes. The patients exhibited improvement in the eyelids edema and swelling and hyperemia of the caruncle and plica. His CAS was reduced to 2 points. Postoperative CT scans demonstrated relief of bilateral crowding in the orbital apex (Fig. 2d–f).

Discussion and conclusion

DON is a rare and severe complication of TED that can lead to definite visual loss [3]. Compression of the optic nerve at the orbital apex due to extraocular muscles enlargement and inflammatory reaction are the main causes of DON [2]. The diagnosis of DON is made based on the presence of a decreased visual function due to optic neuropathy secondary to TED [3, 4]. The European Group on Graves' Orbitopathy (EUGOGO) reported a prospective case series of 47 patients to identify clinical manifestations of DON [5]. The EUGOGO study found that patients with DON may not have severe proptosis and orbital inflammation. Evidence of optic nerve compression on imaging was one of the most sensitive clinical features, consistent with the findings in our patient. In our patient, the proptosis was 32 mm in the right eye and 30 mm in the left eye, which is far greater than the mean proptosis of 22.1 mm in both eyes

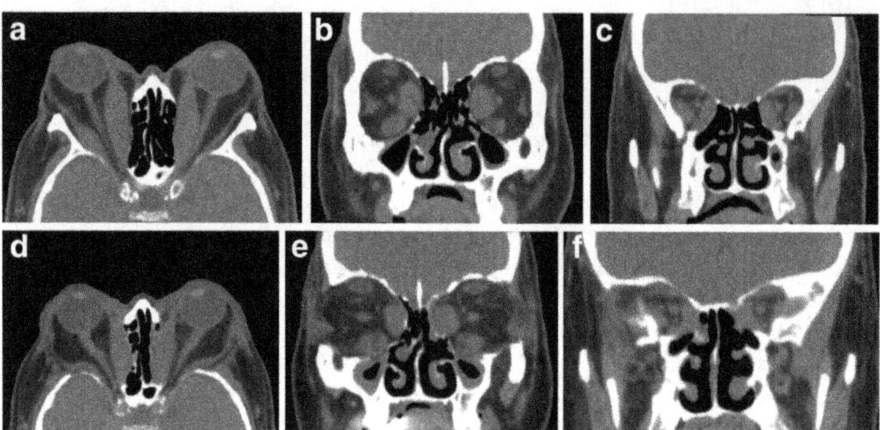

Fig. 2 Preoperative and postoperative computed tomography (CT) of the orbit. Preoperative axial (**a**) and coronal (**b** and **c**) CT images showing proptosis, enlargement of extraocular muscles and apical crowding. Postoperative axial (**d**) and coronal (**e** and **f**) CT images showing the reduction in proptosis and relief of apical crowding

reported in the EUGOGO study. To the authors' knowledge, this is the first case of a patient with such severe chemosis and conjunctival prolapse, which made the treatment more perplexing and challenging.

Glucocorticoids, orbital radiotherapy, orbital decompression, immunosuppressive therapy and biological drugs are available for the management of TED [3]. Iv-MP and prompt orbital decompression, if necessary, are is still considered to be the standard treatment for DON [3]. A randomized trial including 15 patients with active TED and DON suggested that immediate surgery does not result in better outcomes, and systemic glucocorticoids appeared to be the optimal first-line treatment [6]. To the best of our knowledge, no reports are available regarding the treatment of patients with DON with contraindications to steroids and surgical intolerance. Orbital radiotherapy plays an important role in controlling the inflammatory process of TED by inducing apoptosis or disrupting the functions of B and T lymphocytes, macrophages, or orbital fibroblasts and therefore reducing the secretion of proinflammatory cytokines from activated lymphocytes [7, 8]. A total dose of 20 Gy is commonly used [9, 10]. Grassi et al. reported significant early reduction in CAS and ocular motility disturbances after orbital radiotherapy in patients without DON [8]. Another study demonstrated that all patients with TED showed regression of the disease with combined iv-MP and orbital radiotherapy or iv-MP therapy alone. Two of fifty-nine patients undergoing iv-MP therapy developed DON during the follow-up period, but no patients receiving combined iv-MP and orbital radiotherapy developed DON [11]. In addition, some studies have indicated that the high incidence of IgE elevation in Graves' disease suggested a difference in the autoimmune processes of the disease with and without IgE elevation [12, 13]. We found elevated serum IgE levels in our case, suggesting that IgE may also participate in the immunopathogenesis of TED. The patient's IgE level decreased after orbital radiotherapy. The existing literature provides evidence of the efficacy of radiotherapy and its protective role against TED. Therefore, we advocate orbital radiation as the ideal therapy in patients with DON who have contraindications to steroids and cannot tolerate surgery, especially those with elevated IgE levels.

The reported effects of radiotherapy on visual acuity have been variable [8, 14]. In our case, no significant improvement in visual acuity was found after radiotherapy. Since the recovery of visual acuity is the main goal of treatment in patients with DON, additional orbital decompression is often required. Decompression is the only definitive treatment to relieve apical crowding, save the vision and reduce considerable exophthalmos [3]. Medial and inferior wall decompression led to marked improvement in visual acuity [15]. Balanced medial and lateral wall decompression has shown equal efficacy in terms of saving vision and lowering the rate of postoperative diplopia [16]. Kikkawa et al. proposed graded orbital decompression based on the severity of exophthalmometry, and a mean proptosis reduction of 8.9 ± 3.4 mm was obtained in the three-wall decompression group [17]. In the present case, a proptosis reduction of 10 mm in the right eye and 7 mm in the left eye was achieved. Orbital radiotherapy ameliorated the inflammatory reactions in the orbit and offered time to prepare for orbital decompression surgery.

Preoperative radiotherapy does not interfere with the outcomes of orbital decompression [18], and may prevent and control relapses in DON [19].

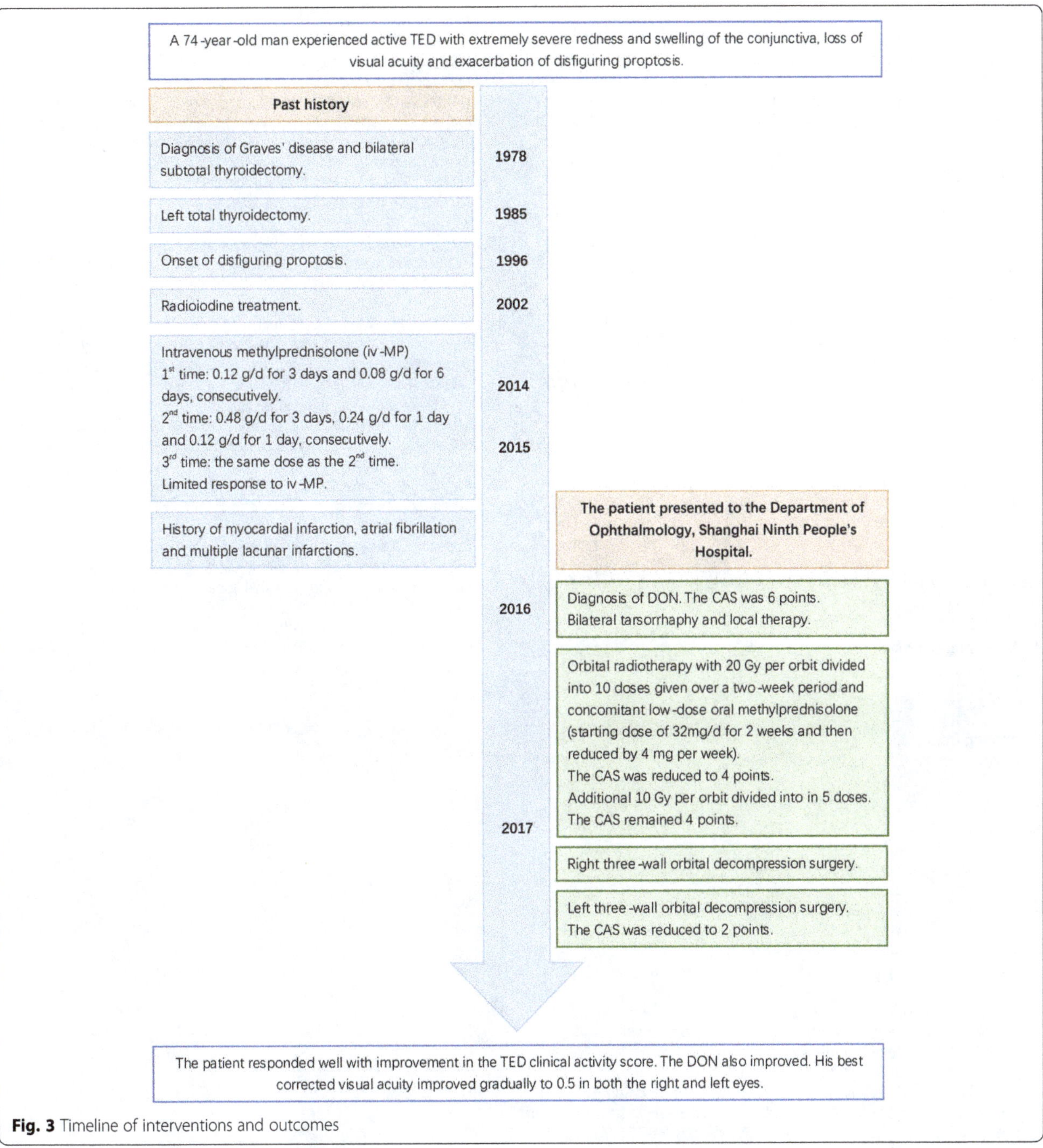

Fig. 3 Timeline of interventions and outcomes

Shams et al. reported that the rate of DON was significantly reduced in patients receiving orbital radiotherapy in addition to corticosteroids in their study [19]. In our case, preoperative radiotherapy offered optimal operating conditions for orbital decompression surgery and eased the surgery.

In conclusion, DON is a rare disease in patients with TED. Apart from the well-known ocular manifestations of TED, severe conjunctival prolapse and apical crowding can occur, resulting in devastating sight loss. We suggest that orbital radiotherapy can be a temporizing treatment for patients with DON in poor general condition and with contraindications to steroids until the patients are well prepared for orbital decompression. Patients with elevated IgE levels are especially likely to benefit from radiotherapy. The efficacy of orbital radiation for DON has not been well investigated and further studies and clinical trials are needed.

Abbreviations

CRP: C-reactive protein; DON: Dysthyroid optic neuropathy; FT3: Free triiodothyronine; FT4: Free thyroxin; Ig: Immunoglobulin; IL-6: Interleukin-6; TED: Thyroid eye disease; TgAb: Thyroglobulin antibody; TNF-α: Tumor necrosis factor-α; TPOAb: Thyroid peroxidase antibody; TRAb: Thyroid stimulating hormone receptor antibody; TSH: Thyroid-stimulating hormone

Acknowledgements

The authors would like to thank all staff involved in the care of the patient presented in this case report.

Funding

This study was supported in part by the National Natural Science Foundation of China (81170876, 31600971, 81320108010), Shanghai Municipal Education Commission-Gaofeng Clinical Medicine Grant Suppport (20152228), National High Technology Research and Development Program (863 Program) (2015AA020311); Shanghai Municipal Hospital Emerging Frontier Technology Joint Project (SHDC12012107), and Shanghai Science and Technology Commission Research Project (16411950600, 14411968000).

Authors' contributions

SZ drafted the manuscript and performed the literature review. YW, SSZ, XL, YH, SF and AZ performed the ophthalmic assessments and participated in data collection. YL, JS and HZ managed the patient's ophthalmic conditions and performed the decompression surgery. HZ and XF reviewed and revised the manuscript. All authors read and approved the final manuscript.

Authors' information

Not applicable.

Competing interests

The authors declare that they have no competing interests.

References

1. Bahn RS. Graves' ophthalmopathy. N Engl J Med. 2010;362(8):726–38.
2. Bartalena L, Pinchera A, Marcocci C. Management of Graves' ophthalmopathy: reality and perspectives. Endocr Rev. 2000;21(2):168–99.
3. Bartalena L, Baldeschi L, Boboridis K, Eckstein A, Kahaly GJ, Marcocci C, Perros P, Salvi M, Wiersinga WM. European group on graves O: the 2016 European thyroid association/European group on graves' Orbitopathy guidelines for the Management of Graves' Orbitopathy. Eur Thyroid J. 2016; 5(1):9–26.
4. Weis E, Heran MK, Jhamb A, Chan AK, Chiu JP, Hurley MC, Rootman J. Quantitative computed tomographic predictors of compressive optic neuropathy in patients with thyroid orbitopathy: a volumetric analysis. Ophthalmology. 2012;119(10):2174–8.
5. McKeag D, Lane C, Lazarus JH, Baldeschi L, Boboridis K, Dickinson AJ, Hullo AI, Kahaly G, Krassas G, Marcocci C, et al. Clinical features of dysthyroid optic neuropathy: a European group on Graves' Orbitopathy (EUGOGO) survey. Br J Ophthalmol. 2007;91(4):455–8.
6. Wakelkamp IM, Baldeschi L, Saeed P, Mourits MP, Prummel MF, Wiersinga WM. Surgical or medical decompression as a first-line treatment of optic neuropathy in Graves' ophthalmopathy? A randomized controlled trial. Clin Endocrinol. 2005;63(3):323–8.
7. Dolman PJ, Rath S. Orbital radiotherapy for thyroid eye disease. Curr Opin Ophthalmol. 2012;23(5):427–32.
8. Grassi P, Strianese D, Piscopo R, Pacelli R, Bonavolonta G. Radiotherapy for the treatment of thyroid eye disease-a prospective comparison: is orbital radiotherapy a suitable alternative to steroids? Ir J Med Sci. 2017;186(3):647–52.
9. Bartalena L, Baldeschi L, Dickinson AJ, Eckstein A, Kendall-Taylor P, Marcocci C, Mourits MP, Perros P, Boboridis K, Boschi A, et al. Consensus statement of the European group on Graves' orbitopathy (EUGOGO) on management of Graves' orbitopathy. Thyroid. 2008;18(3):333–46.
10. Prummel MF, Terwee CB, Gerding MN, Baldeschi L, Mourits MP, Blank L, Dekker FW, Wiersinga WM. A randomized controlled trial of orbital radiotherapy versus sham irradiation in patients with mild Graves' ophthalmopathy. J Clin Endocrinol Metab. 2004;89(1):15–20.
11. Kim JW, Han SH, Son BJ, Rim TH, Keum KC, Yoon JS. Efficacy of combined orbital radiation and systemic steroids in the management of Graves' orbitopathy. Albrecht Von Graefes Arch Klin Exp Ophthalmol. 2016;254(5):991–8.
12. Sato A, Takemura Y, Yamada T, Ohtsuka H, Sakai H, Miyahara Y, Aizawa T, Terao A, Onuma S, Junen K, et al. A possible role of immunoglobulin E in patients with hyperthyroid Graves' disease. J Clin Endocrinol Metab. 1999; 84(10):3602–5.
13. Komiya I, Yamada T, Sato A, Kouki T, Nishimori T, Takasu N. Remission and recurrence of hyperthyroid Graves' disease during and after methimazole treatment when assessed by IgE and interleukin 13. J Clin Endocrinol Metab. 2001;86(8):3540–4.
14. Hutchison BM, Kyle PM. Long-term visual outcome following orbital decompression for dysthyroid eye disease. Eye. 1995;9(Pt 5):578–81.
15. Liao SL, Chang TC, Lin LL. Transcaruncular orbital decompression: an alternate procedure for graves ophthalmopathy with compressive optic neuropathy. Am J Ophthalmol. 2006;141(5):810–8.
16. Graham SM, Brown CL, Carter KD, Song A, Nerad JA. Medial and lateral orbital wall surgery for balanced decompression in thyroid eye disease. Laryngoscope. 2003;113(7):1206–9.
17. Kikkawa DO, Pornpanich K, Cruz RC Jr, Levi L, Granet DB. Graded orbital decompression based on severity of proptosis. Ophthalmology. 2002;109(7): 1219–24.
18. Baldeschi L, MacAndie K, Koetsier E, Blank LE, Wiersinga WM. The influence of previous orbital irradiation on the outcome of rehabilitative decompression surgery in graves orbitopathy. Am J Ophthalmol. 2008; 145(3):534–40.
19. Shams PN, Ma R, Pickles T, Rootman J, Dolman PJ. Reduced risk of compressive optic neuropathy using orbital radiotherapy in patients with active thyroid eye disease. Am J Ophthalmol. 2014;157(6):1299–305.

22

Reference intervals for thyroid stimulating hormone and free thyroxine derived from neonates undergoing routine screening for congenital hypothyroidism at a university teaching hospital in Nairobi, Kenya

Geoffrey Omuse[1*], Ali Kassim[1], Francis Kiigu[1], Syeda Ra'ana Hussain[2] and Mary Limbe[2]

Abstract

Background: In order to accurately interpret neonatal thyroid function tests (TFTs), it is necessary to have population specific reference intervals (RIs) as there is significant variation across different populations possibly due to genetic, environmental or analytical issues. Despite the importance of RIs, globally there are very few publications on RIs for neonatal TFTs primarily due to ethical and technical issues surrounding recruitment of neonates for a prospective study. To the best of our knowledge, this is the first report from Africa on neonatal RIs for TFTs.

Methods: We used hospital based data largely derived from neonates attending the wellness clinic at the Aga Khan University Hospital Nairobi (AKUHN) where screening for congenital hypothyroidism is routinely done. Specifically we derived age and gender stratified RIs for free thyroxine (fT4) and thyroid stimulating hormone (TSH) which had been analyzed on a Roche e601 analyzer from 2011 to 2013. Determination of reference intervals was done using a non-parametric method.

Results: A total of 1639 and 1329 non duplicate TSH and fT4 values respectively were used to derive RIs. There was a decline in TSH and fT4 levels with increase in age. Compared to the Roche RIs, the derived RIs for TSH in neonates aged 0–6 days and those aged 7–30 days had lower upper limits and narrower RIs. The fT4 lower limits for neonates less than 7 days and those aged 7–30 days were higher than those proposed by Roche. There was a significant difference in TSH RIs between male and female neonates aged less than 15 days. No gender differences were seen for all other age stratifications for both TSH and fT4. Appropriate age and gender specific RIs were subsequently determined.

Conclusion: The AKUHN derived RIs for fT4 and TSH revealed similar age related trends to what has been published. However, the differences seen in upper and lower limits across different age stratifications when compared to the Roche RIs highlight the need for population specific RIs for TFTs especially when setting up a screening programme for congenital hypothyroidism. We subsequently recommend the adoption of the derived RIs by the AKUHN laboratory and hope that the RIs obtained can serve as a reference for the African population.

Keywords: Neonatal reference intervals, free thyroxine (fT4), Thyroid stimulating hormone (TSH), Congenital hypothyroidism (CH)

* Correspondence: g_omuse@yahoo.com
[1]Department of Pathology, Aga Khan University Hospital, P.O. Box 30270-00100, Nairobi, Kenya
Full list of author information is available at the end of the article

Background

Several pediatric reference intervals (RIs) for thyroid function tests (TFTs) have been published [1–7]. The neonatal RIs described in some of these studies were established on the basis of relatively small numbers of subjects or using analyzers with diverse measurement principles and analytical performance. For example, in earlier studies ultrasensitive immunoassays were not used to measure thyroid stimulating hormone (TSH) [3]. The use of TSH immunoassays that can accurately determine very low concentrations has resulted in a change in published RIs and resulted in the introduction of diagnoses such as subclinical hyperthyroidism. Use of TSH assays with different test methodologies has been shown to influence reported incidence of congenital hypothyroidism (CH) [8]. Despite the importance of screening for CH in the neonatal period, there are very few studies that specifically address RIs in this age group.

CH is one of the most common preventable causes of mental retardation. Its overall incidence ranges from 1 in 3000 to 1 in 4000 newborn infants [9, 10]. The most common cause of CH is a primary disorder of the thyroid gland where reduced function from dysgenesis or dyshormonogenesis results in an increase in TSH concentration [11]. TFTs play an important role in screening for CH before the onset of symptoms hence enabling the institution of early treatment which has been associated with better clinical outcomes [12]. The prevalence of CH has been reported to have increased after the introduction of screening tests [13–15]. Several factors could contribute to a variation in reported prevalence of CH across different populations. Some of these factors include race and ethnicity [15]. Furthermore, the testing algorithm adopted when screening for CH as well as the RIs used can contribute to the variation in CH prevalence. Initially, many screening programs performed a thyroxine (T4) test, with a follow-up TSH test on infants with values below a specified T4 cutoff. This strategy not only identified primary CH but was able to identify neonates with secondary hypothyroidism. However, with advancements in the sensitivity of TSH assays, there has been a move towards the use of TSH as a screening test [12]. This is because serum TSH has a log-linear relationship with circulating thyroid hormone levels with a 2-fold change in free thyroxine (fT4) producing a 100-fold change in TSH [16]. Some programs have undertaken pilot programs measuring both fT4 and TSH on all newborns resulting in a higher diagnostic rate of congenital hypothyroidism [17].

It is recommended by the international federation of clinical chemistry (IFCC) that RIs should be population-specific and derived from a set of reference individuals representative of a reference population [18]. The clinical laboratory standards institute (CLSI) also recommends derivation of RIs through a formal study where samples are collected from a reference group comprising a minimum of 120 individuals identified from a reference population through probability sampling and use of non-parametric statistical methods to derive RIs. It also recommends transference or verification of RIs as an option in the event that establishing population specific RIs is not possible [19]. For a CH screening program, the laboratory carrying out testing should use TFT cut offs derived from the local population to ensure that they are appropriate since misdiagnosis can easily result from the adoption of inappropriate RIs.

At the Aga Khan University Hospital Nairobi (AKUHN), TFTs are performed on the Roche e601 analyzer. The cut offs recommended by Roche for fT4 and TSH in babies less than 3 months of age were derived from only 223 and 222 babies respectively from Leipzig, Germany [20]. This population was comprised of primarily a Caucasian population which was quite different from the AKUHN population which is largely comprised of black Africans.

We therefore set out to derive age and gender specific neonatal RIs for fT4 and TSH at AKUHN and compare them with the manufacturer's intervals to determine whether any differences existed.

Methods

Study site

The study was carried out at AKUHN which is a Joint Commission International accredited (JCIA) 300 bed private hospital. It is a not-for-profit institution that provides both primary and tertiary health care services. It has state of the art intensive care and high dependency units for children and adults as well as a laboratory that has attained International Organization for Standardization (ISO) 15189:2007 accreditation since July 2011. The hospital also runs a number of general and specialized outpatient clinics. Among these is the Well Baby Clinic where infants are followed up. Since newborn screening is not yet a policy in Kenya, the hospital routinely encourages parents to have their babies screened for CH and have blood samples drawn on the fourth or fifth day of life, though some babies get screened later than this, but still within the newborn period, for different reasons. For pre-terms, routine screening for CH is only performed on attainment of an age equivalent to a term baby. Data on TSH and fT4 for neonates was obtained from the hospital health management system from February 2011 to December 2013. Specifically, we extracted consecutive data for all neonates who had fT4 or TSH done during the specified time period. Most of the neonatal TFTs are done as part of routine screening for CH and it was thought that this would serve as an ideal reference population assuming that neonates attending a wellness clinic will most likely be healthy. A neonate was defined as any newborn

30 days of age and below. This was used as a criterion when extracting data from the hospital health management system. File reviews were carried out only for neonates with TSH or fT4 outside the Roche RIs so as to identify and exclude from statistical analysis those with a diagnosis of a thyroid disorder or an acute illness. Neonates with both fT4 and TSH values outside Roche RIs were excluded from the study.

Ethical approval

Informed consent from the patients whose laboratory data was used was not required as this study was classified as a clinical audit according to the hospitals research guidelines. Ethical waiver was obtained from the AKUHNs health research ethics committee (2013/REC-15).

Thyroid function test determination

TFTs were carried out on the Roche e601 analyzer (Roche diagnostic GmbH, Mannheim, Germany) which uses the electro-chemiluminescence immunoassay principle to determine the concentrations of fT4 and TSH. Samples used were serum or plasma. The e601 TSH assay is a third generation immunoassay according to the definition by Spencer et al. [21]. Its functional sensitivity is 0.014 μIU/mL and limit of detection 0.005 μIU/mL. The coefficient of variation (CV) for fT4 was 1.97 % and 2.98 % at concentrations of 15.4 pmol/L and 55.3 pmol/L respectively. For TSH, the CVs were 2.64 % and 2.42 % at concentrations of 3.4 μIU/mL and 13.6 μIU/mL respectively. Both the assays are enrolled for the Randox International Quality Assessment Scheme (RIQAS) and performance has been satisfactory over the period for which the data was obtained.

Data analysis

Reference interval determination was performed using Reference Value Advisor v2.1 (National Veterinary School, Toulouse, France) [22]. This is a free set of Excel macros that compute reference intervals from data contained in a spreadsheet. It carries out both parametric and non-parametric analysis for all data sets provided. The non-parametric derived RIs that capture the mid 95 % of reference values were used to determine RIs for this study. Initially, the data was stratified into 2 age groups 0–6 days and 7–30 days to enable comparison with Roche RIs. Subsequently, further age and gender stratification was done and comparisons using Mann–Whitney *U* test or Kruskal-Wallis H test were performed to determine differences between groups. Median or mean rank values were compared as appropriate. The age-wise stratification for determining RIs was 0–7 days, 8–14 days, 15–22 days and 23–30 days. Comparisons that showed no statistically significant difference after the independent samples median test were grouped together. Inferential statistical analysis was performed using IBM International Business Machines Statistical Package for the Social Sciences (IBM SPSS) Statistics for Windows, Version 21.0. (Armonk, NewYork, IBM Corporation). For all RIs, 90 % confidence limits were calculated for both the lower (2.5th percentile) and upper limits (97.5th percentile). RIs were also determined using standard and robust parametric methods to compare with the non-parametrically derived RIs. This was done on both untransformed data and data transformed using the Box-Cox method. Testing for normality was done using Anderson-Darling and a test for symmetry was performed for the robust method. Outliers and suspect data were determined using the Tukey's method depending on whether values were less or greater than 3 times the inter-quartile range (IQR) or 1.5–3 times the IQR relative to the first and third quartiles. The Clinical Laboratory Standards Institute (CLSI) guidelines for determining reference intervals were used for this analysis [19]. P-values less than 0.05 were considered significant.

Results

A total of 1673 and 1359 non duplicate values for TSH and fT4 respectively were obtained, however 34 TSH and 30 fT4 values respectively were excluded after review of 119 medical records and all TFT results. A total of 29 patients had both fT4 and TSH values excluded. The main reasons for exclusion included presence of an acute illness such as neonatal sepsis or jaundice, both fT4 and TSH values outside the Roche RIs and discrepancies in age. Subsequently, 1639 TSH and 1329 fT4 values were used in determining RIs.

There was a general decline in TSH with increase in age as shown in Fig. 1. The proposed Roche RIs for neonates in the age group 0–6 days is 0.7–15.2 μIU/ml and 0.72–11.0 μIU/ml for the age group 7–30 days. Out of 632 neonates in the age group 0–6 days, 38 (6.0 %) fell outside the Roche RIs, with 9 (1.4 %) having values above the upper limit. In the age group 7 to 30 days, out of 1009 neonates, 15 (1.5 %) fell outside the Roche reference limits with only 1 (0.1 %) having a value above the upper limit.

Compared to the Roche RIs, the derived RI for TSH in the 0–6 day age group was lower with narrower confidence limits around the upper and lower limits as shown in Fig. 2. For the 7–30 day old neonates, the derived RI had a narrower spread and lower upper limit with narrower confidence limits around the upper and lower limits as shown in Fig. 2. Age stratified comparison of medians showed no statistically significant difference between neonates aged 0–7 days and 8–14 days as well as those aged 15–22 days and 23–30 days. These were subsequently grouped into 0–14 days and 15–30 days respectively for further analysis. There was a statistically

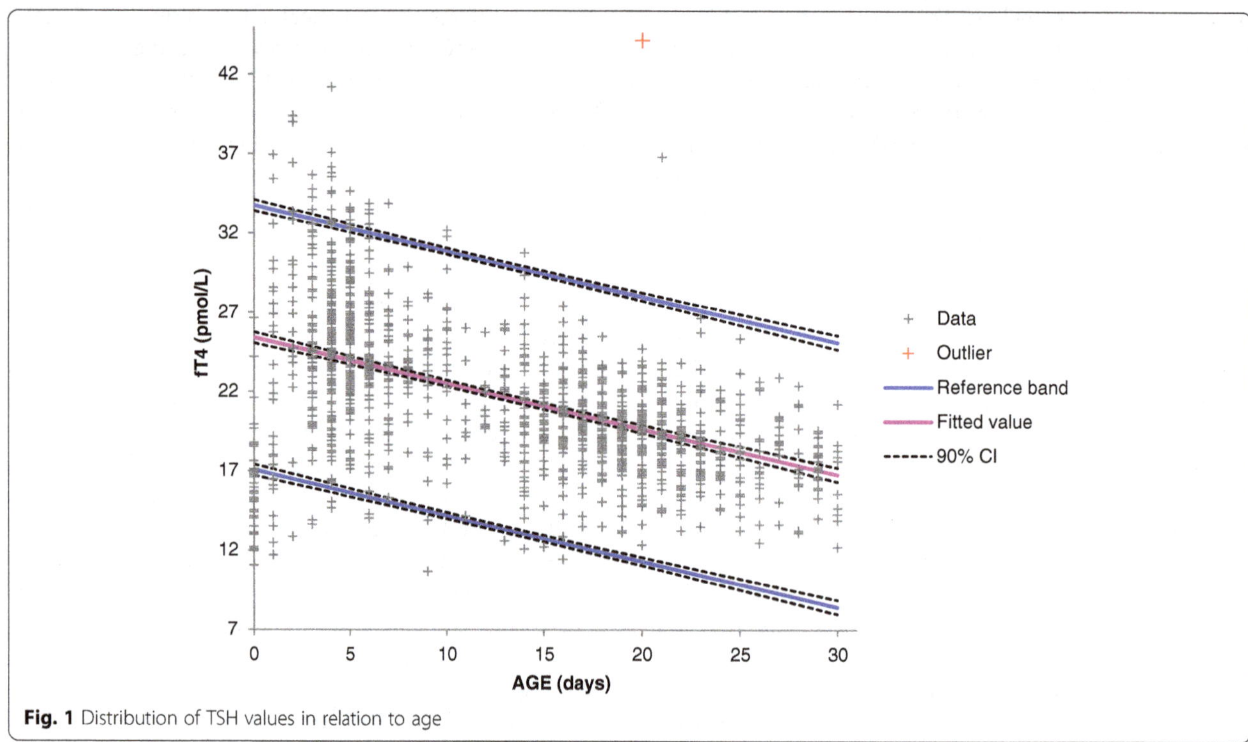

Fig. 1 Distribution of TSH values in relation to age

significant difference in TSH mean ranks between neonates aged 0–14 days and those aged 15–30 days (U = 312129, p = .029). There was a statistically significant difference in TSH mean ranks between male and female neonates aged 0–14 days (U = 87542, p = .002). Age and gender stratified TSH RIs are shown in Table 1.

The TSH RIs derived parametrically after data transformation and exclusion of outliers were similar to the non-parametrically derived RIs. However, most of the data failed to normalize after Box-Cox transformation hence the non-parametrically derived RIs were deemed most appropriate.

For fT4, the suggested Roche RIs are 11.0–32.0 pmol/L and 11.5–28.3 pmol/L for neonates in the age groups 0–6 days and 7–30 days respectively. Out of 515 neonates in the age group 0–6 days, 43 (8.3 %) had values outside the Roche RIs with all of them being above the upper limit. In neonates aged 7–30 days, 6 out of 814 (0.7 %) had fT4 values outside the Roche RIs with 2 (0.6 %) having values below the lower limit. Four of the

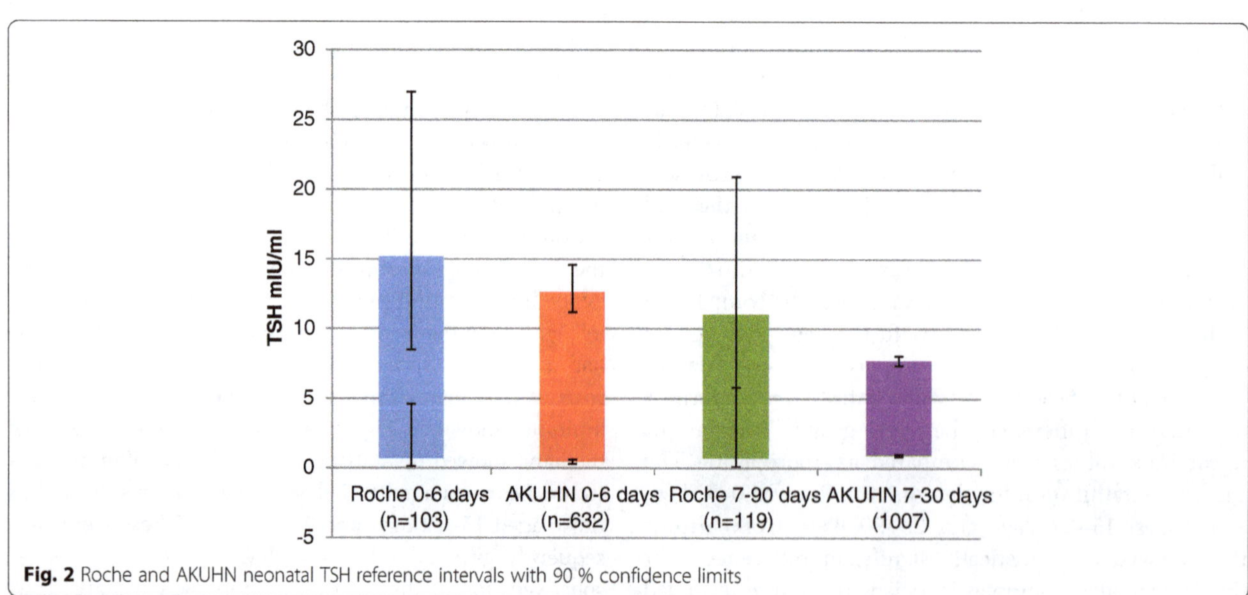

Fig. 2 Roche and AKUHN neonatal TSH reference intervals with 90 % confidence limits

Table 1 AKUHN non-parametrically derived neonatal reference intervals for thyroid stimulating hormone (TSH)

Age (days)	Number(gender)	Lower Limit (μIU/mL) (90 % confidence limits)	Median	Upper Limit (μIU/mL) (90 % confidence limits)
0 to 14	415 (M)	0.59 (0.42–0.77)	3.31	12.84 (10.62–14.44)
0 to 14	479 (F)	0.56 (0.42–0.69)	2.74	11.00 (9.56–12.33)
15 to 30	359 (M)	0.90 (0.83–0.97-0.94)	2.71	7.46 (7.01–7.83)
	386 (F)			

Key: *M* Male, *F* Female

5 had corresponding TSH results with only 1 being above the Roche upper limit.

There was a decline in fT4 levels with increase in age as shown in Fig. 3. The upper and lower limits of the derived RI for neonates less than 7 days old were higher than the ones proposed by Roche. For neonates aged 7–30 days, the derived RI had a higher lower limit and a narrower interval compared to the one proposed by Roche as shown in Fig. 4.

There was a statistically significant difference in the fT4 means across the 4 age stratifications. Gender-wise comparisons in the different age strata were not statistically significant ($x^2(3) = 379.601$, $p = 0.000$). RIs were subsequently derived for the different age strata as shown in Table 2.

Discussion

There is scanty data on the prevalence of CH in Africa most likely due to a greater focus on infectious diseases which are major causes of morbidity and mortality in children [23]. It is therefore not surprising that there is scarce data on RIs for neonatal TFTs from the African continent. To the best of our knowledge, this is the first study to publish neonatal RIs for TFTs from Africa.

In order to avoid the lengthy and expensive process of establishing RIs, many clinical laboratories adopt values from in-vitro diagnostic company kit inserts, text books or published literature. This is despite the possibility that the populations used in deriving such RIs may be different from the populations served by the respective laboratories. There are very few published studies on neonatal RIs for TFTs partly due to the difficulty in enrolling neonates. The CALIPER study which was carried out in Canada and has so far enrolled 8500 children from birth to 18 years of age has established RIs for many analytes including TFTs [24]. Carrying out a formal RI study is extremely challenging given the need to standardize all phases of the laboratory testing cycle and the significant cost involved. In the absence of a formal RI study, hospital data especially from a primary care setting can be used as an alternative especially for tests

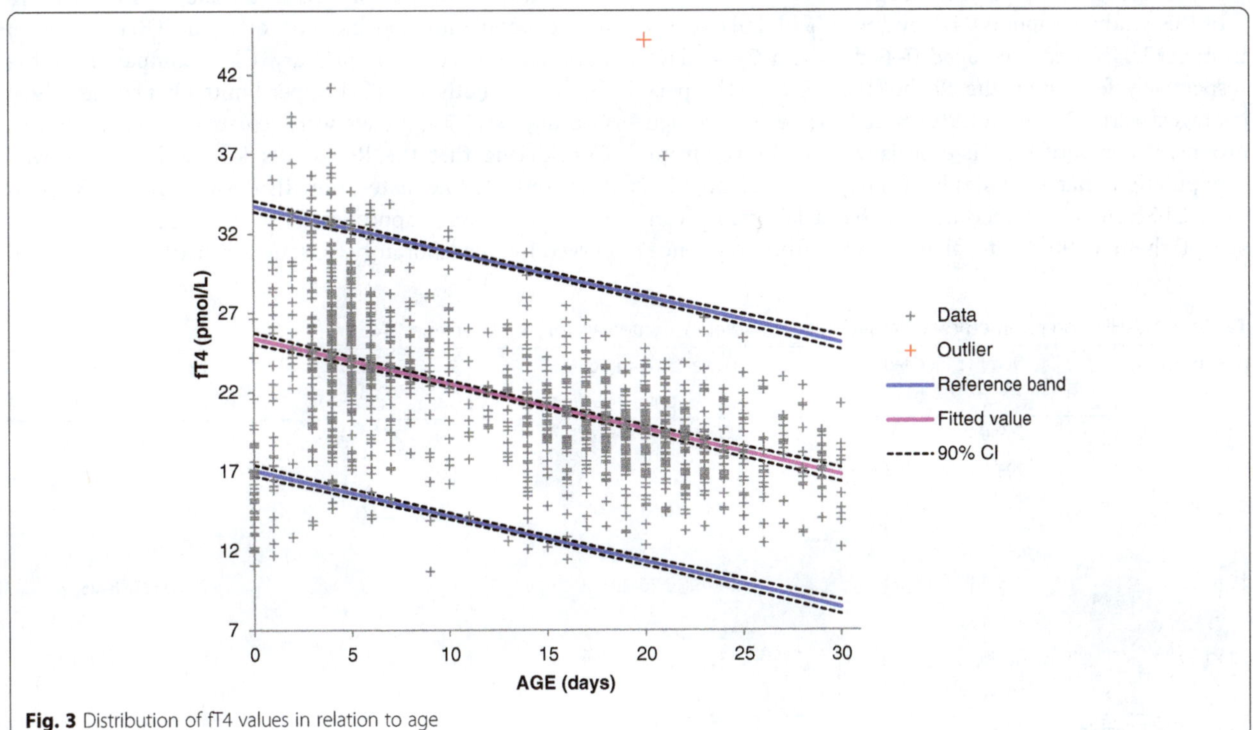

Fig. 3 Distribution of fT4 values in relation to age

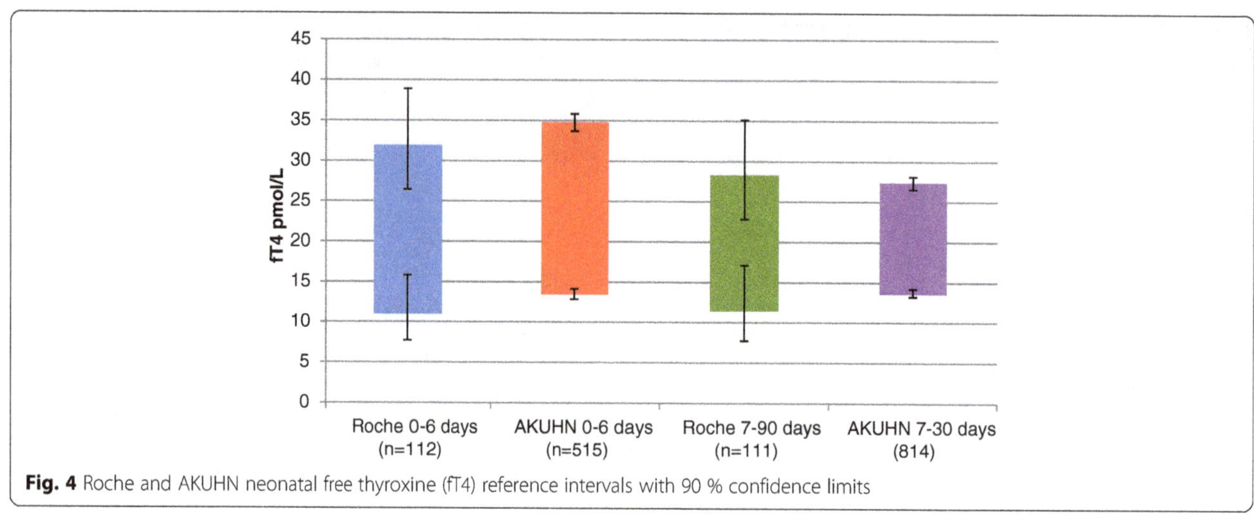

Fig. 4 Roche and AKUHN neonatal free thyroxine (fT4) reference intervals with 90 % confidence limits

that are performed routinely to screen for conditions whose prevalence is not high [25–27]. Given that the prevalence of CH is between 1 in 3000 to 1 in 10000 new born infants [9, 10, 28], most neonates screened for CH would most likely be healthy and serve as appropriate reference individuals. Zurakowski et al. used hospital data collected between January 1993 and August 1996 to derive RIs for T4, T3, TSH, and fT4. This data was obtained from outpatient records at Children's Hospital in Boston for patients 1 month through 20 years of age [3]. Kapelari et al. carried out a similar study more recently using hospital data from the Medical University Innsbruck in Austria for children aged 1 day to 18 years of age [4].

In this study, we found 94 % and 98.5 % of TSH values from AKUHN neonates aged 0–6 days and 7–30 days respectively fell within the Roche RIs. For fT4, the percentages were 91.7 % and 99.3 % for the respective age groups. When verifying RIs especially those derived from a population that is dissimilar from your local population, CLSI guidelines recommend that a laboratory can accept them if 90 % of values derived from reference individuals from the population served by the laboratory fall within the RIs being verified [19].

The intent of CH screening programs is biased towards detection of primary CH. Given the log linear relationship of fT4 with TSH, measurement of TSH is preferred as a cost effective approach to screening for primary CH. A slight decline in fT4 results in a significant rise in TSH allowing for the diagnosis of subclinical hypothyroidism and possibly early intervention before development of overt symptoms. There is marked variability in published neonatal TSH RIs most likely due to differences in reference populations arising from genetic or environmental factors. It is, therefore, important to adopt population-specific cut offs for TSH so as to optimize detection of primary CH. Compared to the Roche RIs, both our TSH upper limits for neonates aged 0–6 days and 7–30 days were lower with narrower RIs. Considering that the Roche RIs for TSH were derived from only 223 neonates, our RIs derived from 1639 neonates are more appropriate to the local population served by our laboratory. A standard textbook of clinical

Table 2 AKUHN non-parametrically derived neonatal reference intervals for free thyroxine (fT4)

Age (days)	Number (gender)	Lower Limit (pmol/L) (90 % confidence limits)	Median	Upper Limit (pmol/L) (90 % confidence limits)
0 to 7	259 (M) 293 (F)	13.62 (12.98–14.16)	25.10	34.75 (33.64–35.67)
8 to 14	73 (M) 72 (F)	13.45 (10.68–15.44)	22.27	30.17 (27.93–32.18)
15 to 22	215 (M) 250 (F)	14.16 (13.26–14.63)	19.56	24.80 (23.98–25.48)
23 to 30	87 (M) 80 (F)	13.26 (12.23–13.90)	18.15	23.37 (22.39–26.64)

Key: *M* Male, *F* Female

chemistry has proposed a TSH RI of 1.0–39 μIU/mL for neonates less than 5 days of age and 1.7–9.1 μIU/mL for those aged 2–20 weeks [5]. These are significantly different from what we have derived and would therefore not be ideal for our population. The TSH RI derived from the CALIPER study for babies aged 4 days to 6 months is 0.73–4.77 μIU/mL. This was obtained from 278 babies with equal numbers of males and females and analysis done on the Abbott Architect i2000 [24]. The low upper limit for TSH published from the CALIPER study most likely is a consequence of including babies as old as 6 months of age in the same group as neonates despite the known decline in TSH and fT4 with increase in age within the first year of life. Kapelari et al. determined a TSH RI for neonates of 0.7–18.1 μIU/mL and demonstrated a marked decline in TSH values in the neonatal period very similar to what we have observed [4]. Unexpectedly, we found a significant difference in the distribution and mean rank values between male and female neonates aged 14 days and below. The female neonates had a lower RI which is in keeping with a trend observed by Zurakowski et al. for babies aged 1 year and above [3]. Kapelari et al. found that males had higher mean fT3 concentrations but no sex-differences were found for TSH and fT4 between age-matched serum samples. The observation of a significant gender wise difference in mean rank values for TSH is therefore unique and needs to be further investigated as an obvious explanation is not forthcoming.

There was a general decline in fT4 values with increase in age within the neonatal period which is in keeping with what has been published previously [1, 2, 4, 24]. However, compared to the RIs provided by Roche, our fT4 upper and lower limits for the age group 0–6 days are higher and more precise. For the age group 7–30 days, the lower limit is higher and upper limit lower giving a narrower interval than what is provided by Roche [20]. As mentioned earlier, the Roche study that determined fT4 RIs only included 223 babies compared to 1329 in our study. Burtis et al. has published fT4 RIs for neonates aged 1–4 days as 28.4–68.4 pmol/L and 10.3–25.8 pmol/L for those aged more than 2 weeks [5]. For neonates less than 7 days of age, the fT4 lower limit was 13.62 pmol/L. This is significantly lower than what is proposed by Burtis et al. and potentially would reduce the number of neonates that would require unnecessary follow up. In the CALIPER study, the fT4 RI for both male and female neonates aged 5–14 days was 13.47–41.32 pmol/L and 8.71–32.53 pmol/L for those aged 15–29 days. The CALIPER study used values from 264 neonates with equal numbers of males and females [24]. In our study, the lower limit for fT4 for neonates aged 8–14 days is 13.45 pmol/L which is very similar to the CALIPER study. For neonates aged 15–22 days and 23–30 days, the lower limits of 14.16 pmol/L and 13.26 pmol/L respectively are higher than that derived for the CALIPER study. We found no significant difference in RIs between male and female neonates across all age stratifications. Zurakowski et al. found a significant difference between males and females in T4 but not fT4 levels though their study did not include neonates [3]. Djemli et al. found a significant difference in fT4 levels between males and females in the age group 15–17 years [1].

We do recommend the adoption of our derived RIs by our laboratory and anticipate an increase in the number of neonates found to have elevated TSH given the lower upper limits. The age and gender wise stratification of RIs will ensure that the interpretation of fT4 and TSH is based on appropriate cut-offs that are sensitive to the dynamic nature of TFTs within the neonatal period and hopefully this will result in higher sensitivity for detection of CH.

Our study is limited by the fact that we used hospital data without having well defined exclusion criteria to ensure that sick neonates or those with thyroid disorders were not included. However, most of our data is from neonates attending the wellness clinic which largely comprises healthy neonates. We also reviewed medical records for neonates with out-of-range values and excluded those with acute illnesses. None of the neonates had a confirmed diagnosis of CH at the time of carrying out the study though the follow up data was limited to a maximum of 3 years as the review of medical records was done in 2014. We also carried out parametric analysis to determine RIs after excluding outliers but found no significant change. We therefore believe the non-parametrically derived RIs are appropriate for our neonatal population.

Conclusion

This is the first study from Africa that has published TSH and fT4 RIs for neonates and will go a long way in providing a guide for the interpretation of TFTs especially when setting up a CH screening programme where the target population is largely a black African population. The differences seen when compared to other published RIs may be reflective of a difference in reference populations or analytical methodologies. More studies from a similar population across the African continent will help verify the findings of this study.

Abbreviations

AKUHN: Aga Khan University Hospital Nairobi; ANOVA: Analysis of variance; CH: Congenital hypothyridism; CLSI: Clinical Laboratory Standards Institute; fT3: free triiodothyronine; fT4: free thyroxine; IFCC: International Federation of Clinical Chemistry; IQR: Inter Quartile Range; RI: Reference interval; SPSS: Statistical Package for the Social Sciences; T4: Thyroxine; TFT: Thyroid function test; TSH: Thyroid stimulating hormone.

Acknowledgement
None.

Funding
None.

Authors' contributions
GO conceived and designed the study, performed the data analysis and drafted the manuscript. AK helped in the design of the study, data collection, data analysis and drafting of the manuscript. FK helped in the design of the study, data collection, data analysis and critical revision of the manuscript. SH participated in data collection and critical revision of the manuscript. ML participated in its design, coordination and critical revision of the manuscript. All authors read and approved the final manuscript.

Competing interests
The authors declare that they have no competing interests.

Author details
[1]Department of Pathology, Aga Khan University Hospital, P.O. Box 30270-00100, Nairobi, Kenya. [2]Department of Paediatrics, Aga Khan University Hospital, P.O. Box 30270-00100, Nairobi, Kenya.

References
1. Djemli A, Van Vliet G, Belgoudi J, Lambert M, Delvin EE. Reference intervals for free thyroxine, total triiodothyronine, thyrotropin and thyroglobulin for Quebec newborns, children and teenagers. Clin Biochem. 2004;37:328–30.
2. Lott JA, Sardovia-Iyer M, Speakman KS, Lee KK. Age-dependent cutoff values in screening newborns for hypothyroidism. Clin Biochem. 2004;37:791–7.
3. Zurakowski D, Di Canzio J, Majzoub JA. Pediatric reference intervals for serum thyroxine, triiodothyronine, thyrotropin, and free thyroxine. Clin Chem. 1999;45:1087–91.
4. Kapelari K, Kirchlechner C, Hogler W, Schweitzer K, Virgolini I, Moncayo R. Pediatric reference intervals for thyroid hormone levels from birth to adulthood: a retrospective study. BMC Endocr Disord. 2008;8:15.
5. Burtis CA, Ashwood ER, Bruns DE. Tietz Textbook of Clinical Chemistry and Molecular Diagnostics. 4th ed. Missouri: Elsevier Inc.; 2006.
6. Elmlinger MW, Kuhnel W, Lambrecht HG, Ranke MB. Reference intervals from birth to adulthood for serum thyroxine (T4), triiodothyronine (T3), free T3, free T4, thyroxine binding globulin (TBG) and thyrotropin (TSH). Clin Chem Lab Med. 2001;39:973–9.
7. Hubner U, Englisch C, Werkmann H, Butz H, Georgs T, Zabransky S, Herrmann W. Continuous age-dependent reference ranges for thyroid hormones in neonates, infants, children and adolescents established using the ADVIA Centaur Analyzer. Clin Chem Lab Med. 2002;40:1040–7.
8. Hertzberg V, Mei J, Therrell BL. Effect of laboratory practices on the incidence rate of congenital hypothyroidism. Pediatrics. 2010;125 Suppl 2:S48–53.
9. Haddow JE, Palomaki GE, Allan WC, Williams JR, Knight GJ, Gagnon J, O'Heir CE, Mitchell ML, Hermos RJ, Waisbren SE, et al. Maternal thyroid deficiency during pregnancy and subsequent neuropsychological development of the child. N Engl J Med. 1999;341:549–55.
10. Waller DK, Anderson JL, Lorey F, Cunningham GC. Risk factors for congenital hypothyroidism: an investigation of infant's birth weight, ethnicity, and gender in California, 1990–1998. Teratology. 2000;62:36–41.
11. Rastogi MV, LaFranchi SH. Congenital hypothyroidism. Orphanet J Rare Dis. 2010;5:17.
12. LaFranchi SH. Approach to the diagnosis and treatment of neonatal hypothyroidism. J Clin Endocrinol Metab. 2011;96:2959–67.
13. Alm J, Larsson A, Zetterstrom R. Congenital hypothyroidism in Sweden. Incidence and age at diagnosis. Acta Paediatr Scand. 1978;67:1–3.
14. Fisher DA. Second International Conference on Neonatal Thyroid Screening: progress report. J Pediatr. 1983;102:653–4.
15. Harris KB, Pass KA. Increase in congenital hypothyroidism in New York State and in the United States. Mol Genet Metab. 2007;91:268–77.
16. Andersen S, Bruun NH, Pedersen KM, Laurberg P. Biologic variation is important for interpretation of thyroid function tests. Thyroid. 2003;13: 1069 78.
17. van Tijn DA, de Vijlder JJ, Verbeeten Jr B, Verkerk PH, Vulsma T. Neonatal detection of congenital hypothyroidism of central origin. J Clin Endocrinol Metab. 2005;90:3350–9.
18. Solberg HE. International Federation of Clinical Chemistry. Scientific committee, Clinical Section. Expert Panel on Theory of Reference Values and International Committee for Standardization in Haematology Standing Committee on Reference Values. Approved recommendation (1986) on the theory of reference values. Part 1. The concept of reference values. Clin Chim Acta. 1987;165:111–8.
19. CLSI. Defining, establishing, and verifying reference intervals in the clinical laboratory; approved guideline. In: Book Defining, establishing, and verifying reference intervals in the clinical laboratory; approved guideline, vol. 28. 3rd ed. 2008.
20. Roche Diagnostics GmbH: Reference intervals for children and adults. Elecsys Thyroid Tests. 2008
21. Spencer CA, Takeuchi M, Kazarosyan M. Current status and performance goals for serum thyrotropin (TSH) assays. Clin Chem. 1996;42:140–5.
22. Geffre A, Concordet D, Braun JP, Trumel C. Reference Value Advisor: a new freeware set of macroinstructions to calculate reference intervals with Microsoft Excel. Vet Clin Pathol. 2011;40:107–12.
23. Child mortality, Millenium Development Goal (MDG) 4. [http://www.who.int/pmnch/media/press_materials/fs/fs_mdg4_childmortality/en/]. Accessed 07 Dec 2015.
24. Bailey D, Colantonio D, Kyriakopoulou L, Cohen AH, Chan MK, Armbruster D, Adeli K. Marked biological variance in endocrine and biochemical markers in childhood: establishment of pediatric reference intervals using healthy community children from the CALIPER cohort. Clin Chem. 2013;59:1393–405.
25. Harwood SJ, Cole GW. Reference values based on hospital admission laboratory data. JAMA. 1978;240:270–4.
26. Kouri T, Kairisto V, Virtanen A, Uusipaikka E, Rajamaki A, Finneman H, Juva K, Koivula T, Nanto V. Reference intervals developed from data for hospitalized patients: computerized method based on combination of laboratory and diagnostic data. Clin Chem. 1994;40:2209–15.
27. Yamakado M, Ichihara K, Matsumoto Y, Ishikawa Y, Kato K, Komatsubara Y, Takaya N, Tomita S, Kawano R, Takada K, Watanabe K. Derivation of gender and age-specific reference intervals from fully normal Japanese individuals and the implications for health screening. Clin Chim Acta. 2015;447:105–14.
28. Zilka LJ, Lott JA, Baker LC, Linard SM. Finding blunders in thyroid testing: experience in newborns. J Clin Lab Anal. 2008;22:254–6.

23

Complicated Gitelman syndrome and autoimmune thyroid disease: a case report with a new homozygous mutation in the SLC12A3 gene

Haiyang Zhou†, Xinhuan Liang†, Yingfen Qing, Bihui Meng, Jia Zhou, Song Huang, Shurong Lu, Zhenxing Huang, Haiyan Yang, Yan Ma* and Zuojie Luo*

Abstract

Background: Gitelman syndrome (GS) is an inherited autosomal recessive renal tubular disorder characterized by low levels of potassium and magnesium in the blood, decreased excretion of calcium in the urine, and elevated blood pH. GS is caused by an inactivating mutation in the SLC12A3 gene, which is located on the long arm of chromosome 16 (16q13) and encodes a thiazide-sensitive sodium chloride cotransporter (NCCT).

Case presentation: A 45-year-old man with Graves' disease complicated by paroxysmal limb paralysis had a diagnosis of thyrotoxic periodic paralysis for 12 years. However, his serum potassium level remained low despite sufficiently large doses of potassium supplementation. Finally, gene analysis revealed a homozygous mutation in the SLC12A3 gene. After his thyroid function gradually returned to normal, his serum potassium level remained low, but his paroxysmal limb paralysis resolved.

Conclusions: GS combined with hyperthyroidism can manifest as frequent episodes of periodic paralysis; to date, this comorbidity has been reported only in eastern Asian populations. This case prompted us to more seriously consider the possibility of GS associated with thyroid dysfunction.

Keywords: Gitelman syndrome, Graves' disease, Hypokalemia

Background

Gitelman syndrome (GS) is an inherited autosomal recessive renal tubular disorder characterized by low levels of potassium and magnesium in the blood, decreased excretion of calcium in the urine, and elevated blood pH. GS is caused by an inactivating mutation in the SLC12A3 gene, which is located on the long arm of chromosome 16 (16q13) and encodes a thiazide-sensitive sodium chloride cotransporter (NCCT). Graves' disease (GD) is a common cause of hyperthyroidism. In our department, we diagnosed a patient with GD and GS.

* Correspondence: luoma628@163.com; zhouhaiyang4000@163.com
†Haiyang Zhou and Xinhuan Liang contributed equally to this work.
The Department of Endocrinology, The First Affiliated Hospital of Guangxi Medical University, Nanning 530021, China

Case presentation

The patient was a 45-year-old male with a 12-year history of paroxysmal weakness of the limbs. He was diagnosed with hypokalemic periodic paralysis in 2005 and hyperthyroidism in 2008. He had taken antithyroid drugs on an irregular basis since 2008 but had not undergone proper biochemical examination. Whenever he felt that his weakness was becoming severe, he would self-prescribe potassium chloride. In June 2017, the extent of his lower limb weakness increased such that he could no longer walk. He took potassium chloride without improvement. Subsequently, he was admitted to another hospital. His temperature was 36.7 °C, and his pulse was 96 beats/min. The muscle strength in his lower limbs was grade II [1], and that in his upper limbs was grade III. His limb muscle tone was normal. His electrolyte and blood marker levels were as follows: K^+, 1.4 mmol/l; Na^+, 138 mmol/l, Cl^-, 97 mmol/l; Ca^{2+}, 2.61 mmol/l; free triiodothyronine (FT3) 6.96 pmol/l (1.86–6.44); free thyroxine (FT4) 38.96 mIU/l (11.45–22.14); thyroid-stimulating hormone (TSH) < 0.01 mIU/l (0.4–4.5); thyroglobulin antibody (TgAb) 16.61 IU/ml (0–150); and thyrotropin receptor antibody (TRAb) 22.36 mIU/l (0–5). Thyroid ultrasound demonstrated diffuse thyromegaly with a rich blood supply. The patient was diagnosed with GD and hypokalemic periodic paralysis and was treated with propylthiouracil (PTU) and potassium chloride. However, 2 days later, despite improvement of his weakness, his temperature increased to 41 °C, and he experienced cough and expectoration. Computed tomography (CT) imaging of his lungs revealed pneumonia. He was subsequently treated with cefazolin and transferred to our hospital 2 days later.

When the patient was admitted to our department, his limb weakness had significantly improved. He had a temperature of 38.8 °C, a pulse of 96 beats/min, a breathing rate of 20 respirations/min, a blood pressure of 106/68 mmHg, and grade II thyroid enlargement. Vascular murmur was audible in the thyroid. The muscle strength in his limbs was grade V, and his limb muscle tone was normal. The patient's biochemical parameters were as follows (the reference values are different from those used in the previous department): [blood count] leukocytes 13.10×10^9/l, neutrophils 11.99×10^9/l and hemoglobin 13.3 g/dl; [serum electrolytes] K^+ 2.110 mmol/l, Na^+ 131.6 mmol/l, Cl^- 91.1 mmol/l, Ca^{2+} 1.850 mmol/l, and Mg^{2+} 0.540 mmol/l; [thyroid function and thyroid antibodies] triiodothyronine (T3) 1.40 mmol/l (1.34–2.75), thyroxine (T4) > 300 nmol/l (78.38–157.40), FT3 5.32 pmol/l (3.60–6.00), FT4 51.23 pmol/l (7.86–14.41), TSH 0.01 mIU/l (0.34–5.65), thyroid peroxidase antibody (TPOAb) 36.33 IU/ml (0–30), TRAb 9.011 IU/ml (0–30), TgAb 6.04% (< 30%), and thyroid microsomal antibody (TMAB) 6.48% (< 20%); and creatine kinase (CK) 1398 U/l (38–174) and CK-MB 29 U/l (0.0–25.0). The patient's liver and kidney functions were normal. We treated him with cefazolin, propranolol, PTU and potassium chloride. The patient's vital signs and strength normalized after 3 days, and his leukocyte count had decreased to 5.97×10^9/l, his neutrophils had decreased to 3.59×10^9/l, and his CK had decreased to 40 U/l. However, his serum potassium level remained low despite 24 g/d of potassium supplementation. Additionally, the patient had hypomagnesemia and metabolic alkalosis (the results are shown in Tables 1 and 2). Further testing showed that his renin activity (supine) was 5.17 ng/ml/h (reference value 0.15–2.33), his aldosterone level was 436.10 pg/ml (10–160), his random urinary calcium/creatinine ratio was 0.23, his osteocalcin level was 1.06 ng/ml (6.00–48.00), his parathyroid hormone level was 11.22 pg/ml (6.0–80.0) and his calcitonin level was 4.87 pg/ml (0.00–18.00).

Based on these results, we suspected that the patient did not have thyrotoxic periodic paralysis (TPP) but rather GS. Therefore, we sent a blood sample to Beijing Huada Company for sequencing. The Next Generation Sequencing (NGS) was used. The sequencing protocol was based on the Roche Nimblegen SeqCap EZ Choice XL Library for exon trapping. A total of 25 genes (Table 3) known to be associated with hypokalemia were targeted and the total size of target regions was 11.8 M. Libraries were prepared with the Kapa Hyper Prep kit and sequencing was carried out by Illumina NextSeq500 System. The sequencing data were compared to the human genome by BWA (0.7.12-r1039) software (http://bio-bwa.sourceforge.net/), and ANNOVAR (Date: 2015-06-17) was used to annotate the mutation sites based on dbSNP, Clinvar, ExAC, and 1000 genomes, among others. We found a homozygous mutation in the SLC12A3 gene (Exon12 1562-1564delTCA) with an amino acid change of 522delIle, which was first reported as a compound heterozygous mutation.by Vargas-Poussou [2]. The mutation was confirmed by sanger sequencing. No other phenotypes were found, including those for Bartter syndrome, hypokalemic periodic paralysis,Liddle syndrome, hyperaldosteronism, and apparent mineralocorticoid excess. The diagnosis was changed to GD with GS. Moreover, we obtained blood samples from the patient's mother and son (his father had passed away) who did not have hypokalemia and hyperthyroidism. Both of them were proved as heterozygous mutation carriers by sanger sequencing. The sequencing chromatograms are shown in Figs. 1 and 2. The patient had three brothers and one sister, but we were unable to obtain blood samples from them.

In addition to antithyroid drugs (methimazole 30 mg/d), we gave the patient potassium chloride (3 g/d), potassium citrate (6 g/d), and magnesium potassium aspartate (1.788 g/d). At the follow-up

Table 1 Serum and urine electrolyte levels on admission

	24th July		5th August	
	Urine electrolytes	Serum electrolytes	Urine electrolytes	Serum electrolytes
K (mmol/l)	214.05	2.850	245.71	3.550
Ca (mmol/l)	4.80	2.303	2.91	2.309
Mg (mmol/l)	6.40	0.720	3.35	0.54
Urine volume (ml)	3200	–	3100	–

Table 2 Blood gas analysis on admission

	22nd Jul	24th Jul	4th Aug
pH	7.602	7.499	7.447
PCO_2	26.1	31.9	37.7
PO_2	78.3	91.3	93.0
HCO_3^-	25.2	24.3	25.4
BE	5.0	1.8	1.6
K^+	1.92	2.72	2.67
Ca^{2+}	1.03	0.97	1.03
Cl^-	93	102	100

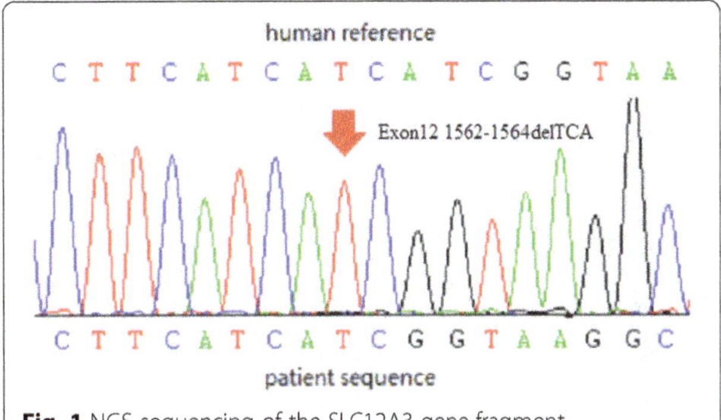

Fig. 1 NGS sequencing of the SLC12A3 gene fragment encompassing homozygous mutation c.1562_1564delTCA in patient

visit, we found that the patient often forgot to take his medicine. The results for thyroid function and electrolyte levels before and after treatment are listed in Table 4, which indicated that the patient's thyroid function had improved. Hypothyroidism occurred during the course of treatment, but the patient's thyroid function returned to normal after we reduced the dose of methimazole. The patient refused the recommendation to undergo I^{131} therapy. His serum potassium level remained low despite a sufficiently large daily dose of potassium, but no paroxysmal paralysis occurred after discharge.

Discussion and conclusions

More than 400 SLC12A3 variations have been identified to date. The prevalence of GS among Japanese populations is 10.3/10000 [3, 4]. The incidence rates of GD and Hashimoto's thyroiditis (HT) among the Chinese population are 120/100000/year and 100/100000/year, respectively [5]. The prevalence rates of both autoimmune thyroid disease (AITD) and GS among East Asian populations are higher than those among European populations [6]. Through a Chinese and English literature review, we identified 17 cases of AITD complicated with GS from nine papers (18 cases including ours) [7–17]. The cases included seven males (aged 20~45 years) and 11 females (aged 14~50 years). Among the patients, 13 had GD, 3 had HT, and two had antibody-positive AITD. All patients with GD and HT developed hypokalemic periodic paralysis. Twelve patients underwent genetic analysis, and all mutations were located in the SLC12A3 gene; four patients were homozygotes, one was a heterozygote, and five were complex heterozygotes. One patient did not have any detectable mutation, and the mutation type for one patient was not mentioned. The details of these cases are listed in Tables 5 and 6. Except for our case, the mutations in all cases were single base substitutions; two of the mutations were T60 M [18], which is a common variation among Chinese individuals. Six patients underwent renal biopsy, and all of the patients had juxtaglomerular complex (JGC) hyperplasia. Patient 6 had clinical and pathological features of GS but a wild-type SLC12A3 gene; therefore, the patient may have had acquired GS caused by autoimmune disease [19, 20]. Interestingly, we noticed that all the reported cases were from eastern Asia, possibly because of the high prevalence of GS and AITD in East Asian populations.

Table 3 The list of genes in the panel

SLC12A3	SCN4A	KCNJ2
SLC12A1	HSD11B2	ATP6V0A4
KCNJ1	KCNJ5	KCNJ10
CLCNKB	SCCN1B-exon13	SLC34A1
BSND	SCCN1G-exon13	EHHADH
CLCNKA	CYP11B1	HNF4A
CASR	CTP17A1	SLC4A1
CACNA1S	NR3C1	
KCNE3	CACNA1D	

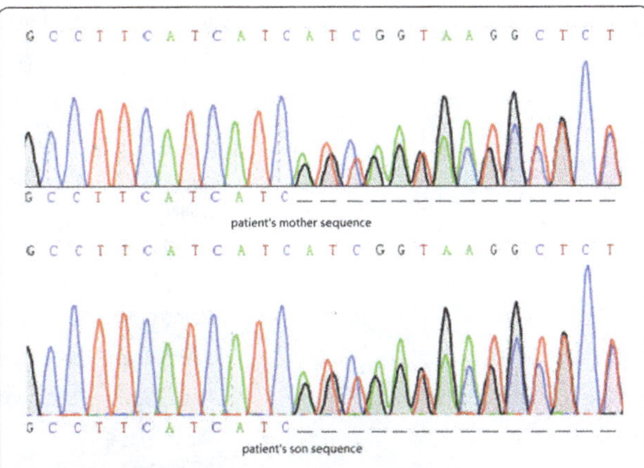

Fig. 2 Sanger sequencing of the SLC12A3 gene fragment encompassing heterozygous mutation c.1562_1564delTCA in patient mother(above) and

Table 4 Most recent re-examination results

	SerumK$^+$ (mmol)	Serum Mg^{2+} (mmol)	T3 (nmol/l)	T4 (nmol/l)	FT3 (pmol/l)	FT4 (pmol/l)	TSH (mIU/l)
2017.22nd Jul (admission)	2.110↓	0.540↓	1.40	> 300↑	5.32	51.23↑	0.01↓
5th.Aug	3.550	0.520↓	–	–	–	–	–
18th Aug (discharge)	2.580↓	0.540↓	2.75↑	189.53↑	8.88↑	20.77↑	0.01↓
19th Sep	2.810↓	0.700↓	2.63↑	114.75↑	6.69↑	15.81↑	0.01↓
27th Oct	2.530↓	0.700↓	–	–	4.33	3.85	1.39↓
12th.Dec	2.360↓	0.700↓	–	–	2.64↓	1.87↓	38.87↑
2018.8th.Feb	2.440↓	0.680↓	–	–	4.00	8.46	5.23↑
28th.Mar	–	–	–	–	4.45	9.59	5.43↑

Table 5 Pathology and gene information for the reported cases to date

No	Sex	Age	Thyroid disease	Diagnosis method	Pathology	Mutation type	Variation site	Change in nucleotide base	Change in amino acid
1	Male	45	GD	Gene analysis	No mention	Homozygote	Exon 12	1562-1564delTCA	522delIle
2 [7]	Male	39	GD	Gene analysis	No mention	Compound heterozygote	Exon 15	1841C-T	Ser614Phe
							Exon 26	2968G-A	Arg990Lys
3 [7]	Female	41	Antibody-positive	Gene analysis	No mention	Compound heterozygote	Intron 7	964 + 2 T-C	
							Exon 1	179C-T	Thr60Met
4 [8]	Female	40	Antibody-positive	Gene analysis	No mention	Compound heterozygote	Exon 22	2552 T-A	Leu849His
							Exon 22	2561G-A	Arg852His
5 [8]	Female	28	GD	Gene analysis	No mention	Homozygote	Exon 22	2552 T-A	Leu849His
6 [9]	Male	20	HT	Pathology and Gene analysis	JGC hyperplasia	Wild-type	–	–	–
7 [9]	Female	46	GD	Gene analysis	No mention	Heterozygote	Exon 1	185C-T	Thr60Met
8 [9]	Male	21	GD	Gene analysis	No mention	Homozygote	Exon 23	2744G-A	Arg913Gln
9 [10]	Female	18	GD	Gene analysis	No mention	Compound heterozygote	Exon 12	1015A-C	Thr339Pro
							Exon 22	2573 T-A	Leu858His
10 [10]	Female	50	GD	Gene analysis	No mention	Compound heterozygote	Exon 4	539C-A	Thr180Lys
							Exon 8	1045C-T	Pro349Ser
11 [10]	Female	56	GD	Gene analysis	No mention	Homozygote	Exon 14	1706C-T	Ala569Val
12 [11]	Female	14	GD	Gene analysis	No mention	No mention	Exon 6	791G-C	Gly264Ala
13 [12]	Female	20	GD	Pathology	JGA hyperplasia	–	–	–	–
14 [13, 14]	Male	21	GD	Pathology	JGA hyperplasia		–	–	–
15 [14]	Male	18	GD	Pathology	JGA hyperplasia			–	–
16 [15]	Female	39	HT	Biochemical analysis	–			–	–
17 [16]	Male	22	GD	Pathology	JGC hyperplasia				
18 [17]	Female	29	HT	Pathology	JGC hyperplasia				

Table 6 Chemical indicators of the reported cases to date

No	Serum potassium (mmol/l)	Serum magnesium (mmol/l)	Urinary calcium/ creatinine	pH	HCO_3-	FT3	FT4	T3	T4	TSH (mIU/l)	TPOAb	TRAb
1	1.4	0.54	0.23	7.602	25.2	↑	↑	↑	↑	0.1	↑	↑
2	1.9	0.52	0.08			↑	↑	↑	↑	0.01	–	↑
3	2.6	0.4	0.01			normal	normal			2.22	↑	
4	3.3	1.8	0.029	7.458	29.3	normal	normal			2.02	↑	
5	1.7	1.5	0.02	7.506	35.4	↑	↑			0.01		↑
6	2.67	0.56	0.05		29	↓	↓			75.4	↑	
7	2.3	0.43	0		33	↑	↑			0.01	↑	↑
8	2.64	0.36	0.07		35	↑	↑			<0.005	↑	↑
9	3.2	0.86	<0.003			–	↑			0.01		normal
10	3	0.66	<0.003			–	↑			<0.005		↑
11	2.8	0.49	0.03			–	↑			0.007		↑
12	2.2	0.53				↑	↑			0.01	↑	↑
13	2.46	0.73		7.47								
14	1.87			7.45	27	↑	normal	↑	normal	–		
15	2.02	0.5		7.55	28	↑	↑	↑	↑	–		
16	2.44	0.45		7.488	27.3			normal		4.28		
17	1.8	0.49–0.53		7.46	26.6	↑	↑			0.01	normal	
18	2.65	0.55		7.45	32.6	normal	normal			66.78	↑	

Nevertheless, we still lack sufficient data to demonstrate whether AITD is more likely to occur in patients with GS. Patients with GS may undergo more extensive testing, including thyroid functional analysis, compared to healthy individuals, which may facilitate the identification of additional abnormalities. Although sufficient data are available regarding the induction of hypokalemia and hypomagnesemia by hyperthyroidism, research on the long-term effects of hypokalemia and hypomagnesemia on the thyroid is lacking. Iodine and magnesium metabolism have been found to be closely linked [21]. One study showed that long-term high dietary magnesium can lead to abnormal thyroid function. Another study suggested that hypomagnesemia may lead to rapid relapse of GD [22]. In contrast, increasing magnesium supplementation has also been shown to promote normalization of thyroid morphology and function [23].

Autoimmune thyroid diseases (AITDs) are complex genetic diseases. The genes contributing to AITD can be divided into two categories: immunomodulatory genes, including the human leukocyte antigen (HLA), cytotoxic T lymphocyte-related antigen 4 (CTLA-4), protein tyrosine phosphatase, nonreceptor type 22 (PTPN22), CD40, CD25, and Fc receptor-like 3 (FCRL3) genes, and thyroid-specific genes, including the thyroid-stimulating hormone receptor (TSHR) gene and the thyroglobulin (Tg) gene. However, no studies have indicated that a correlation exists between these genes and the SLC12A3 gene.

In conclusion, GS combined with hyperthyroidism (or other AITDs) can cause hypokalemic periodic paralysis. Our patient was misdiagnosed with hypokalemic TPP for a long time, indicating that the possibility of GS should be considered in clinical cases with hyperthyroidism and persistent hypokalemia.

Abbreviations

AITD: autoimmune thyroid disease; CT: computed tomography; FT3: free triiodothyronine; GD: Graves' disease; GS: Gitelman syndrome; HT: Hashimoto's thyroiditis; JGC: juxtaglomerular complex; PTU: propylthiouracil; TgAb: thyroglobulin antibody; TMAB: thyroid microsomal antibody; TPOAb: thyroid peroxidase antibody; TRAb: thyrotropin receptor antibody; TSH: thyroid-stimulating hormone; WBC: white blood cell

Acknowledgments

The authors thank the patient and his family for their participation.

Funding

This work was supported by the National Natural Science Foundation of China (Grant No. 81660138).

Authors' contributions

HZ, XL, YQ, BM, JZ, and SH diagnosed the patient and performed the investigations and the follow-up. HZ, XL, SL, ZH, and HY analyzed the data. HZ and XL reviewed the literature, drafted the manuscript, and reviewed the manuscript for final publication. YM and ZL critically revised the manuscript. All authors read and approved the final manuscript.

Competing interest

The authors declare that they have no competing interests.

References

1. Frese E, Brown M, Norton BJ. Clinical reliability of manual muscle testing. Middle trapezius and gluteus medius muscles Phys Ther. 1987;67(7):1072–6.
2. Vargas-Poussou R, Dahan K, Kahila D, Venisse A, Riveira-Munoz E, Debaix H, et al. Spectrum of mutations in Gitelman syndrome. J Am Soc Nephrol. 2011;22(4):693–703.
3. Tago N, Kokubo Y, Inamoto N, et al. A high prevalence of Gitelman's syndrome mutations in Japanese. Hyperten Res. 2004;27:327–31.
4. Melander O, Orhomelander M, Bengtsson K, et al. Genetic variants of thiazide-sensitive NaCl-cotransporter in Gitelman's syndrome and primary hypertension. Hypertension. 2000;36:389–94.
5. McLeod DS, Cooper DS. The incidence and prevalence of thyroid autoimmunity. Endocrine. 2012;42:252–65.
6. Nyström HF, Jansson S, Berg G. Incidence rate and clinical features of hyperthyroidism in a long-term iodine sufficient area of Sweden (Gothenburg) 2003-2005. Clin Endocrinol. 2013;78:768–76.
7. Dong H, Lang Y, Shao Z, Lin L, Shao L. Coexistence of Gitelman's syndrome and thyroid disease:SLCl2A3 gene analysis in two patients. Chin J Endocrinol Metab. 2010;26:395–8 (in Chinese).
8. Aoi N, Nakayama T, Tahira Y, et al. Two novel genotypes of the thiazide-sensitive Na-cl cotransporter (SLC12A3) gene in patients with Gitelman's syndrome. Endocrine. 2007;31:149–53.
9. Xinyu Xu, Min sun, Xiaoyun Liu, et al. clinical feature and genetic analysis of Gitelman's syndrome accompanied by autoimmune thyroid disease. Chin J Endocrinol Metab. 2013;29:50–54. (in Chinese).
10. Mizokami T, Hishinuma A, Kogai T, et al. Graves' disease and Gitelman syndrome. Clin Endocrinol. 2016;84:149–50.
11. Zha B, Zheng P, Liu J, Huang X. Coexistence of Graves' disease in a 14-year-old young girl with Gitelman syndrome. Clin Endocrinol. 2015;83:995.
12. Xiao X, Liao E, Zhang H, Mao J, Pingan H. Gitelman syndrome with Graves's disease: a case report. Chin J Endocrinol Metab. 2006;22:91–2 (in Chinese).
13. Yayi He, Bingyin Shi, Xiaoyan Wu, et al. Gitelman syndrome complicated with hyperthyroidism and IgA nephropathy patients. Chin J Nephrol 2010; 26:70. (in Chinese).
14. Li M, Li T, He Y, Shi B. Nursing care of 2 patients with Gitelman syndrome comlicated with hyperthyroidism and IgA nephropathy. J Nurs Sci. 2015;30:33–4.
15. Shuiyu Ji, Xiang Zhao. Hashimoto's thyroiditis complicated with Gitelman syndrome: a case report. Chin J Nephrol. 2013;29:76. (in Chinese).
16. Zhenwen Zhang, Yan Zhu, Yan Wang, et al. A case of hyperthyroidism complicated with Gitelman syndrome. Chin J Postgraduates of Med 2010; 33:76–77. (in Chinese).
17. Yu Duan, Lan Luo, Chunyu Zhang, et al. Gitelman syndrome combined with primary hypothyroidism. Chin J General Practitioners 2009;8:269–270. (in Chinese).
18. Ma J, Ren H, Lin L, et al. Genetic features of Chinese patients with Gitelman syndrome: sixteen novel SLC12A3 mutations identified in a new cohort. Am J Nephrol. 2016;44:113–21.
19. Ren H, Wang WM, Chen XN, et al. Renal involvement and followup of 130 patients with primary Sjogren's syndrome. J Rheumatol. 2008;35:278–84.
20. Schwarz C, Barisani T, Bauer E, Druml W. A woman with red eyes and hypokalemia: a case of acquired Gitelman syndrome. Wien Klin Wochenschr. 2006;118:239–42.
21. Chandra AK, Goswami H, Sengupta P. Effects of magnesium on cytomorphology and enzyme activities in thyroid of rats. Indian J Exp Biol. 2014;52:787–92.
22. Klatka M, Grywalska E, Partyka M, Charytanowicz M, Rolinski J. Impact of methimazole treatment on magnesium concentration and lymphocytes activation in adolescents with Graves' disease. Biol Trace Elem Res. 2013;153:155–70.
23. Moncayo R, Moncayo H. The WOMED model of benign thyroid disease: acquired magnesium deficiency due to physical and psychological stressors relates to dysfunction of oxidative phosphorylation. BBA Clin. 2015;3:44–64.

Thyroid function and metabolic syndrome in the population-based LifeLines cohort study

Bruce H. R. Wolffenbuttel[1*], Hanneke J. C. M. Wouters[1], Sandra N. Slagter[1], Robert P. van Waateringe[1], Anneke C. Muller Kobold[2], Jana V. van Vliet-Ostaptchouk[1], Thera P. Links[1] and Melanie M. van der Klauw[1]

Abstract

Background: The metabolic syndrome (MetS) is a combination of unfavourable health factors which includes abdominal obesity, dyslipidaemia, elevated blood pressure and impaired fasting glucose. Earlier studies have reported a relationship between thyroid function and some MetS components or suggested that serum free thyroxine (FT4) or free triiodothyronine (FT3) levels within the normal range were independently associated with insulin resistance. We assessed how thyroid function relates to MetS prevalence in a large population-based study.

Methods: Data of 26,719 people of western European descent, aged 18–80 years from the Dutch LifeLines Cohort study, all with normal thyroid stimulating hormone (TSH), FT4 and FT3 levels (electrochemiluminescent immunoassay, Roche Modular E170 Analyzer), were available. MetS was defined with the revised National Cholesterol Education Programs Adults Treatment Panel III (NCEP ATP III) criteria. We calculated prevalence of all MetS components according to TSH, FT4 and FT3 quartiles.

Results: At similar TSH levels and age (mean 45 yrs), men had significantly higher levels of FT4, FT3, blood pressure (BP), heart rate, total and LDL-cholesterol, triglycerides (TG), and creatinine, but lower HDL-cholesterol compared to women (all $p < 0.001$). In total, 11.8% of women and 20.7% of men had MetS. In men, lower FT4 levels were associated with higher prevalence of MetS and all MetS components. In women, lower FT4 quartile was only associated with a higher prevalence of elevated TG, waist circumference, and MetS. However, when corrected for confounding factors like age, BMI, current smoking and alcohol consumption, a significant relationship was found between FT3 and three MetS components in men, and all five components in women. Moreover, the highest quartiles of FT3 and the FT3FT4 ratio predicted a 49% and 67% higher prevalence of MetS in men, and a 62 and 80% higher prevalence in women.

Conclusions: When corrected for possible confounding factors, higher plasma levels of FT3 are associated with several components of the MetS. Only in men, lower FT4 is related to MetS. In the highest FT3 and FT3FT4 quartiles, there is a 50–80% increased risk of having MetS compared to the lowest quartile. Further studies are needed to assess the possible causality of this relationship.

Keywords: Metabolic syndrome, Thyroid, Triiodothyronine, Epidemiology

* Correspondence: bwo@umcg.nl
[1]Department of Endocrinology, University of Groningen, University Medical Center Groningen, HPC AA31, P.O. Box 30001, 9700 RB Groningen, The Netherlands
Full list of author information is available at the end of the article

Background

The metabolic syndrome (MetS) is a clustering of medical conditions that reflects overnutrition, sedentary lifestyles, and resultant adiposity. Metabolic abnormalities such as abdominal obesity, hyperglycaemia, hypertension and dyslipidaemia often are present together, suggesting that they are not independent of one another and that they may share underlying causes and mechanisms [1]. Having MetS places a subject at a substantially increased risk to develop serious diseases like type 2 diabetes (T2D) and cardiovascular disease (CVD) [2].

In an earlier paper we described results from the population-based PREVEND study, and reported that low normal free thyroxine (FT4) levels were significantly related to a higher prevalence of all five MetS components in a group of almost 2300 people from the general population [3]. From this, we concluded that subjects with thyroid function in the low normal range already are at increased cardiovascular risk.

In recent years, there have been confusing results on the relationship between thyroid hormone levels within the normal range and cardiovascular risk factors and MetS. Several papers have described a relationship between thyroid hormone parameters and components of MetS [3–7]. However, some authors have reported an association between thyroid stimulating hormone (TSH) levels and metabolic risk factors, whereas others have observed that high normal free triiodothyronine (FT3) levels, and the FT3FT4-ratio were related to MetS. One of the largest study until now [4] evaluated 44,196 individuals (of whom 25,147 men), and reported that FT4 in men was significantly associated with blood pressure (BP), HDL-cholesterol (HDL-C), fasting blood glucose (FBG), and triglycerides (TG), and in women was associated with BP, HDL-C, FBG, waist circumference (WC). The authors however did not see an association with MetS, when adjusted for age. They did not adjust for smoking or alcohol, two important factors which influence the prevalence of MetS components, like low HDL-C, elevated triglycerides (TG), and -in women- increased WC [8]. Another study from Korea evaluated data from 13,496 middle-aged individuals, and found a relationship between higher T3 and T3/T4 and an unfavourable metabolic profile [6]. And a very recent paper reported in over 132,000 subjects that higher FT3/FT4 ratio was associated with increased risk of metabolic syndrome parameters and insulin resistance, adjusted for age, body mass index, smoking status and menopausal status (in women) [7].

For the current study, we used data of 26,719 participants from the population-based LifeLines Cohort Study to address the discrepancies in the literature. We aimed to investigate the relationship between thyroid hormone parameters and components of the MetS in this large sample of euthyroid subjects in the general population. As differences in MetS prevalence and thyroid hormone parameters have been demonstrated between men and women, we analysed these relationship separately for both sexes.

Methods

Subjects

For this cross-sectional study, we obtained data from subjects participating in the LifeLines Cohort Study. LifeLines is a multi-disciplinary prospective population-based cohort study examining in a unique three-generation design the health and health-related behaviours of persons living in the North of The Netherlands. It started in 2007, and employs a broad range of investigative procedures in assessing the biomedical, socio-demographic, behavioural, physical and psychological factors which contribute to the health and disease of the general population, with a special focus on multi-morbidity and complex genetics. The methodology has been described previously [9, 10]. All participants provided written informed consent before entering the study. The study protocol was approved by the medical ethical review committee of the University Medical Center Groningen. For the present study, we included subjects with an age between 18 and 80 years, who were of Western European descent, in whom thyroid hormone parameters were measured, and found to be within the normal range. We excluded participants who were treated because of a thyroid disorder, or who were current users of drugs known to influence thyroid hormone parameters, like lithium, amiodarone, and corticosteroids. Also, participants with a CRP level > 10 mg/L were excluded, because inflammation may disturb the activity of the deiodinase enzymes and alter thyroid hormone levels.

Clinical examination

Subjects completed a self-administered questionnaire on medical history, past and current diseases, use of medication and health behaviour at home. Medication use was verified by a certified research assistant, and scored by ATC code. The number of different medications used by a participant was considered as a proxy for multimorbidity [11]. Participants were defined as never smoker, current smoker or former smoker. Alcohol intake was calculated as the average number of units of alcohol based on the response to specific questions regarding intake frequency. Individuals who reported that they had not consumed alcohol during the previous month were considered non-drinkers.

BP and anthropometric measurements were obtained using a standardized protocol [9, 10]. BP was measured every minute during a period of 10 min with an automated DINAMAP Monitor (GE Healthcare, Freiburg, Germany). The average of the final three readings was recorded for systolic and diastolic BP. Height, weight, and waist and hip circumference were measured with the participant in light clothing and without shoes [8].

Biochemical measurements

Blood samples were collected between 8 and 10 a.m. after an overnight fast, directly into tubes containing heparin, and centrifuged. Total cholesterol (TC) and HDL-cholesterol (HDL-C) were measured with an enzymatic colorimetric method, triglycerides (TG) with UV colorometry, and LDL-cholesterol (LDL-C) using an enzymatic method (Roche Modular P chemistry analyser, Roche, Basel, Switzerland). HbA1c was measured with a turbidimetric inhibition immunoassay (Cobas Integra 800 CTS analyser, Roche Diagnostics Nederland BV, Almere, the Netherlands). Fasting blood glucose was measured using a hexokinase method. Levels of thyroid stimulating hormone (TSH), as well as free thyroxine (FT4) and free triiodothyronine (FT3) were assayed by electrochemiluminescent immunoassay (Roche Modular E170, Roche, Switzerland) [12]. Normal values for TSH are 0.4–4.5 mU/l, FT4 are 11–20 pmol/L, for FT3 4.4–6.7 pmol/l. The general Dutch population is iodine sufficient. Tests to measure anti-thyroid peroxidase antibody levels were not performed.

Calculations, definitions and statistical analysis

Body mass index (BMI) was calculated as weight (kg)/height (m^2), and categorized as normal weight (<25 kg/m^2), overweight (25–30 kg/m^2) and obesity (≥ 30 kg/m^2). Diagnosis of type 2 diabetes was based either on self-report (known diabetes), or on the finding of a fasting blood glucose ≥7.0 mmol/l at LifeLines' screening (newly-diagnosed diabetes) [13]. Diagnosis of MetS was established if a subject satisfied at least three out of five criteria according to the modified guidelines of the National Cholesterol Education Programs Adults Treatment Panel III (NCEP ATPIII criteria) [1, 8]. Relevant parameters were calculated according to FT4 and FT3 quartiles. As it is known that women and men differ regarding cardiovascular parameters, as well as MetS and thyroid hormone parameters, all calculations were made for both sexes separately.

Analyses were carried out with PASW Statistics (Version 24, IBM, Armonk, NY, USA). Data are presented as mean ± SD, or median and interquartile range when not normally distributed. Means were compared between groups with analysis of variance. In case of non-normal distribution, medians were compared with the nonparametric Kruskal-Wallis test. Chi-square test was used to analyse categorical variables. Both smoking and alcohol alter various components of the MetS [8]. Multiple linear regression models were therefore created to assess the associations of thyroid hormone parameters with the components of the MetS, with and without correction for factors known to influence either thyroid hormone parameters and MetS components: age, BMI, current smoking, and alcohol consumption. We subsequently used logistic regression analysis to estimate the odds ratios (ORs) and 95% confidence intervals (CI) for quartiles of thyroid hormone parameters to predict the presence of MetS, again adjusted for age, BMI, as well as smoking and alcohol consumption. To allow adjustment for multiple comparisons, a *P*-value <0.001 was considered statistically significant.

Results

The characteristics of the participants are given for men and women separately in Table 1. At similar TSH levels and age (mean 45 yrs), men had significantly higher levels of FT4, FT3, BP, heart rate, total and LDL-C, TG, and creatinine, but lower HDL-C compared to women (all $p < 0.001$). In total, 11.8% of women and 20.7% of men had MetS.

In men, lower FT4 levels were associated with lower levels of FT3 and higher TSH levels, higher levels of BMI, WC, waist-to-hip ratio, BP, FBG, total and LDL-C and TG levels, but lower HDL-C. In the lowest FT4 quartile, there were also fewer current smokers. In contrast, lower FT3 quartiles were only associated with lower FT4, higher TSH, and higher age, and also with higher levels of TC, HDL-C and LDL-C, and with a lower percentage of current smokers. As a consequence, lower FT4 levels were associated with higher prevalence of all MetS components. The lowest FT4 quartile (Additional file 1: Table S1) was associated with the highest prevalence of elevated BP (60%), elevated FBG (22.7%), WC (33.4%) and TG (30.2%), low HDL-cholesterol (26.5%), and MetS (27.7%). In contrast, higher FT3 levels were associated only with low HDL-C.

In women, the lowest FT4 quartile was associated with lower FT3 and higher TSH, higher BMI and waist circumference, but not with age, or with differences in blood pressure or cholesterol levels, while triglyceride levels were slightly higher. As a consequence, low FT4 levels (Additional file 2: Table 2) were only associated with elevated TG (11.2%), WC (47.4%), and MetS (13.8%). In contrast, higher FT3 levels were associated only with low HDL-C, and with a higher percentage of participants with ≥3 MetS components.

It became apparent that age, BMI and current smoking were confounders in all analyses: higher age was associated with lower FT3, and the lower FT4 and FT3 quartiles contained fewer current smokers. Also, age, BMI, smoking and alcohol consumption are known to influence several MetS components. Therefore, we performed four models within linear regression analyses, in which model 4 corrects for all these confounders. The

Table 1 Baseline characteristics of the participants

	Men N = 11.819	Women N = 14.900	P-value
Age (years)	46 ± 13	45 ± 13	<0.001
BMI (kg/m2)	26.5 ± 3.5	25.7 ± 4.4	<0.001
Waist (cm)	96 ± 10	87 ± 12	<0.001
Waist-hip ratio	0.97 ± 0.07	0.87 ± 0.07	<0.001
FT3	5.46 ± 0.53	5.10 ± 0.52	<0.001
FT4	16.1 ± 1.9	15.5 ± 1.8	<0.001
TSH	2.11 ± 0.85	2.20 ± 0.90	<0.001
Normal weight/overweight			
/obesity (n,%)	35.1/51.0/13.9	37.2/47.9/14.9	NS
Current/never smokers (%)	17.5/42.3	33.1/43.4	<0.001/NS
Systolic BP (mmHg)	131 ± 14	122 ± 15	<0.001
Diastolic BP (mmHg)	77 ± 9	72 ± 9	<0.001
Heart rate (b/min)	70 ± 11	72 ± 10	<0.001
Creatinine (mcmol/l)	83 ± 12	68 ± 9	<0.001
Fasting glucose (mmol/l)	5.2 ± 0.8	4.9 ± 0.7	<0.001
HbA1c (%)	5.6 ± 0.4	5.6 ± 0.4	<0.001
Total cholesterol (mmol/l)	5.16 ± 1.00	5.01 ± 0.98	<0.001
HDL-cholesterol (mmol/l)	1.29 ± 0.31	1.60 ± 0.39	<0.001
LDL-cholesterol (mmol/l)	3.38 ± 0.89	3.06 ± 0.88	<0.001
Triglycerides (mmol/l)	1.15 (0.84–1.66)	0.86 (0.65–1.18)	<0.001
% with metabolic syndrome	20.7	11.8	<0.001
% with type 2 diabetes	2.9	1.7	<0.001

results of these analyses are depicted in Tables 2 and 3, and show some differences between men and women. In men, only the association between FT4 and TG remained significant after correcting for all confounders, while FT3 correlated with 3 of 5 MetS components (BP, HDL-C, WC). In women, FT3 was associated with all MetS components after correction for the confounders. In both men and women, the FT3FT4-ratio was associated 4 of the 5 components of MetS, but not with FBG.

Finally, Tables 4 and 5 depicts the results of the logistic regression analyses, in which we have correlated the thyroid parameters (divided in quartiles again) with the presence of MetS. In both men and women, higher levels of FT3 and the FT3FT4-ratio, adjusted for age, BMI, current smoking and alcohol consumption, were associated with a higher risk MetS, while FT4 was associated with higher risk of MetS in men only. Both for men and women, we observed a 1.67–1.80 higher OR for the highest FT3FT4-ratio quartile compared to the lowest quartile to predict the presence of MetS.

Discussion

In this large population-based study in subjects with thyroid hormone levels in the normal range, we have shown that higher levels of FT3 and the FT3FT4 ratio and lower levels of FT4 (in men only) are associated with components of MetS, when corrected for important confounders like age, BMI, current smoking and alcohol consumption. A significant relationship was found for FT3 and three MetS components in men, and all five components in women. Moreover, the highest quartiles of FT3 and the FT3FT4 ratio predicted a 49% and 67% higher prevalence of MetS in men, and a 62 and 80% higher prevalence in women.

From our uncorrected analyses, FT4 levels appeared the most strongly related to MetS. However, it has been known that both age and BMI can influence thyroid hormone parameters and MetS. In the current study, we observed a gradual decrease of plasma FT3 levels with increasing age, while TSH and FT4 levels did not change significantly. Furthermore, it is known that FT4 levels are lower and TSH levels are higher in obese individuals compared to those with normal weight. This was the reason we included both parameters as confounders in our linear regression models. In addition, both smoking and alcohol consumption have a profound effect on some MetS components. Smoking lowers HDL-C levels, and is associated with increased WC, as we have

Table 2 Associations of thyroid function with components of the metabolic syndrome in men

		FT4		FT3		TSH		FT3FT4	
	Model	β	P	β	P	β	P	β	P
SBP	1	**−0.048**	**<0.001**	0.008	0.385	0.009	0.330	0.049	**<0.001**
	2	−0.013	0.147	**0.096**	**<0.001**	0.003	0.705	**0.074**	**<0.001**
	3	−0.016	0.084	**0.093**	**<0.001**	0.003	0.741	**0.075**	**<0.001**
	4	0.015	0.098	**0.081**	**<0.001**	0.005	0.576	**0.040**	**<0.001**
DBP	1	**−0.048**	**<0.001**	**−0.047**	**<0.001**	−0.017	0.066	0.009	0.304
	2	−0.005	0.584	**0.054**	**<0.001**	−0.024	0.007	**0.039**	**<0.001**
	3	−0.006	0.486	**0.052**	**<0.001**	−0.027	0.002	**0.039**	**<0.001**
	4	0.020	0.023	**0.041**	**<0.001**	−0.026	0.003	0.009	0.312
HDL-C	1	**0.044**	**<0.001**	**−0.097**	**<0.001**	−0.016	0.086	**−0.112**	**<0.001**
	2	**0.060**	**<0.001**	**−0.072**	**<0.001**	−0.018	0.048	**−0.103**	**<0.001**
	3	**0.065**	**<0.001**	**−0.063**	**<0.001**	**−0.032**	**<0.001**	**−0.100**	**<0.001**
	4	0.023	0.008	**−0.045**	**<0.001**	**−0.035**	**<0.001**	**−0.051**	**<0.001**
TG	1	**−0.084**	**<0.001**	0.011	0.246	**0.057**	**<0.001**	**0.083**	**<0.001**
	2	**−0.074**	**<0.001**	0.040	**<0.001**	**0.076**	**<0.001**	**0.092**	**<0.001**
	3	**−0.081**	**<0.001**	0.027	0.005	**0.068**	**<0.001**	**0.090**	**<0.001**
	4	**−0.040**	**<0.001**	0.010	0.286	**0.070**	**<0.001**	**0.041**	**<0.001**
FBG	1	**−0.074**	**<0.001**	**−0.040**	**<0.001**	−0.003	0.710	**0.038**	**<0.001**
	2	**−0.042**	**<0.001**	**0.037**	**<0.001**	−0.009	0.333	**0.062**	**<0.001**
	3	**−0.043**	**<0.001**	**0.036**	**<0.001**	−0.008	0.353	**0.062**	**<0.001**
	4	−0.014	0.112	0.024	0.010	−0.007	0.456	0.028	**0.001**
Waist	1	**−0.143**	**<0.001**	−0.018	0.051	−0.015	0.106	**0.119**	**<0.001**
	2	**−0.105**	**<0.001**	**0.079**	**<0.001**	−0.021	0.016	**0.148**	**<0.001**
	3	**−0.106**	**<0.001**	**0.079**	**<0.001**	−0.021	0.017	**0.148**	**<0.001**
	4	−0.002	0.657	**0.036**	**<0.001**	−0.015	0.001	**0.0125**	**<0.001**

Values of β are standardized regression coefficients
Regression for triglycerides was performed after logarithmic transformation. Significant associations are shown in bold
Model 1: crude
Model 2: after adjustment for age
Model 3: after adjustment for age, current smoking, alcohol consumption
Model 4: after adjustment for age, BMI, current smoking, alcohol consumption

demonstrated earlier within the LifeLines population [8]. Alcohol consumption may increase HDL-C levels, but also levels of BP [8, 14, 15]. As our initial data analyses revealed that there were fewer smokers and users of alcohol in the lowest FT4 and FT3 quartiles, both in men and in women, we have corrected in our regression models for these factors as well. And only with these important adjustments, we were able to demonstrate that FT3 levels and the FT3FT4 ratio were significantly associated with MetS components, and having MetS.

Several papers have described the relationship between thyroid hormone parameters and components of MetS. In 2007, our group has demonstrated in the population-based PREVEND study the association between levels of FT4 (within the normal reference range) and plasma lipids; these findings were in accordance with the earlier observed association between (sub)clinical hypothyroidism and hyperlipidaemia [3]. Low normal FT4 levels proved to be significantly associated with MetS (four of five components) and increased insulin resistance. From our data, we concluded that this suggested an increased risk of cardiovascular events in subjects with low normal thyroid function [3]. Several additional papers, as summarized in Table 6, have been published the last decade which have assessed the relationship between thyroid hormone levels and cardiovascular risk factors, including the MetS. These studies have been performed in populations with different ethnic background. As can be seen in Table 6, there are significant differences between these studies, not only related to study setting and population, but also related to the results. One of the striking differences is that several papers have not separated between women and men, as it is known (which

Table 3 Associations of thyroid function with components of the metabolic syndrome in women

		FT4		FT3		TSH		FT3FT4	
	Model	β	P	β	P	β	P	β	P
SBP	1	**0.034**	**<0.001**	**0.040**	**<0.001**	**0.033**	**<0.001**	0.006	0.455
	2	**0.027**	**<0.001**	**0.131**	**<0.001**	0.025	0.001	**0.081**	**<0.001**
	3	**0.028**	**<0.001**	**0.137**	**<0.001**	0.023	0.002	**0.083**	**<0.001**
	4	**0.054**	**<0.001**	**0.130**	**<0.001**	0.018	0.015	**0.054**	**<0.001**
DBP	1	−0.003	0.754	0.015	0.06	0.007	0.426	0.017	0.044
	2	−0.007	0.400	**0.064**	**<0.001**	0.002	0.823	**0.058**	**<0.001**
	3	−0.006	0.461	**0.068**	**<0.001**	0.000	0.962	**0.059**	**<0.001**
	4	0.014	0.078	**0.063**	**<0.001**	−0.004	0.658	**0.037**	**<0.001**
HDL-C	1	0.016	0.046	**−0.112**	**<0.001**	0.020	0.016	**−0.106**	**<0.001**
	2	0.013	0.107	**−0.079**	**<0.001**	0.016	0.047	−0.078	<0.001
	3	0.023	0.005	**−0.062**	**<0.001**	0.001	0.877	**−0.071**	**<0.001**
	4	−0.016	0.034	**−0.052**	**<0.001**	0.009	0.240	−0.027	<0.001
TG	1	**−0.068**	**<0.001**	**0.046**	**<0.001**	**0.078**	**<0.001**	**0.105**	**<0.001**
	2	**−0.073**	**<0.001**	**0.101**	**<0.001**	**0.073**	**<0.001**	**0.154**	**<0.001**
	3	**−0.083**	**<0.001**	**0.086**	**<0.001**	**0.087**	**<0.001**	**0.150**	**<0.001**
	4	**−0.051**	**<0.001**	**0.078**	**<0.001**	**0.080**	**<0.001**	**0.113**	**<0.001**
FBG	1	0.000	0.964	−0.011	0.161	**0.036**	**<0.001**	−0.003	0.731
	2	−0.007	0.405	**0.059**	**<0.001**	**0.029**	**<0.001**	**0.057**	**<0.001**
	3	−0.007	0.405	**0.059**	**<0.001**	**0.029**	**<0.001**	**0.056**	**<0.001**
	4	0.025	0.001	**0.051**	**<0.001**	0.023	0.002	0.020	0.011
Waist	1	**−0.091**	**<0.001**	−0.011	0.175	0.018	0.032	**0.081**	**<0.001**
	2	**−0.096**	**<0.001**	**0.048**	**<0.001**	0.012	0.137	**0.134**	**<0.001**
	3	**−0.097**	**<0.001**	**0.047**	**<0.001**	0.014	0.084	**0.133**	**<0.001**
	4	−0.004	0.380	**0.024**	**<0.001**	−0.005	0.284	**0.024**	**<0.001**

Values of β are standardized regression coefficients
Regression for triglycerides was performed after logarithmic transformation. Significant associations are shown in bold
Model 1: crude
Model 2: after adjustment for age
Model 3: after adjustment for age, current smoking, alcohol consumption
Model 4: after adjustment for age, BMI, current smoking, alcohol consumption

is also apparent from the current paper) that the prevalence of the individual MetS components differs considerably between women and men [16–19]. For instance, we have recently demonstrated that increased waist circumference is a common features of MetS among women while men have often an elevated blood pressure [20]. Moreover, FT4 and FT3 levels differ between men and women as well. Therefore, simply adjusting for sex may obscure possible differences between sexes. In addition, no study has reported data on smoking and alcohol consumption, or corrected for these important confounders. Interestingly, our data indicate a dysbalance of smoking and alcohol consumption in the different FT4 and FT3 quartiles, which causes a warning regarding the proper interpretation of earlier studies. With the exception of recent studies by Kim et al. [4], Park et al. [5] and by Kim et al. [6, 21], earlier studies have incorporated a limited number of participants.

There are a number of possible explanations for the relationship between FT3 and the different MetS components, c.q. insulin resistance. One may be that a small increase of T3 may directly influence insulin sensitivity. Recent data have supported this with the notion that overproduction of thyroid hormones may have a negative effect on peripheral insulin action [22]. Indeed, it has been shown that in obese individuals, who more frequently are insulin-resistant, FT4 levels are lower, and TSH and FT3 levels are higher. This has been postulated to be the consequence of an excess of nutrition, especially when consuming a diet high in fat. Obesity may directly influence tissue type 2 deiodinase activity -which converts T4 into T3- in order to compensate for this. It has also been argued that in the brain T3 may have a stimulatory effect on food intake behaviour, which can be considered a compensation for the increase of

Table 4 Risk of having metabolic syndrome according to quartiles of thyroid hormone parameters, in men

	Quartile	MetS/Total, n (%)	model 1	model 2	model 3	model 4
TSH	1	578/2923 (19.8)	1	1	1	1
	2	595/2975 (20.0)	1.014 (0.893–1.153)	1.015 (0.892–1.155)	1.030 (0.904–1.174)	1.000 (0.861–1.161)
	3	618 (2946 (21.0)	1.077 (0.948–1.223)	1.072 (0.943–1.219)	1.116 (0.980–1.271)	1.101 (0.949–1.276)
	4	650/2975 (21.8)	1.134 (1.000–1.286)	1.110 (0.977–1.261)	1.155 (1.015–1.314)	1.214 (1.047–1.407)
FT4	1	796/2877 (27.7)	1	1	1	1
	2	635/3000 (21.2)	**0.702 (0.623–0.791) #**	**0.717 (0.635–0.809) #**	**0.704 (0.623–0.796) #**	**0.816 (0.709–0.939) #**
	3	532/3014 (17.7)	**0.560 (0.495–0.635) #**	**0.596 (0.525–0.675) #**	**0.579 (0.509–0.657) #**	**0.733 (0.634–0.848) #**
	4	478/2928 (16.3)	**0.510 (0.449–0.579) #**	**0.567 (0.498–0.646) #**	**0.545 (0.478–0.622) #**	**0.722 (0.621–0.839) #**
FT3	1	516/2655 (19.4)	1	1	1	1
	2	652/3300 (19.8)	1.021 (0.897–1.161)	1.192 (1.045–1.360)	**1.172 (1.026–1.339) #**	1.174 (1.010–1.366)
	3	695/3185 (21.8)	1.157 (1.018–1.315)	**1.487 (1.302–1.699) #**	**1.458 (1.275–1.668) #**	**1.360 (1.167–1.586) #**
	4	578/2679 (21.6)	1.140 (0.998–1.303)	**1.652 (1.434–1.904) #**	**1.577 (1.366–1.821) #**	**1.491 (1.266–1.756) #**
FT3FT4	1	457/2945 (15.5)	1	1	1	1
	2	528/2958 (17.8)	1.183 (1.031–1.357)	1.241 (1.080–1.426)	**1.220 (1.060–1.405) #**	1.234 (1.054–1.445)
	3	667/2960 (22.5)	**1.584 (1.388–1.807) #**	**1.753 (1.533–2.005) #**	**1.731 (1.512–1.983) #**	**1.537 (1.318–1.791) #**
	4	789/2956 (26.7)	**1.982 (1.743–2.255) #**	**2.263 (1.984–2.582) #**	**2.267 (1.984–2.590) #**	**1.674 (1.438–1.948) #**

Model 1: crude; model 2: adjusted for age; model 3: adjusted for age, current smoking and alcohol consumption
model 4: adjusted for age, BMI, current smoking and alcohol consumption
OR and 95% CI for metabolic syndrome were calculated using logistic regression models
Significant associations ($P < 0.001$) are shown in bold

Table 5 Risk of having metabolic syndrome according to quartiles of thyroid hormone parameters, in women

	Quartile	MetS/Total, n (%)	model 1	model 2	model 3	model 4
TSH	1	388/3726 (10.4)	1	1	1	1
	2	428/3710 (11.5)	1.122 (0.970–1.298)	1.149 (0.989–1.334)	1.192 (1.025–1.386)	1.162 (0.984–1.372)
	3	451/3729 (12.1)	1.184 (1.025–1.367)	1.165 (1.005–1.351)	1.219 (1.049–1.417)	1.046 (0.885–1.236)
	4	493/3735 (13.2)	1.308 (1.136–1.507) #	1.212 (1.053–1.061)	1.288 (1.110–1.494)	1.167 (0.990–1.375)
FT4	1	523/3784 (13.8)	1	1	1	1
	2	417/3707 (11.2)	0.790 (0.689–0.907)	**0.761 (0.660–0.876) #**	**0.757 (0.656–0.874) #**	0.854 (0.728–1.002)
	3	423/3624 (11.7)	0.824 (0.718–0.945)	**0.762 (0.661–0.877) #**	**0.758 (0.657–0.874) #**	0.900 (0.767–1.057)
	4	397/3785 (10.5)	**0.731 (0.636–0.840) #**	**0.651 (0.564–0.752) #**	**0.620 (0.535–0.717) #**	0.819 (0.696–0.964)
FT3	1	317/3104 (10.2)	1	1	1	1
	2	482/4361 (11.1)	1.095 (0.943–1.272)	1.179 (1.011–1.375)	1.154 (0.988–1.348)	1.095 (0.923–1.299)
	3	521/3897 (13.4)	**1.357 (1.170–1.574) #**	**1.644 (1.410–1.916) #**	**1.558 (1.334–1.819) #**	**1.515 (1.276–1.798) #**
	4	439/3538 (12.4)	1.245 (1.068–1.452)	**1.819 (1.550–2.134) #**	**1.707 (1.451–2.008) #**	**1.622 (1.354–1.942) #**
FT3FT4	1	374/3724 (10.0)	1	1	1	1
	2	392/3718 (10.5)	1.056 (0.909–1.226)	1.227 (1.051–1.432)	1.217 (1.041–1.423)	1.241 (1.045–1.473)
	3	438/3726 (11.8)	1.193 (1.031–1.381)	**1.557 (1.337–1.813) #**	**1.539 (1.319–1.795) #**	**1.423 (1.201–1.687) #**
	4	556/3732 (14.9)	**1.568 (1.364–1.803) #**	**2.372 (2.045–2.751) #**	**2.329 (2.004–2.705) #**	**1.798 (1.522–2.125) #**

Model 1: crude; model 2: adjusted for age; model 3: adjusted for age, current smoking and alcohol consumption
model 4: adjusted for age, BMI, current smoking and alcohol consumption
OR and 95% CI for metabolic syndrome were calculated using logistic regression models
Significant associations ($P < 0.001$) are shown in bold

Table 6 Studies evaluating the relationship between thyroid hormone levels and components of the metabolic syndrome

Author, year	N	Subjects' age	Gender separation?	Corrections for confounders	Major findings	Ref
Roos, 2007	1581, 716 M	28–75 yrs	No	Age, sex, HOMA-IR	FT4 negative association with TC, LDL-C, TG and waist, positive association with HDL-C, FT3 negative association with TC, LDL-C, TG	[3]
Park, 2009	949	Postmenopausal women	Women only	Age, BMI, HOMA-IR, FT4, exercise (3 levels), alcohol (3 levels)	TSH associated with TC, LDL-C, DBP and TG, MetS	[30]
Kim, 2009	44,196, 25,147 M	25–70 yrs	Yes	Age	Men: FT4 associated with BP, HDL-C, FBG, TG, and with WC in those over 50; Women: associated with BP, HDL-C, FBG, WC; no association with MetS, when adjusted for age	[4]
Garduno-Garcia, 2010	3033	18–70 yrs	No	Age, sex	TSH associated with TC, TG, WC; FT4 associated with HDL-C, WC, HOMA-IR; 10% had SCH.	[31]
Ruhla, 2010	1333, 481 M	>18 yrs	No	Age	TSH positively associated with BMI, TG, MetS; no data on FT4 or FT3	[32]
Park, 2011	5998, 3469 M	>18 yrs	No	Age, sex, BMI, smoking (y/n), alcohol (y/n), exercise (y/n)	TSH and FT4 associated with WC, FBG, HDL-C, FT4 also with DBP; higher TSH predicted MetS at follow-up	[5]
Tarcin, 2012	211, 24 M	Obesity, 18–73 yrs	No	Age	FT3/FT4 negatively associated with FBG, TG, BP, TT3 positively with HOMA-IR, FBG, WC	[33]
Waring, 2012	2119	70–79 yrs	No	Age, sex, race, BMI, smoking, HOMA-IR	TSH associated with MetS prevalence, in entire cohort with broad range of TSH levels, and in euthyroid range	[34]
Oh, 2013	2760	18–39	Women only	Age, BMI, HOMA-IR	TSH between 2.5 and 4.5 associated with BMI, WC, BP, TG	[35]
Roef, 2014	2315, 1177 M	Middle-aged	No	Age, sex, height, current smoking	FT3 and FT3/FT4 ratio positively associated with BMI, WC, TG, BP, FBG, negatively with HDL-C; FT4 negatively associated with BMI, WC, TG	[36]
Mehran, 2014	3755, 1709 M	≥20 yrs	No	Age, sex, smoking, BMI, HOMA-IR	FT4 associated with HDL-C, LDL-C, TG, WC, BP, but not fasting glucose; no FT3 data	[37]
Minami, 2015	283, 161 M	Children, 6–15 yrs	Yes	None	Higher FT3/FT4 ratio in boys with MetS; no difference thyroid function in girls with MetS	[38]
Laclaustra, 2015	3533 M	20–65 yrs	Men only	Age, alcohol consumption, smoking (never, former, current)	Higher TSH & lowest FT4 quintiles associated with higher MetS prevalence	[39]
Kim, 2016	13,496, 8168 M	Middle-aged, 35–65 yrs	No	Age, sex, % body fat, smoking, HOMA-IR	Higher quartiles of T3 and T3/T4 ratio associated with MetS; only measured total T4 and T3 levels; modified MetS criteria	[6]
Kim, 2017	12,037, 6950 M	Middle-aged, 35–65 yrs	No	Age, sex, smoking	Highest T3 quartile associated with highest 6-year MetS incidence; only measured total T4 and T3 levels; modified MetS criteria	[21]
Ferrannini, 2017	940	30–60 yrs	No	Age, sex, BMI, WHR, family history of diabetes	Higher FT3 associated with decreased insulin sensitivity (insulin clamp), predicted follow-up increases in glycaemia	[22]
Park, 2017	132,346, 66,991 M	>18 yrs	Yes	Age, BMI, smoking status, menopausal status (in women)	FT3FT4 ratio associated with increased risk of MetS parameters and insulin resistance	[7]

BMI body mass index, *BP* blood pressure, *DBP* diastolic blood pressure, *FBG* fasting blood glucose, *HDL-C* high-density-lipoprotein-cholesterol, *HOMA-IR* homeostasis-model assessment - insulin resistance, *LDL-C* low-density-lipoprotein-cholesterol, *M* males, *MetS* metabolic syndrome, *SCH* subclinical hypothyroidism, *TC* total cholesterol, *TG* triglycerides, *WC* waist circumference, *WHR* waist-to-hip ratio, *yrs.* years, *y/n* yes/no

metabolic rate which is induced by the thyroid hormone itself [23]. This author suggested that T3 may stimulate specific neurons that influence appetite-increasing neuropeptides. However, in our data we did observe lower FT4 and higher TSH levels with increasing BMI, but no significant changes of FT3. However, changes in brain T3 production may not be mirrored by similar changes in plasma FT3. Another explanation may be that MetS or insulin resistance itself may lead to a relative higher intracellular production of T3 as a way to compensate -on a local tissue level- for the disturbances in the metabolic state [24, 25]. The increase in local T3 production may be intended to limit nutrient overload by inducing tissue thermogenesis and simulating metabolic activity [25, 26]. It has also been postulated that 3,5-diiodo-l-thyronine (T2) has marked effects on energy metabolism in order to protect skeletal muscle against excessive intramyocellular lipid storage [27], that may occur in MetS. A positive energy balance both as a consequence of caloric excess and due to insufficient physical activity may contribute to this. In contrast, caloric restriction and prolonged fasting have been associated with lower type 2 deiodinase activity, which will reduce the conversion of T4 to T3 and lower plasma (F)T3 levels, and an increase in the conversion to reverse T3. In addition, the slightly lower (F)T4 levels observed in obesity themselves may upregulate tissue type 2 deiodinase activity, thereby leading to a relative increase of T3. Other factors which may influence tissue deiodinase activity and thereby resulting T3 levels are changes in circadian rhythm. Indeed, it has been shown that disturbances in sleep pattern may play a role in the development of obesity and diabetes [28, 29].

Our study has several strengths, but also some weaknesses. It comprises a large dataset of participants from the general population with available thyroid hormone parameters. Also, all subjects have been uniformly characterized, with well-standardized BP measurements and blood drawing in the fasting state, thereby minimizing the effect of possible circadian changes in thyroid hormone parameters. The large number of participants allowed to assess all relationships for men and women separately, which is of importance considering the significant differences between sexes for a large number of baseline characteristics (Table 1). As mentioned, this is one of the few studies in which confounding factors like smoking and alcohol have been taken into account. Currently, we lack information regarding menopausal status of the female participants, which may influence the possible difference between sexes. Also, data on physical activity could not be taken into account, and it is known that this factor may directly influence some MetS components, and is an important factor in maintaining an optimal energy balance. Tests to measure anti-thyroid peroxidase antibody levels were not available. Due to the cross-sectional design, we can not evaluate the effects of thyroid hormone parameters on future development of MetS. This also relates to the fact that the LifeLines study did not systematically collect medication use during follow-up investigations.

Conclusions

In conclusion, plasma levels of both FT4 and FT3 are associated with several components of the MetS, after correction for possible important confounding factors. In the highest FT3 and FT3FT4 quartiles there is a 50–80% increased risk of having MetS compared to the lowest quartile. Further studies are needed to assess the possible causality of this relationship.

Abbreviations

BMI: Body mass index; BP: Blood pressure; FBG: Fasting blood glucose; HbA1c: Glycated haemoglobin; HDL-C: High-density lipoprotein cholesterol; LDL-C: Low density lipoprotein cholesterol; MetS: Metabolic syndrome; OR: Odds ratio; TC: Total cholesterol; TG: Triglycerides; WC: Waist circumference

Acknowledgements

The authors wish to acknowledge all participants of the LifeLines Cohort Study and everybody involved in the set-up and implementation of the study.

Funding

Lifelines has been funded by a number of public sources, notably the Dutch Government, The Netherlands Organization of Scientific Research NOW [grant 175.010.2007.006], the Northern Netherlands Collaboration of Provinces (SNN), the European fund for regional development, Dutch Ministry of Economie Affairs, Pieken in de Delta, Provinces of Groningen and Drenthe, the Target project, BBMRI-NL, the University of Groningen, and the University Medical Center Groningen, The Netherlands. This work was supported by the National Consortium for Healthy Ageing, and funds from the European Union's Seventh Framework program (FP7/2007–2013) through the BioSHaRE-EU (Biobank Standardisation and Harmonisation for Research Excellence in the European Union) project, grant agreement 261,433. LifeLines (BRIF4568) is engaged in a Bioresource research impact factor (BRIF) policy pilot study, details of which can be found at: http://www.bioshare.eu/content/bioresource-impact-factor

Authors' contributions

BHRW was the primary investigator. SNS, MMvdK and BHRW contributed to the study design. SNS and BHRW performed the statistical analyses. HJCMW, SNS, RPvW, ACMK, JVVVO, TPL, MMvdK contributed to interpretation of the data and analyses. BHRW drafted the manuscript. All authors read and approved the final manuscript.

Competing interests

The authors declare that they have no competing interests.

Author details

[1]Department of Endocrinology, University of Groningen, University Medical Center Groningen, HPC AA31, P.O. Box 30001, 9700 RB Groningen, The Netherlands. [2]Department of Clinical Chemistry, University of Groningen, University Medical Center Groningen, HPC AA31, P.O. Box 30001, 9700 RB Groningen, The Netherlands.

References

1. Alberti KG, Eckel RH, Grundy SM, Zimmet PZ, Cleeman JI, Donato KA, et al. Harmonizing the metabolic syndrome: a joint interim statement of the international diabetes federation task force on epidemiology and prevention; National Heart, Lung, and Blood Institute; American Heart Association; world heart federation; international atherosclerosis society; and International Association for the Study of obesity. Circulation. 2009;120: 1640–5.

2. Cornier MA, Dabelea D, Hernandez TL, Lindstrom RC, Steig AJ, Stob NR, et al. The metabolic syndrome. Endocr Rev. 2008;29:777–822.
3. Roos A, Bakker SJ, Links TP, Gans RO, Wolffenbuttel BH. Thyroid function is associated with components of the metabolic syndrome in euthyroid subjects. J Clin Endocrinol Metab. 2007;92:491–6.
4. Kim BJ, Kim TY, Koh JM, Kim HK, Park JY, Lee KU, et al. Relationship between serum free T4 (FT4) levels and metabolic syndrome (MS) and its components in healthy euthyroid subjects. Clin Endocrinol. 2009;70:152–60.
5. Park SB, Choi HC, Joo NS. The relation of thyroid function to components of the metabolic syndrome in Korean men and women. J Korean Med Sci. 2011;26:540–5.
6. Kim HJ, Bae JC, Park HK, Byun DW, Suh K, Yoo MH, et al. Triiodothyronine levels are independently associated with metabolic syndrome in Euthyroid middle-aged subjects. Endocrinol Metab (Seoul). 2016;31:311–9.
7. Park SY, Park SE, Jung SW, Jin HS, Park IB, Ahn SV, et al. Free triiodothyronine/free thyroxine ratio rather than thyrotropin is more associated with metabolic parameters in healthy euthyroid adult subjects. Clin Endocrinol. 2017;87:87–96.
8. Slagter SN, van Vliet-Ostaptchouk JV, Vonk JM, Boezen HM, Dullaart RP, Kobold AC, et al. Combined effects of smoking and alcohol on metabolic syndrome: the LifeLines cohort study. PLoS One. 2014;9:e96406.
9. Stolk RP, Rosmalen JG, Postma DS, de Boer RA, Navis G, Slaets JP, et al. Universal risk factors for multifactorial diseases: LifeLines: a three-generation population-based study. Eur J Epidemiol. 2008;23:67–74.
10. Scholtens S, Smidt N, Swertz MA, Bakker SJ, Dotinga A, Vonk JM, et al. Cohort profile: LifeLines, a three-generation cohort study and biobank. Int J Epidemiol. 2015;44:1172–80.
11. Schubert CC, Boustani M, Callahan CM, Perkins AJ, Carney CP, Fox C, et al. Comorbidity profile of dementia patients in primary care: are they sicker? J Am Geriatr Soc. 2006;54:104–9.
12. Klaver EI, van Loon HC, Stienstra R, Links TP, Keers JC, Kema IP, et al. Thyroid hormone status and health-related quality of life in the LifeLines cohort study. Thyroid. 2013;23:1066–73.
13. American Diabetes A. Diagnosis and classification of diabetes mellitus. Diabetes Care. 2010;33(Suppl 1):S62–9.
14. Lee K. Gender-specific relationships between alcohol drinking patterns and metabolic syndrome: the Korea National Health and nutrition examination survey 2008. Public Health Nutr. 2012;15:1917–24.
15. Marchi KC, Muniz JJ, Tirapelli CR. Hypertension and chronic ethanol consumption: what do we know after a century of study? World J Cardiol. 2014;6:283–94.
16. Grundy SM. Metabolic syndrome pandemic. Arterioscler Thromb Vasc Biol. 2008;28:629–36.
17. Lee YJ, Woo SY, Ahn JH, Cho S, Kim SR. Health-related quality of life in adults with metabolic syndrome: the Korea national health and nutrition examination survey, 2007-2008. Ann Nutr Metab. 2012;61:275–80.
18. van Vliet-Ostaptchouk JV, Nuotio ML, Slagter SN, Doiron D, Fischer K, Foco L, et al. The prevalence of metabolic syndrome and metabolically healthy obesity in Europe: a collaborative analysis of ten large cohort studies. BMC Endocr Disord. 2014;14:9.
19. Slagter SN, van Vliet-Ostaptchouk JV, van Beek AP, Keers JC, Lutgers HL, van der Klauw MM, et al. Health-related quality of life in relation to obesity grade, type 2 diabetes, metabolic syndrome and inflammation. PloS one 2015;10:e0140599.
20. Slagter SN, van Waateringe RP, van Beek AP, van der Klauw MM, Wolffenbuttel BHR, van Vliet-Ostaptchouk JV. Sex, BMI and age differences in metabolic syndrome: the Dutch Lifelines cohort study. Endocr Connect. 2017;6:278–88.
21. Kim HJ, Bae JC, Park HK, Byun DW, Suh K, Yoo MH, et al. Association of triiodothyronine levels with future development of metabolic syndrome in euthyroid middle-aged subjects: a 6-year retrospective longitudinal study. Eur J Endocrinol. 2017;176:441–50.
22. Ferrannini E, Iervasi G, Cobb J, Ndreu R, Nannipieri M. Insulin resistance and normal thyroid hormone levels: prospective study and metabolomic analysis. Am J Physiol Endocrinol Metab. 2017;312:E429–E36.
23. Oliveira RM. Role of type 2 deiodinase in hypothalamic control of feeding behavior. J Endocrinology, Diabetes & Obesity. 2014;2:1048.
24. Bianco AC, Silva JE. Intracellular conversion of thyroxine to triiodothyronine is required for the optimal thermogenic function of brown adipose tissue. J Clin Invest. 1987;79:295–300.
25. Silva JE. The thermogenic effect of thyroid hormone and its clinical implications. Ann Intern Med. 2003;139:205–13.
26. Silvestri E, Schiavo L, Lombardi A, Goglia F. Thyroid hormones as molecular determinants of thermogenesis. Acta Physiol Scand. 2005;184:265–83.
27. Lombardi A, de Lange P, Silvestri E, Busiello RA, Lanni A, Goglia F, et al. 3,5-Diiodo-L-thyronine rapidly enhances mitochondrial fatty acid oxidation rate and thermogenesis in rat skeletal muscle: AMP-activated protein kinase involvement. Am J Physiol Endocrinol Metab. 2009;296: E497–502.
28. St-Onge MP, Grandner MA, Brown D, Conroy MB, Jean-Louis G, Coons M, et al. Sleep duration and quality: impact on lifestyle behaviors and cardiometabolic health: a scientific statement from the American Heart Association. Circulation. 2016;134:e367–e86.
29. Dutil C, Chaput JP. Inadequate sleep as a contributor to type 2 diabetes in children and adolescents. Nutr Diabetes. 2017;7:e266.
30. Park HT, Cho GJ, Ahn KH, Shin JH, Hong SC, Kim T, et al. Thyroid stimulating hormone is associated with metabolic syndrome in euthyroid postmenopausal women. Maturitas. 2009;62:301–5.
31. Garduno-Garcia Jde J, Alvirde-Garcia U, Lopez-Carrasco G, Padilla Mendoza ME, Mehta R, Arellano-Campos O, et al. TSH and free thyroxine concentrations are associated with differing metabolic markers in euthyroid subjects. Eur J Endocrinol. 2010;163:273–8.
32. Ruhla S, Weickert MO, Arafat AM, Osterhoff M, Isken F, Spranger J, et al. A high normal TSH is associated with the metabolic syndrome. Clin Endocrinol. 2010; 72:696–701.
33. Tarcin O, Abanonu GB, Yazici D, Tarcin O. Association of metabolic syndrome parameters with TT3 and FT3/FT4 ratio in obese Turkish population. Metab Syndr Relat Disord. 2012;10:137–42.
34. Waring AC, Rodondi N, Harrison S, Kanaya AM, Simonsick EM, Miljkovic I, et al. Thyroid function and prevalent and incident metabolic syndrome in older adults: the health, ageing and body composition study. Clin Endocrinol. 2012; 76:911–8.
35. Oh JY, Sung YA, Lee HJ. Elevated thyroid stimulating hormone levels are associated with metabolic syndrome in euthyroid young women. Korean J Intern Med. 2013;28:180–6.
36. Roef GL, Rietzschel ER, Van Daele CM, Taes YE, De Buyzere ML, Gillebert TC, et al. Triiodothyronine and free thyroxine levels are differentially associated with metabolic profile and adiposity-related cardiovascular risk markers in euthyroid middle-aged subjects. Thyroid. 2014;24:223–31.
37. Mehran L, Amouzegar A, Tohidi M, Moayedi M, Azizi F. Serum free thyroxine concentration is associated with metabolic syndrome in euthyroid subjects. Thyroid. 2014;24:1566–74.
38. Minami Y, Takaya R, Takitani K, Ishiro M, Okasora K, Niegawa T, et al. Association of thyroid hormones with obesity and metabolic syndrome in Japanese children. J Clin Biochem Nutr. 2015;57:121–8.
39. Laclaustra M, Hurtado-Roca Y, Sendin M, Leon M, Ledesma M, Andres E, et al. Lower-normal TSH is associated with better metabolic risk factors: a cross-sectional study on Spanish men. Nutr Metab Cardiovasc Dis. 2015;25: 1095–103.

25

Usefulness of core needle biopsy for the diagnosis of thyroid Burkitt's lymphoma

Stella Bernardi[1,2*], Andrea Michelli[1], Deborah Bonazza[1,3], Veronica Calabrò[2], Fabrizio Zanconati[1,3], Gabriele Pozzato[1,4] and Bruno Fabris[1,2]

Abstract

Background: Thyroid lymphomas are an exceptional finding in patients with thyroid nodules. Burkitt's lymphoma is one of the rarest and most aggressive forms of thyroid lymphomas, and its prognosis depends on the earliness of medical treatment. Given the rarity of this disease, making a prompt diagnosis can be challenging. For instance, fine-needle aspiration (FNA) cytology, which is the first-line diagnostic test that is performed in patients with thyroid nodules, is often not diagnostic in cases of thyroid lymphomas, with subsequent delay of the start of therapy.

Case presentation: Here we report the case of a 52-year-old woman presenting with a rapidly enlarging thyroid mass. Thyroid ultrasonography demonstrated a solid hypoechoic nodule. FNA cytology was only suggestive of a lymphoproliferative disorder and did not provide a definitive diagnosis. It is core needle biopsy (CNB) that helped us to overcome the limitations of routine FNA cytology, showing the presence of thyroid Burkitt's lymphoma. Subsequent staging demonstrated bone marrow involvement. The early start of an intensive multi-agent chemotherapy resulted in complete disease remission. At 60 months after the diagnosis, the patient is alive and has not had any recurrence.

Conclusions: Clinicians should be aware that thyroid Burkitt's lymphoma is an aggressive disease that needs to be treated with multi-agent chemotherapy as soon as possible. To diagnose it promptly, they should consider to order/perform a CNB in any patient with a rapidly enlarging thyroid mass that is suspicious for lymphoma.

Keywords: Thyroid, Burkitt's lymphoma, Thyroid lymphomas, Core needle biopsy, Case report

Background

Thyroid nodules are an extremely common occurrence. It is estimated that up to 67% of the population has a thyroid nodule that could be detected by ultrasonography [1]. Thyroid cancer occurs in 7–15% of cases depending on risk factors such as age, sex, family history, and radiation exposure [2]. Thyroid lymphoma accounts for less than 5% of all thyroid cancers. Nevertheless, clinicians should know how to manage this extremely rare occurrence, as the prognosis of the most aggressive subtypes depends on the earliness of the diagnosis and the subsequent start of multiagent chemotherapy regimens.

Routine medical work-up of patients with thyroid nodules is based on the evidence that fine-needle aspiration (FNA), preferably performed under ultrasonographic guidance and with rapid on-site evaluation by a cytopathologist [3], is the most sensitive and cost-effective method to assess their nature and/or the need for surgery [2, 4–6]. By contrast, FNA has a low accuracy for the diagnosis of thyroid lymphomas [7, 8], often leading to diagnostic surgery. It has been argued that in cases suspicious of thyroid lymphomas, core needle biopsy (CNB) could help to reduce diagnostic surgery [7] and, most importantly, to obtain earlier the diagnosis

* Correspondence: stella.bernardi@asuits.sanita.fvg.it; shiningstella@gmail.com
[1]Department of Medical Surgical and Health Sciences, Università degli Studi di Trieste, Cattinara Teaching Hospital, Strada di Fiume 447, 34149 Trieste, Italy
[2]Endocrinology Unit - Azienda Sanitaria Universitaria Integrata Trieste, Cattinara Teaching Hospital, Strada di Fiume 447, 34149 Trieste, Italy

necessary to start life-saving treatment with multiagent chemotherapy.

Here we report the case of a woman with Burkitt's lymphoma of the thyroid gland, where CNB helped us to overcome the limitations of routine FNA cytology and to prescribe the right medical treatment. We also performed a review of the literature and a search in Pubmed of other clinical cases of adult patients affected by Burkitt's lymphoma of the thyroid gland. For this purpose, we used the combined terms "Burkitt", "thyroid", and "case", and we selected only English written articles [9–24], while we excluded a few reports in other languages, such as Spanish [25–28], French [29, 30], and Japanese [31, 32].

Case presentation

A 52-year-old woman presented to our Endocrinology Unit with a growing thyroid mass, which had enlarged so rapidly she had become unable to wear her motorcycle helmet in the weeks prior to her visit. She suffered from Hashimoto's thyroiditis for which she was taking levothyroxine. There was no history of neck irradiation or family history of thyroid cancer. On examination, there was a large, firm thyroid nodule on the right side of the neck, without palpable cervical lymphadenopathy. TSH was 4.79 μU/mL with FT3 and FT4 within the reference range. Otherwise, there was only a mild thrombocytopenia. Thyroid ultrasonography showed a solid hypoechoic nodule in the right lobe of the gland, with significant internal vascularity and absence of calcifications (Figure 1). FNA cytology with rapid on-site evaluation of the material adequacy showed that there were only atypical lymphoid cells with no thyrocytes and the specimens were considered suggestive of a lymphoproliferative disorder but insufficient to make a diagnosis, such that a CNB was scheduled for the following day.

After checking the blood coagulation profile, the patient underwent a CNB, which allowed histological/morphological tissue analysis. This showed that normal thyrocytes were virtually all replaced by homogeneous medium-sized lymphocytes with scanty blue cytoplasm, round nuclei, coarse chromatin, and multiple small nucleoli. There were frequent mitotic figures and scattered macrophages ingesting apoptotic cells, giving to the tissue section the so-called 'starry sky' appearance (Fig. 1). Overall, these features were consistent with the presence of a thyroid Burkitt's lymphoma, and further investigations were ordered to confirm the diagnosis and evaluate the disease extent. A CT of chest and abdomen showed the 44x43x87 mm thyroid nodule with left tracheal deviation (Figure 1) without other visible masses or lymph nodes. Bone marrow biopsy showed almost 100% lymphoid infiltration, consisting of a population of intermediate-sized blast-like cells, with prominent nucleoli, which were replacing all normal cells. These cells expressed CD10, CD20, and were negative for Bcl2, CD34, and TdT. Altogether these results led us to the final diagnosis of stage IV Burkitt's lymphoma [33].

The patient was admitted to our hospital's Haematology Unit and was successfully treated with 3 cycles of Hyper-CVAD chemotherapy (cyclophosphamide, vincristine, doxorubicin and dexamethasone) completed in five months. The thyroid mass disappeared (Fig. 1) and the platelets returned to baseline levels. At 60 months after diagnosis the patient is alive, and remains disease-free at regular follow-up.

Discussion

Burkitt's lymphoma is one of the rarest [34] and also most aggressive subtypes of thyroid lymphomas [11]. It is considered the fastest growing human tumor, with a cell doubling time of 24–48 h [33]. It arises from B cells, where a chromosomal translocation, more frequently t(8;14)(q24;q32) and less frequently either t(2;8)(p12;q24) or t(8;22)(q24;q11), leads to the deregulated expression of the oncogene C-Myc, which promotes cell cycle progression [35]. As a result, this lymphoma is characterized by the presence of monomorphic medium-sized B cells with a very high proliferation rate and increased apoptosis. To the best of our knowledge, 23 cases of thyroid Burkitt's lymphoma have been described in the English medical literature [9–24] (Table 1). The majority of them (13 out of 23) were cases of Burkitt's lymphoma with disseminated disease (stage III/IV). Among them, at least 5 patients (22%) died within the first 2 years of follow-up [11, 21, 22, 24] (Table 1). These were cases of age greater than 60 years, advanced disease, or disease onset complicated by cavernous sinus thrombosis (Table 1). Consistent with this, advanced age, poor performance status, advanced stage, and central nervous system or bone marrow involvement are considered the most relevant prognostic factors of a poor outcome in Burkitt's lymphoma [35]. Therefore, starting chemotherapy as soon as possible is key for a complete response.

Unfortunately, given the rarity of this disease, making a prompt diagnosis can be challenging. The first aspect that should raise the suspicion of a thyroid lymphoma should be the presence of a rapidly growing goiter or nodule. It is estimated that 70% of patients with aggressive thyroid lymphomas complain of a rapidly expanding cervical mass that causes obstructive symptoms, such as dyspnea and dysphagia [8, 36]. In line with this figure, these symptoms were reported by 65% (15 out of 23) of patients with thyroid Burkitt's lymphoma (Table 1). However, these symptoms are not specific and they might also be due to other conditions, such as anaplastic carcinoma or Riedel's thyroiditis. Moreover, sometimes,

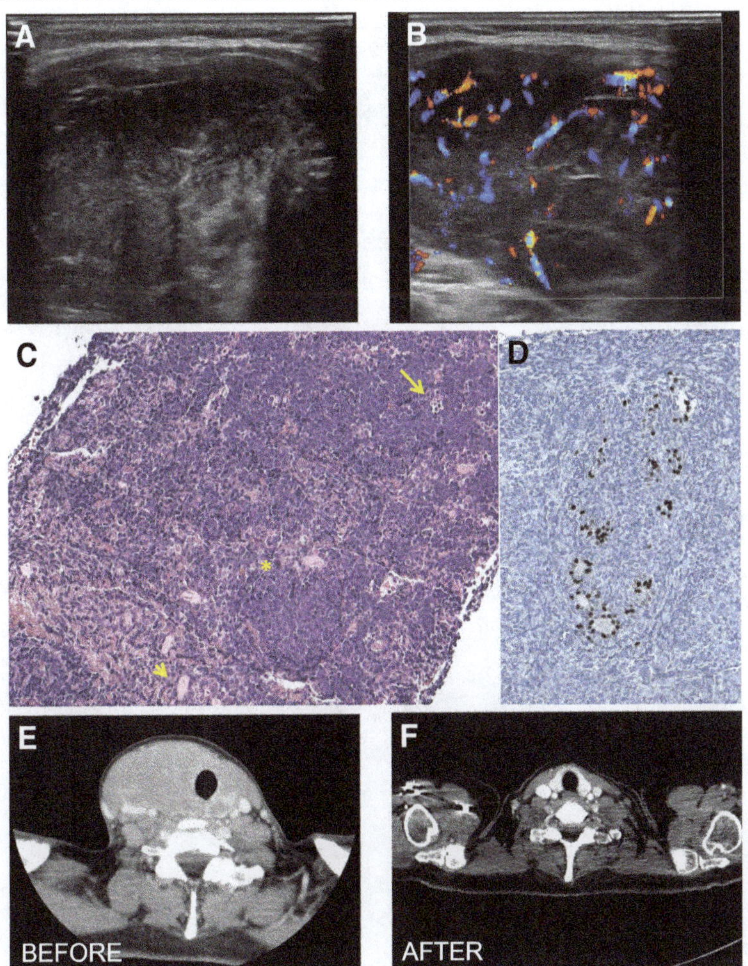

Fig. 1 Endocrine imaging of a patient with Burkitt's lymphoma. Thyroid US showed a solid hypoechoic mass (**a**) with significant internal vascularity (**b**) and no calcifications. Core needle biopsy showed homogeneous medium-sized B cells infiltrating the thyroid (**c**, arrowhead), mitotic figures (**c**, asterisk), and scattered macrophages ingesting apoptotic cells (**c**, arrow), giving a "starry sky" appearance. The extent of thyroid infiltration can be appreciated on (**d**) where follicular cells are only those positively stained for TTF1 (thyroid transcription factor 1). The CT scan performed before treatment showed a 44x43x87 mm thyroid nodule (**e**), which disappeared at the CT scan performed one year after treatment completion (**f**)

the thyroid mass due to a lymphoma can be an incidental occurrence in patients with fever, malaise, weight loss, or hypothyroidism due to Hashimoto's thyroiditis, as reported by [9, 16, 20]. Otherwise, there have been also a few reports of exceptional presentations such as a pathological fracture due to a secondary lytic lesion [13], and the onset of diplopia and headache due to a bilateral cavernous sinus thrombosis [24].

According to current guidelines [2, 6], ultrasonography is the first exam that should be performed in patients with a goiter or a thyroid nodule, and it should be generally followed by FNA cytology, whenever a solid thyroid nodule greater than 1-2 cm is detected. However, in case of a thyroid lymphoma, these procedures are often non-diagnostic. For instance, the ultrasound features of thyroid lymphomas, which include very low echogenicity, enhanced posterior echoes, increased vascularity, and lack of internal calcifications, are all aspecific [36]. In addition, as shown by the rapid on-site evaluation of our specimens, FNA cytology is often suggestive but insufficient to make a diagnosis of thyroid lymphoma. Apart from not providing adequate material, other pitfalls of FNA include the cytological similarities with thyroiditis and the high rate at which both pathologies occur simultaneously in the same gland, as 60–90% of lymphomas arise on a background of thyroiditis [36]. For these reasons, it has been argued that patients with suspected thyroid lymphomas require CNB or excision for diagnosis [8].

Tissue biopsies can provide the material necessary to assess tissue morphology and to perform a panel of immunostains, which should be the first aspects to evaluate when a Burkitt's lymphoma is suspected [37]. In

Table 1 Reported cases of thyroid Burkitt's lymphomas

Authors (ref)	Age (y) Sex	Sites of involvement	Stage	Symptoms (S) Diagnosis (D)	Follow-up (mo)	Outcome
Thieblemont [9]	46 M	Thyroid, cervical and mediastinal nodes, bone marrow, stomach	IV	S: asymptomatic D: CNB	NA	NA
Iqbal [10]	6 M	Thyroid, right atrium, right ventricle, pericardium, abdominal masses, CNS	IV	S: thyroid enlargement, anorexia, weight loss, shortness of breath D: biopsy of suprarenal mass	NA	Alive, CR
Ruggiero [11]	40 F	Thyroid, other sites	IV	S: obstructive symptoms D: FNA + CNB	Died after 3 months	
Kalinyak [12]	53 M	Thyroid, bone marrow	IV	S: obstructive symptoms D: FNA + bone marrow	27	Alive, CR
Camera [13]	56 M	Thyroid, mediastinum, kidneys, right femur	IV	S: pathological fracture D: FNA + open surgery	NA	Reduction of all lesions
Kandil [14]	60 F	Thyroid and cervical nodes	I	S: obstructive symptoms D: FNA + incisional biopsy	NA	Succesfully treated after 1 cycle of CT
Yildiz [15]	31 M	Thyroid, cervical and jugulodigastric nodes	I	S: obstructive symptoms D: open surgery	6	Alive, CR
Bongiovanni [16]	72 F	Thyroid, cervical nodes, liver and skeletal lesions	IV	S: fever D: FNA + CNB	NA	NA
Mweempwa [17]	58 F	Thyroid	I	S: obstructive symptoms D: FNA + CNB	4	Alive, CR
Albert [18]	16 M	Thyroid	I	S: obstructive symptoms D: open surgery	NA	Alive, CR
Zhang [19]	8 M	Thyroid	I	S: obstructive symptoms D: open surgery	48	Alive, CR
Cooper [20]	14 M	Thyroid, lung, kidney and pancreas	IV	S: malaise, lethargy, weight loss D: FNA + OWB	36	Alive, CR
Alloui [21]	70 M	Thyroid	I	S: obstructive symptoms D: CNB	Patient died of septic shock after 17 days	
Quesada [22]	24 NA	Thyroid, cervical, aortcaval, preaortic, and paraortic nodes	III	S: obstructive symptoms 5/7 D: FNA 5/7 + either CNB 4/7, or open surgery 3/7	41	Alive, CR
	28 NA	Thyroid and cervical nodes	I		361	Alive, CR
	47 NA	Thyroid, cervical nodes, CNS	IV		25	Alive, CR
	45 NA	Thyroid	I		12	Alive, PD
	41 NA	Thyroid, cervical, pretracheal and retrocrural nodes, mediastinum, bone marrow	IV		113	Alive, CR
	49 NA	Thyroid, cervical and iliac nodes	III		Died after 12 months	
	19 NA	Thyroid, cervical, jugulodigastric nodes, lumbar vertebrae	IV		Dieta after 23 months	
Akshintala [23]	21 F	Thyroid and cervical nodes	I	S: obstructive symptoms D: CNB + incisional biopsy	NA	Alive, CR
Moghaddasi [24]	47 F	Thyroid and cervical nodes	I	S: diplopia D: incisional biopsy	Died after 30 days	
Claudi [45]	56 F	Thyroid, liver	IV	S: obstructive symptoms D: open surgery	NA	NA

CNB is for core needle biopsy; CNS is for central nervous system; CR is for complete remission; FNA is for fine needle aspiration; NA is for not applicable; PD is for persistent disease; OWB is for open wedge biospy

particular, typical morphological features of this lymphoma include the presence of homogeneous medium-sized lymphocytes with round nuclei, coarse chromatin and multiple small nucleoli, surrounded by a scanty blue cytoplasm with frequent small vacuoles and indistinct edges [38]. Another typical feature is the "starry sky" pattern [16], which is due to the presence of macrophages containing apoptotic tumor cells on a background of proliferating B cells. Then, to reach a final diagnosis of Burkitt's lymphoma, immunohistochemical stainings should provide evidence that lymphomatous cells express CD19, CD20, CD10, and CD79a and no CD3, CD5, Bcl2, and

TdT [37, 38]. Additional diagnostic criteria for Burkitt's lymphoma include Ki67 positivity/proliferation index > 90%, light chain restriction, nuclear c-myc positivity at immunocytochemistry, and t(8;14)(q24;q32) by fluorescence in situ hybridization [38], as reported by [9, 11, 16, 17, 21–23] (Table 1).

Core needle biopsy (CNB) is an exam that is not routinely performed in the work-up of patients with thyroid nodules. This is ascribed to higher cost, technical requirements, and concerns about potential complications as compared to FNA [39]. In addition, also CNB can fail to diagnose follicular carcinomas [40], whose presence is diagnosed based on vascular invasion and/or capsular breakthrough [39]. Consistent with these issues, the AACE/ACE/AME guidelines suggest considering the use of CNB only in solid nodules with persistently inadequate cytology [6], and the ATA guidelines do not even recommend its use [2]. Nevertheless, our case reminds that CNB should not be dismissed as it can become extremely useful in cases of thyroid lymphomas, where it allows to obtain a specimen that is adequate for histological/morphological tissue analysis, as well as for other key diagnostic tests. This is supported also by our literature review showing that CNB (but no FNA) was able to provide the final diagnosis without additional exams [9, 11, 16, 17, 21–23] (Table 1). In particular, in the 23 reports of Burkitt's lymphoma, FNA cytology was performed in 12 patients (52%) and was able to provide the diagnosis without core needle or open surgical biopsy only in one case [12] (Table 1). Overall, in the reported cases of thyroid Burkitt's lymphoma, diagnosis was provided by core needle biospy (43%; 10 cases out of 23), open surgery (35%; 8 cases out of 23), incisional/open wedge biopsy (17%; 4 cases out of 23), rarely by FNA (1 case out of 23) [12] or biopsy of other sites of involvement, such as a renal mass (1 cases out of 23) [10] (Table 1).

In line with the concept that CNB should be the advised modality for thyroid lymphoma diagnosis, Sharma and colleagues have recently shown that CNB diagnostic sensitivity for detecting thyroid lymphomas is 93% [41]. This is in line with the results of Ha and colleagues, who found that CNB sensitivity for thyroid lymphoma was 94.7% with a positive predictive value of 100%, such that CNB was able to significantly reduce the rate of diagnostic surgery from 37.9 to 5.3%, as compared to FNA [7]. Interestingly, in a work comparing CNB to open surgical biopsy in patients with lymphoadenopathies, CNB turned out to have greater sensitivity for detecting malignancy, and it was also faster, cheaper and safer than the conventional surgical approach [42].

Having said that, current treatment of Burkitts lymphoma in adults is based on the delivery of short-duration, dose-intensive, multi-agent chemotherapy with minimization of treatment delays, and maintenance of serum drug concentrations over at least 48 to 72 h [35]. Some protocols, like the French LMB, the German BFM, and the CODOX-M/IVAC [43], have been adapted from pediatric regimens. Others, such the Hyper-CVAD regimen [44], which is the one we used, have been evaluated primarily in adults, but incorporate the principles found to be effective in pediatric populations [35]. Overall, with these regimens, 65 to 100% of patients achieve a complete response and 47 to 86% of patients maintain these remissions at least 1 year after treatment completion [35].

Conclusions

This case describes a patient with thyroid Burkitt's lymphoma, which is a rare and highly aggressive thyroid malignancy that requires a prompt diagnosis in order to start as soon as possible life-saving multi-agent chemotherapy. In particular, our case highlights the usefulness of CNB for the diagnosis of thyroid lymphomas and reminds clinicians to order/perform it in any patient with a rapidly enlarging thyroid mass that is suspicious for lymphoma.

Abbreviations

AACE/ACE/AME: American association of clinical endocrinologists/Association of clinical endocrinologists/Associazione medici endocrinologi; ATA: American thyroid association; BFM: Berlin-Frankfurt-Münster; CNB: core needle biopsy; CODOX-M/IVAC: cyclophosphamide, vincristine, doxorubicin, high-dose methotrexate/ifosfamide, etoposide, and high-dose cytarabine; CVAD: cyclophosphamide, vincristine, doxorubicin, and dexamethasone; FNA: fine needle biopsy; FT3: free triiodothyronine; FT4: free thyroxine; LMB: lymphoma malignancy B; TSH: thyroid stimulating hormone

Acknowledgments

Not applicable.

Funding

No funding was received for this study.

Authors' contributions

SB, BF examined the patient and contributed to manuscript conception, preparation, and editing. AM contributed to manuscript preparation and editing. DB and FZ performed the tissue sections readings, and contributed to image preparation and manuscript editing. VC examined the patient and contributed to manuscript editing. GP examined the patient and contributed to manuscript preparation and editing. All authors read and approved the final manuscript.

Competing interests

The authors declare that they have no competing interests.

Author details

[1]Department of Medical Surgical and Health Sciences, Università degli Studi di Trieste, Cattinara Teaching Hospital, Strada di Fiume 447, 34149 Trieste, Italy. [2]Endocrinology Unit - Azienda Sanitaria Universitaria Integrata Trieste, Cattinara Teaching Hospital, Strada di Fiume 447, 34149 Trieste, Italy. [3]Pathology Unit - Azienda Sanitaria Universitaria Integrata Trieste, Cattinara Teaching Hospital, Strada di Fiume 447, 34149 Trieste, Italy. [4]Haematology Unit - Azienda Sanitaria Universitaria Integrata Trieste, Cattinara Teaching Hospital, Strada di Fiume 447, 34149 Trieste, Italy.

References

1. Tan GH, Gharib H. Thyroid incidentalomas: management approaches to nonpalpable nodules discovered incidentally on thyroid imaging. Ann Intern Med. 1997;126(3):226–31.
2. Haugen BR, Alexander EK, Bible KC, Doherty GM, Mandel SJ, Nikiforov YE, Pacini F, Randolph GW, Sawka AM, Schlumberger M, et al. 2015 American Thyroid Association management guidelines for adult patients with thyroid nodules and differentiated thyroid Cancer the American Thyroid Association guidelines task force on thyroid nodules and differentiated thyroid Cancer. Thyroid. 2016;26(1):1–133.
3. Witt BL, Schmidt RL. Rapid onsite evaluation improves the adequacy of fine-needle aspiration for thyroid lesions: a systematic review and meta-analysis. Thyroid. 2013;23(4):428–35.
4. Burman KD, Wartofsky L. CLINICAL PRACTICE. *Thyroid Nodules N Engl J Med.* 2015;373(24):2347–56.
5. Frates MC, Benson CB, Charboneau JW, Cibas ES, Clark OH, Coleman BG, Cronan JJ, Doubilet PM, Evans DB, Goellner JR, et al. Management of thyroid nodules detected at US: Society of Radiologists in ultrasound consensus conference statement. Radiology. 2005;237(3):794–800.
6. Gharib H, Papini E, Garber JR, Duick DS, Harrell RM, Hegedus L, Paschke R, Valcavi R, Vitti P. No AAATFT: American Association of Clinical Endocrinologists, American College of Endocrinology, and Associazione Medici Endocrinologi medical guidelines for clinical Practice for the diagnosis and Management of Thyroid Nodules-2016 update. Endocr Pract. 2016;22:1–60.
7. Ha EJ, Baek JH, Lee JH, Kim JK, Song DE, Kim WB, Hong SJ. Core needle biopsy could reduce diagnostic surgery in patients with anaplastic thyroid cancer or thyroid lymphoma. Eur Radiol. 2016;26(4):1031–6.
8. Graff-Baker A, Sosa JA, Roman SA. Primary thyroid lymphoma: a review of recent developments in diagnosis and histology-driven treatment. Curr Opin Oncol. 2010;22(1):17–22.
9. Thieblemont C, Mayer A, Dumontet C, Barbier Y, Callet-Bauchu E, Felman P, Berger F, Ducottet X, Martin C, Salles G, et al. Primary thyroid lymphoma is a heterogeneous disease. J Clin Endocrinol Metab. 2002;87(1):105–11.
10. Iqbal Y, Al-Sudairy R, Abdullah MF, Al-Omari A, Crankson S. Non-Hodgkin lymphoma manifesting as thyroid nodules and cardiac involvement. J Pediatr Hematol Oncol. 2003;25(12):987–8.
11. Ruggiero FP, Frauenhoffer E, Stack BC Jr. Thyroid lymphoma: a single institution's experience. Otolaryngol Head Neck Surg. 2005;133(6):888–96.
12. Kalinyak JE, Kong CS, McDougall IR. Burkitt's lymphoma presenting as a rapidly growing thyroid mass. Thyroid. 2006;16(10):1053–7.
13. Camera A, Magri F, Fonte R, Villani L, Della Porta MG, Fregoni V, Manna LL, Chiovato L. Burkitt-like lymphoma infiltrating a hyperfunctioning thyroid adenoma and presenting as a hot nodule. Thyroid. 2010;20(9):1033–6.
14. Kandil E, Safah H, Noureldine S, Abdel Khalek M, Waddadar J, Goswami M, Friedlander P. Burkitt-like lymphoma arising in the thyroid gland. Am J Med Sci. 2012;343(1):103–5.
15. Yildiz I, Sen F, Toz B, Kilic L, Agan M, Basaran M. Primary Burkitt's lymphoma presenting as a rapidly growing thyroid mass. Case Rep Oncol. 2012;5(2): 388–93.
16. Bongiovanni M, Mazzucchelli L, Martin V, Crippa S, Bolli M, Suriano S, Giovanella L. Images in endocrine pathology: a starry-sky in the thyroid. Endocr Pathol. 2012;23(1):79–81.
17. Mweempwa A, Prasad J, Islam S. A rare neoplasm of the thyroid gland. N Z Med J. 2013;126(1369):75 8.
18. Albert S. Primary Burkitt lymphoma of the thyroid. Ear Nose Throat J. 2013; 92(12):E1–2.
19. Zhang L, Gao L, Liu G, Wang L, Xu C, Li L, Tian Y, Feng H, Guo Z. Primary Burkitt's lymphoma of the thyroid without Epstein-Barr virus infection: a case report and literature review. Oncol Lett. 2014;7(5):1519–24.
20. Cooper K, Gangadharan A, Arora RS, Shukla R, Pizer B. Burkitt lymphoma of thyroid gland in an adolescent. Case Rep Pediatr. 2014;2014:187467.
21. Allaoui M, Benchafai I, Mahtat el M, Regragui S, Boudhas A, Azzakhmam M, Boukhechba M, Al Bouzidi A, Oukabli M. Primary Burkitt lymphoma of the thyroid gland: case report of an exceptional type of thyroid neoplasm and review of the literature. *BMC Clin Pathol.* 2016;16:6.
22. Quesada AE, Liu H, Miranda RN, Golardi N, Billah S, Medeiros LJ, Jaso JM. Burkitt lymphoma presenting as a mass in the thyroid gland: a clinicopathologic study of 7 cases and review of the literature. Hum Pathol. 2016;56:101–8.
23. Akshintala D, Paturi BT, Liu J, Emani VK. A rare diagnosis of a thyroid mass. Am J Med. 2016;129(9):e191–2.
24. Moghaddasi M, Nabowati M, Razmeh S. Bilateral cavernous sinus thrombosis as first manifestation of primary Burkitt lymphoma of the thyroid gland. Neurol Int. 2017;9(2):7133.
25. Garcia Calzado MC, Ruiz Buendia A, Lopez Aranda JF, Martin Villacanas JA: [Burkitt's lymphoma with onset in the thyroid gland. A case report]. *Med Clin (Barc)* 1997, 108(14):556–557.
26. Hernandez JA, Reth P, Ballestar E. primary thyroid lymphoma with bone marrow and central nervous system infiltration at presentation. Med Clin (Barc). 2001;116(9):357–8.
27. Duran HJ, Diaz-Morfa M, Garcia-Parrenoa J, Bellon JM. Burkitt's lymphoma affecting only the thyroid. Med Clin (Barc). 2008;131(1):38–9.
28. Pereyra Zenklusen A, Burgesser MV. thyroid Burkitt lymphoma. Rev Fac Cien Med Univ Nac Cordoba. 2011;68(2):70–1.
29. Bouges S, Daures JP, Hebrard M. incidence of acute leukemias, lymphomas and thyroid cancers in children under 15 years, living around the Marcoule nuclear site from 1985 to 1995. Rev Epidemiol Sante Publique. 1999;47(3):205–17.
30. Mongalgi MA, Chakroun D, el Bez M, Boussen H, Debabbi A. thyroid goiter revealing Burkitt's lymphoma. Arch Fr Pediatr. 1992;49(6):594–5.
31. Matsuo T, Murase K, Wago M, Matsuo S, Ikeda T, Yamaguchi T. acute B-cell lymphoblastic leukemia with Burkitt's lyphoma cells--a case report. Gan No Rinsho. 1983;29(9):1035–9.
32. Fujii H, Maekawa T, Kamezaki H, Ohno H, Nishida K, Urata Y. Burkitt's lymphoma with an initial symptom of thyroid tumor during pregnancy. Rinsho Ketsueki. 1986;27(10):1957–63.
33. Molyneux EM, Rochford R, Griffin B, Newton R, Jackson G, Menon G, Harrison CJ, Israels T, Bailey S. Burkitt's lymphoma. Lancet. 2012;379(9822):1234–44.
34. Graff-Baker A, Roman SA, Thomas DC, Udelsman R, Sosa JA. Prognosis of primary thyroid lymphoma: demographic, clinical, and pathologic predictors of survival in 1,408 cases. Surgery. 2009;146(6):1105–15.
35. Blum KA, Lozanski G, Byrd JC. Adult Burkitt leukemia and lymphoma. Blood. 2004;104(10):3009–20.
36. Stein SA, Wartofsky L. Primary thyroid lymphoma: a clinical review. J Clin Endocrinol Metab. 2013;98(8):3131–8.
37. Naresh KN, Ibrahim HA, Lazzi S, Rince P, Onorati M, Ambrosio MR, Bilhou-Nabera C, Amen F, Reid A, Mawanda M, et al. Diagnosis of Burkitt lymphoma using an algorithmic approach--applicable in both resource-poor and resource-rich countries. Br J Haematol. 2011;154(6):770–6.
38. Zeppa P, Cozzolino I. Non-Hodgkin lymphoma. Monogr Clin Cytol. 2018; 23:34–51.
39. Paja M, del Cura JL, Zabala R, Corta I, Lizarraga A, Oleaga A, Exposito A, Gutierrez MT, Ugalde A, Lopez JI. Ultrasound-guided core-needle biopsy in thyroid nodules. A study of 676 consecutive cases with surgical correlation. Eur Radiol. 2016;26(1):1–8.
40. Yoon JH, Kim EK, Kwak JY, Moon HJ. Effectiveness and limitations of core needle biopsy in the diagnosis of thyroid nodules: review of current literature. J Pathol Transl Med. 2015;49(3):230–5.
41. Sharma A, Jasim S, Reading CC, Ristow KM, Villasboas Bisneto JC, Habermann TM, Fatourechi V, Stan M. Clinical presentation and diagnostic challenges of thyroid lymphoma: a cohort study. Thyroid. 2016;26(8):1061–7.
42. Pugliese N, Di Perna M, Cozzolino I, Ciancia G, Pettinato G, Zeppa P, Varone V, Masone S, Cerchione C, Della Pepa R, et al. Randomized comparison of

power Doppler ultrasonography-guided core-needle biopsy with open surgical biopsy for the characterization of lymphadenopathies in patients with suspected lymphoma. Ann Hematol. 2017;96(4):627–37.
43. Oosten LEM, Chamuleau MED, Thielen FW, de Wreede LC, Siemes C, Doorduijn JK, Smeekes OS, Kersten MJ, Hardi L, Baars JW, et al. Treatment of sporadic Burkitt lymphoma in adults, a retrospective comparison of four treatment regimens. Ann Hematol. 2018;97(2):255–66.
44. Thomas DA, Faderl S, O'Brien S, Bueso-Ramos C, Cortes J, Garcia-Manero G, Giles FJ, Verstovsek S, Wierda WG, Pierce SA, et al. Chemoimmunotherapy with hyper-CVAD plus rituximab for the treatment of adult Burkitt and Burkitt-type lymphoma or acute lymphoblastic leukemia. Cancer. 2006; 106(7):1569–80.
45. Claudi R, Viola P, Cotellese R, Angelucci R. Atypical primary Burkitt lymphoma of the thyroid gland: a practical approach for differential diagnosis and management. AM J Case Rep. 2010;11:169–73.

26

Using Hashimoto thyroiditis as gold standard to determine the upper limit value of thyroid stimulating hormone in a Chinese cohort

Yu Li[1†], Dong-Ning Chen[1†], Jing Cui[1†], Zhong Xin[2], Guang-Ran Yang[2], Ming-Jia Niu[3] and Jin-Kui Yang[2*]

Abstract

Background: Subclinical hypothyroidism, commonly caused by Hashimoto thyroiditis (HT), is a risk factor for cardiovascular diseases. This disorder is defined as merely having elevated serum thyroid stimulating hormone (TSH) levels. However, the upper limit of reference range for TSH is debated recently. This study was to determine the cutoff value for the upper normal limit of TSH in a cohort using the prevalence of Hashimoto thyroiditis as "gold" calibration standard.

Methods: The research population was medical staff of 2856 individuals who took part in health examination annually. Serum free triiodothyronine (FT3), free thyroxine (FT4), TSH, thyroid peroxidase antibody (TPAb), thyroglobulin antibody (TGAb) and other biochemistry parameters were tested. Meanwhile, thyroid ultrasound examination was performed. The diagnosis of HT was based on presence of thyroid antibodies (TPAb and TGAb) and abnormalities of thyroid ultrasound examination. We used two different methods to estimate the cutoff point of TSH based on the prevalence of HT.

Results: Joinpoint regression showed the prevalence of HT increased significantly at the ninth decile of TSH value corresponding to 2.9 mU/L. ROC curve showed a TSH cutoff value of 2.6 mU/L with the maximized sensitivity and specificity in identifying HT. Using the newly defined cutoff value of TSH can detect patients with hyperlipidemia more efficiently, which may indicate our approach to define the upper limit of TSH can make more sense from the clinical point of view.

Conclusions: A significant increase in the prevalence of HT occurred among individuals with a TSH of 2.6–2.9 mU/L made it possible to determine the cutoff value of normal upper limit of TSH.

Background

Patients with subclinical hypothyroidism have normal level of serum thyroid hormones (T4, T3, FT3, FT4) and elevated TSH. These patienshave a higher incidence of lipid abnormalities, coronary heart disease, psychiatric disorders and pregnancy complications [1–9], although their clinical symptoms are very mild. Proper screening and treatment of these patients may help to improve the adverse outcome of the involving diseases. Therefore, to define the upper limit of TSH precisely had an important role in detecting patients who had mild thyroid dysfunction and might benefit from early intervention.

The upper limit of reference range for "normal" TSH has been the focus of debate in the recent decade. Some authors insisted on the conventional value of 4.0–5.0 mU/L as the upper limit of normal thyroid stimulating hormone (TSH) [10], others suggested it narrowed to 2.5–3.0 mU/L [11]. As mentioned in the National Academy of Clinical Biochemistry (NACB) guideline, more than 95 % of normal individuals had TSH below 2.5 mU/L. There were even data showing that African-Americans had very low incidence of HT

* Correspondence: jkyang@ccmu.edu.cn

†Equal contributors

[2]Department of Endocrinology, Beijing Key Laboratory of Diabetes Research and Care, Beijing Tongren Hospital, Capital Medical University, Beijing 100730, China

Full list of author information is available at the end of the article

with a mean TSH level of 1.18 mU/L This value maybe the "true normal" upper limit for TSH, because African-Americans have very low prevalence of Hashimoto thyroiditis (HT) to elevate TSH [11].

Another question was put forward that which was the true set point of normal upper limit. Which centile (90, 95 or 99th) should be the real normal limit? The approximate questions related to glycemic threshold for diagnosing diabetes were already answered by using diabetic retinopathy (DR) as "gold" calibration standard [12]. Referring to that and based on the correlation between HT (as end-point) and TSH value, we tried using the prevalence of HT as the calibration standard to determine the upper limit of TSH.

Methods

Research population

A total of 2856 medical staffs with age between 20 and 60 years old participated in a health examination in the year of 2013 were included in our research. Questionnaires related to medication history and other health-related behaviors were completed beforehand. Blood sampling was performed in the morning after eight hours of fasting, followed by the detection of height, weight, waist-to-hip ratio (WHR), blood pressure and physical examinations.

The study was conducted with the approval of the Ethics Committee of Beijing Tongren Hospital, Capital Medical University.

Laboratory assessments

Blood samples were collected for testing thyroid function including serum free triiodothyronine (FT3), free thyroxine (FT4) and TSH, thyroid peroxidase antibody (TPAb), thyroglobulin antibody (TGAb) and other biochemistry parameters including total cholesterol (TC), triglyceride (TG), low density lipoprotein cholesterol (LDL),, fasting plasma glucose (FPG), uric acid (UA), alanine aminotransferase (ALT), aspartate aminotransferase (AST), creatinine (Cr) and carbon dioxide combining power (CO_2CP). Appliance for testing the above mentioned biochemistry factors were Immunoassay Systems (Beckman Coulter, UniCel DXI800).

The diagnostic criteria for HT

The diagnosis of HT was established by a combination of presence of thyroid antibodies (TPAb and TGAb) and abnormalities of thyroid sonogram including reduced echo or diffused heterogeneity echo of thyroid with or without nodularity [8]. Ultrasound examination of thyroid was performed by four experienced professional ultrasound physicians. Consistent diagnosis standard was used, including description for the size, nodules and echo of the thyroid.

Framingham score

Framingham score (FS), a 10-year estimated risk of CHD, was calculated by the equation including: age, gender, blood pressure, smoking status and cholesterol levels [13]. FS equaling to or over 9 was considered to be a predictor for the higher CHD risk of over 5 %.

Statistical analysis

Unpaired *t*-test, Mann-Whitney *U* test or Pearson Chi-square test was used to compare the difference between cohorts with or without HT. We used two different methods to estimate the cutoff point of TSH based on the prevalence of HT: Joinpoint regression [14] and ROC curve by maximizing the sensitivity and specificity. All statistical analyses were conducted with the software package SPSS version 13 for windows, and ljr package of R software (http://www.r-project.org). A two-sided p value of less than 0.05 was considered to be statistically significant.

Results

Characteristics of the observed cohort

By the exclusion standard, those with abnormal thyroid function (FT3 and FT4 out of the normal range), being pregnant, taking thyroid related medicine, accepted thyroid operation and patients with personal history of autoimmune disorders were excluded. A total number of 2856 individuals were included in the research, with the average age of 36.0. The proportion of women (75 %) was higher than men (25 %), which was consistent with the gender characteristic of the medical staff in China.

The research population was further divided into HT and non-HT groups. According to the diagnosis standard, 187 (7 %) in the observed cohort had HT (Table 1), which comprised of 14 males and 173 females. The prevalence of HT in females (8 %) was 4 times higher than in males (2 %).

No significant differences between the HT and non-HT groups were found in age, BMI, WHR, blood pressure or biochemical parameters concerning liver function, blood glucose and lipid. However, serum creatinine and uric acid were lower in HT group, which may be related to the high prevalence of HT in females, because females have relatively low level of serum creatinine and uric acid than males.

The distribution of TSH in the total population and subgroups (HT and non-HT group)

Although exclusion standard was used in our research to get a relatively homogeneous cohort without overt thyroid diseases, the distribution of TSH still showed asymmetrical curve with extension to the right side. We then separated HT from the whole population, and the TSH distribution of HT and non-HT groups was described in Fig. 1. Non-HT group showed a more likely Gaussian

Table 1 Characteristics of observed cohort divided by the participants with Hashimoto thyroiditis (HT) or without HT (non-HT)

	Non HT	HT	*P*
No	2669	187	—
Age (year)	35.90 (9.15)	36.99 (9.25)	0.117
Sex (M/F)	704/1965	14/173	**<0.001****
TSH (μIU/l)	1.83 (0.01–26.36)	2.66 (0.01–39.96)	**0.001***
Free triiodothyronine (pmol/l)	4.96 (0.68)	4.95 (0.92)	0.92
Free thyroid hormone (pmol/l)	10.58 (1.72)	10.36 (1.92)	0.12
BMI (kg/m2)	23.23 (3.61)	23.33 (3.31)	0.69
WHR	0.81 (0.07)	0.80 (0.06)	0.14
Systolic blood pressure (mmHg)	114.15 (13.95)	113.66 (13.61)	0.64
Diastolic blood pressure (mmHg)	73.22 (9.39)	72.87 (8.71)	0.60
Alanine aminotransferase (IU/l)	24.26 (17.40)	22.84 (12.04)	0.13
Aspartate aminotransferase (IU/l)	26.53 (9.68)	26.41 (7.73)	0.84
Blood urea nitrogen (mmol/l)	3.80 (1.05)	3.72 (0.99)	0.28
Creatinine (μmol/l)	65.54 (13.99)	60.09 (9.68)	**<0.001***
Total cholesterol (mmol/l)	4.64 (0.84)	4.65 (0.83)	0.87
Triglycerides (mmol/l)	1.10 (0.91)	1.04 (0.73)	0.34
LDL cholesterol (mmol/l)	2.89 (0.89)	2.88 (0.74)	0.87
HDL cholesterol (mmol/l)	1.45 (0.39)	1.47 (0.34)	0.45
Fasting plasma glucose (mmol/L)	5.33 (0.94)	5.24 (0.50)	0.16
Uric acid (mmol/L)	278.90 (74.60)	264.48 (67.47)	**0.010**

Values are mean(SD) or median (range). Comparison between any two groups by unpaired *t*-test, Mann-Whitney *U* test* or Pearson Chi-square test**. Data in bold are statistically significant

curve, and the HT group showed an uneven curve with more rightward trend representing higher TSH values. The different centiles of TSH in both groups were listed in Table 2. By ANOVA analysis, there was no statistically significant influence of age to the upper limit of TSH in our research population ($P = 0.5$).

The prevalence of HT corresponding to each decile of TSH value

A curve was drawn to describe the correlation between HT and TSH value (Fig. 2). Each decile of TSH value was marked in the X-axis, meanwhile the proportion of participants with HT between each decile of TSH was shown in Y-axis. The curve was relatively flat when TSH <2.9 mU/L. Whereas the curve showed a sharp increase at the ninth decile of TSH (corresponding to TSH≧2.9 mU/L) The prevalence of HT in the ninth decile was 21 %, while that in the eighth decile was 8 %. Regression analysis showed a good Joinpoint at the ninth decile ($P = 0.0012$). Logistic regression models adjusted for sex, age, BMI, FT4, systolic blood pressure and biochemical parameters also confirmed a statistically significant difference for the prevalence of HT below vs. above the cutoff point for TSH value (OR 3.07 [95 % CI: 2.24–4.21]; $P = 0.000$).

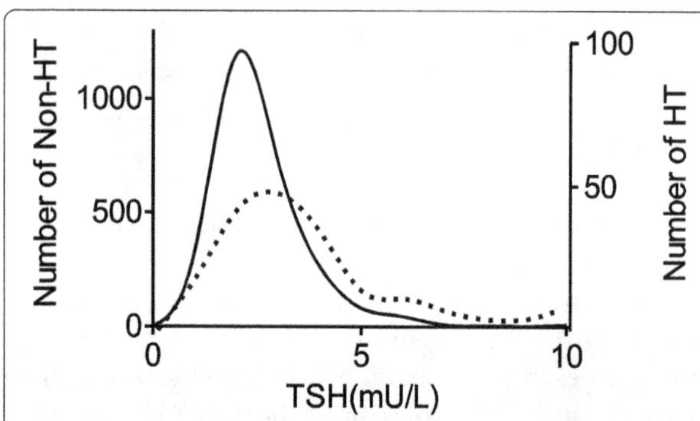

Fig. 1 Distribution of thyroid stimulating hormone (TSH) in both Hashimoto thyroiditis (HT) (– – –) and non-HT (—) participants. Curves were smoothed by the GraphPad Prism 5 software

ROC curve describing the cutoff value of TSH in detecting participants with HT

When maximizing the sensitivity and specificity, the cutoff value of TSH equaled to 2.6 mU/L, with the sensitivity of 52 % and the specificity of 77 %. The area under the ROC curve was 66 % (95 % CI: 61.01–70.51) (Fig. 3). The proportion of participants with HT was 4 % when TSH was below 2.6 mU/L. As compared, when TSH was above 2.6, the proportion of participants with HT was 14 % ($P = 0.000$ by Fisher's exact test).

Table 2 Serum TSH levels (mU/L) in total population and subgroups categorized by age

		Percentile				
Age (yr)	Sample No.	2. 5th	5th	Median	95th	97.5th
A. total						
19–29	845	0.53	0.73	1.80	4.45	5.50
30–39	1060	0.51	0.73	1.85	4.42	4.98
40–49	662	0.61	0.73	1.94	4.99	5.61
50–59	289	0.65	0.70	1.92	5.45	7.49
B. non-HT						
19–29	799	0.56	0.75	1.79	4.33	5.19
30–39	989	0.52	0.74	1,82	4.06	4.62
40–49	616	0.62	0.73	1.91	4.31	5.26
50–59	265	0.65	0.70	1.86	4.58	5.67
C. HT						
19–29	46	0.37	0.74	2.33	8.48	21.67
30–39	71	0.02	0.46	2.43	9.50	18.86
40–49	46	0.03	0.33	3.29	8.34	24.26
50–59	24	0.56	0.73	3.17	14.77	15.50

Comparison of metabolism-related parameters between groups divided by different cutoff values of TSH

As shown in Table 3, the cutoff value of 2.9 mU/L (based on the Joinpoint regression), and 2.6 mU/L (based on the ROC curve analysis), and 4.5 mU/L (conventionally accepted cutoff value) were used to categorize the population. All three grouping methods showed a higher probability of hyperlipidemia and a higher Framingham Score in participants with TSH above the cutoff point, and a relatively younger age in participants with TSH below the cutoff point. As compared to using 4.5 mU/L as the cutoff point, using 2.6 mU/L or 2.9 mU/L as the cutoff value of TSH can detect more patients with abnormal TC and LDL. That may tell us it's more effective to apply the lowered cutoff value of TSH for detecting patients with dyslipidemia.

Discussion

To get a more convincing reference range of TSH, previous researchers used a more stringent standard for screening the reference population proposed by the NHANES III study [2], and more sensitive assays were used to measure TSH of those reference individuals. The upper limit of TSH was lowered to 3.6–3.7 mU/L [3, 15]. It was believed that the skewing right tail of the TSH distribution curve was caused by the inclusion of those with occult thyroid dysfunctions most representatively as HT. Besides, other factors such as gender and age are also critical to the reference range of TSH [16]. In this study, age does not serve as an influence factor to the upper limit of TSH. The reason may be the research population was a homogeneously young cohort. Besides, It is not an iodine deficient area in Beijing. Therefore, the daily iodine intake and total body iodine status should not be a major factor to influence TSH value in our research population. We aimed to clear up the confounding influence of those individuals with HT to determine the cutoff point of TSH in our research population.

If we defined the upper limit of normal TSH as the 95th centile as adopted by previous researchers, the value would be 4.2, which could be comparable to most publications and more approximate to the traditional opinions insisting on 4.0–5.0 mU/L as the upper limit of normal TSH.

However, there were still considerable proportion of people with occult subclinical thyroid disease (mostly HT) within the upper part of the normal TSH range.

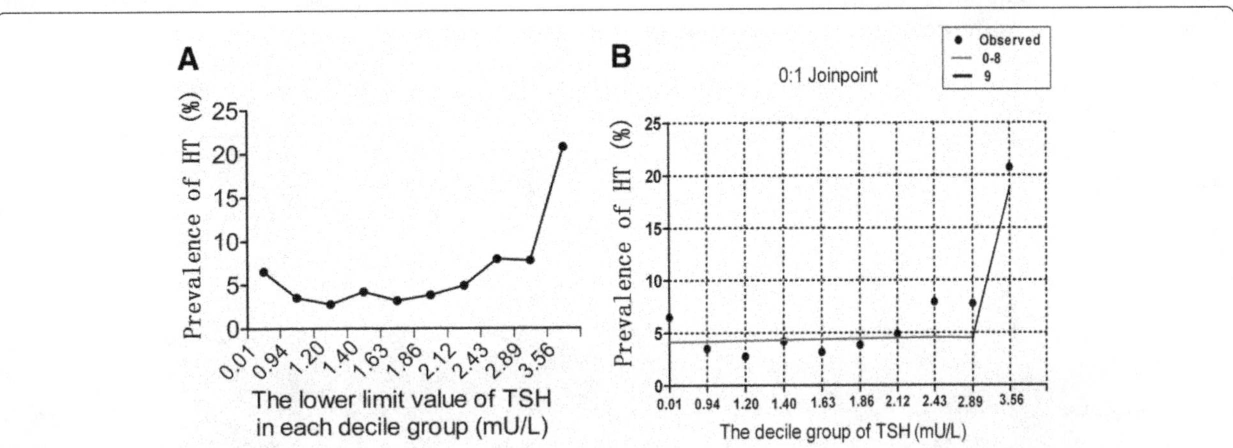

Fig. 2 a The prevalence of HT corresponding to each decile of TSH value (Each point in the chart corresponded to the number labeled in X axis. 2.89 is the cutoff value of TSH revealed by joinpoint analysis). **b** The joinpoint regression analysis showed only one joinpoint was found. This joinpoint presented in the ninth decile group, and the lower limit value of this group of 2.89 was taken as the cutoff

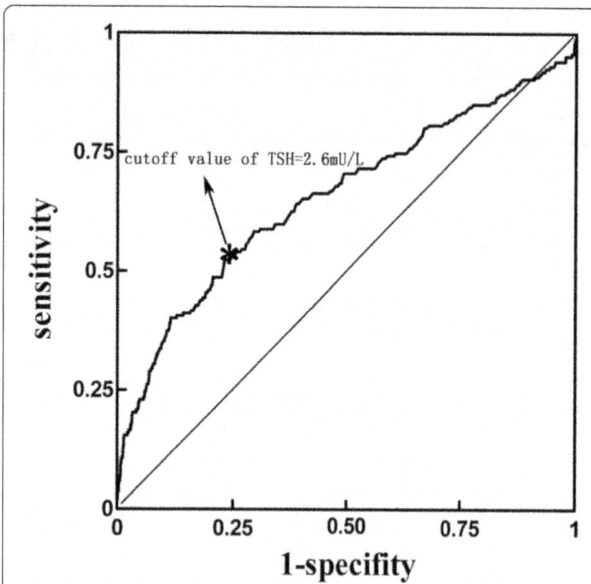

Fig. 3 ROC curve describing the cutoff value of TSH in detecting participants with HT. When maximizing the sensitivity and specificity, the cutoff value of TSH equaled to 2.6 mU/L, with the sensitivity of 52 % and the specificity of 77 %

Whereas we expect the normal range as a tool to screen out abnormal individuals. We tried an alternative approach to exclude the influence to TSH value confounded by individuals with HT. Based on the fact that TSH and the prevalence of HT was well correlated, we used "the prevalence of HT" as a checkout factor to determine the cutoff upper limit of TSH. Mimicking the diagnostic methodology in determining glycemic thresholds using DR as the checkout factor, we drew a curve describing the correlation between the prevalence of HT and TSH value. From this curve we got a turning point at TSH 2.9 mU/L by Joinpoint regression analysis. The prevalence of HT above this point was 14.5 % and much higher than that below the cutoff point (4.6 %). Similarly, ROC curve revealed a cutoff value of 2.6 mU/L, by which we can effectively detect HT with the best sensitivity and specificity.

These two measures showed very close results which are more close to the proposal in recent NACB guideline about narrowing the upper limit of TSH to 2.5 mU/L [11]. As proposed by Surks [16], the normal range for TSH should meet the needs to categorize population into groups 1) normal, 2) those who need to be observed closely and 3) those who need medication. Although the lowered cutoff value of TSH may not be used as a treatment threshold, it can help to find more patients with occult subclinical thyroid diseases. If the limit was increased to 4.5U/L, 2.2 % of individuals with HT would be missed.

It has been indicated by several studies [17–19], that elevated TSH within the normal range was positively related to lipid abnormalities or even to the future occurring of hypertension and hyperlipidemia. Likewise, we used the lowered cutoff value of TSH to categorize population to watch if it made sense concerning the metabolism parameters among groups. As expected, people in the group with higher TSH had a much higher age, higher rate of hyperlipidemia and a higher Framingham score. When the cutoff value of 2.6 mU/L was used, it showed better results with more significant difference between groups concerning hyperlipidemia (hyper-TC, hyper-LDL and hyper-TG). Meanwhile, if a lowered upper limit of TSH was used, we can detect more patients with hyperlipidemia with less missed diagnosis. The Framingham score went higher with the increasing of TSH. This was also consistent with Asvold's observation [9] and suggested increased incidence of coronary heart disease in population with SCH. Therefore, a lowered upper limit of TSH can also help to detect individuals with increased risk of ischemic heart diseases effectively.

Table 3 Comparison of metabolism related parameters between groups divided by cutoff values of TSH based on different method (using Joinpoint regression, ROC curve and conventional accepted value respectively)

Derivation of cutoff values	Group	No	Age (mean(SD))	BMI ≧24	Hyper- TC	Hyper-LDL-c	Hyper-TG	Hyper- FPG	FS≧9
Joinpoint regression	TSH < 2.9	2284	35.7 (9.1)	37 %	22 %	23 %	14 %	7 %	20 %
	TSH≧2.9	572	36.9 (9.5)	35 %	27 %	27 %	18 %	8 %	23 %
	P		0.009	0.49	0.021*	0.07	0.030*	0.46	0.18
ROC curve	TSH < 2.6	2138	35.7 (9.1)	37 %	22 %	23 %	14 %	7 %	20 %
	TSH≧2.6	718	36.8 (9.5)	36 %	28 %	27 %	17 %	8 %	23 %
	P		0.008	0.44	<0.001*	0.007*	0.024*	0.21	0.034*
Conventional accepted	TSH < 4.5	2714	35.9 (9.1)	37 %	23 %	24 %	15 %	7 %	20 %
	TSH≧4.5	142	37.7 (10.2)	38 %	26 %	26 %	20 %	9 %	31 %
	P		0.046	0.77	0.008*	0.50	0.09	0.39	0.003*

Values are means(SD) or probability. Comparison between any two groups by unpaired *t*-test, or Pearson Chi-square test*. Data in bold are statistically significant
FS Framingham score, *LDL-c* low-density lipoprotein cholesterol, *TG* triglyceride, *FPG* fasting plasma glucose

Certainly, there were several limitations in our study, including the higher proportion of females in the research population leading to a bias of TSH value which may be caused by the higher prevalence of HT in females. Secondly, the age of the research population was no older than 60, so the conclusion may not be applied to older people.

Conclusion

This study shows a high prevalence of HT occurred among individuals with a TSH of 2.6–2.9 mU/L. These values are possible to the "true" values of normal upper limit of TSH for Chinese population. From the trend of higher abnormalities in metabolism-related indicators and Framingham score with the elevation of TSH, a proper cutoff value of normal upper limit of TSH will be useful in patients with mild thyroid dysfunction.

Acknowledgements
The authors thank all the participants and staff in the study.

Funding
This work was supported by grants from National Natural Science Foundation of China (81471009, 81561128015).

Authors' contributions
YL and DNC contributed to develop research methodology, coordinate data collection, analysis and discussion, write manuscript and submission revision. CJ coordinated to collect and analyze research data. ZX GRY and MJN contributed to the discussion. YJK contributed to the design of the study, research data analysis and discussion, wrote manuscript and coordinated submission. All authors read and approved the final manuscript.

Competing interests
The authors declare that they have no competing interests.

Author details
[1]Physical Examination Department, Beijing Tongren Hospital, Capital Medical University, Beijing 100730, China. [2]Department of Endocrinology, Beijing Key Laboratory of Diabetes Research and Care, Beijing Tongren Hospital, Capital Medical University, Beijing 100730, China. [3]Department of Endocrinology, First Hospital of Qinghuangdao, Qinghuangdao 066000, China.

References

1. Huber G, Staub JJ, Meier C, Mitrache C, Guglielmetti M, Huber P, Braverman LE. Prospective study of the spontaneous course of subclinical hypothyroidism: prognostic value of thyrotropin, thyroid reserve, and thyroid antibodies. J Clin Endocrinol Metab. 2002;87(7):3221–6.
2. Hollowell JG, Staehling NW, Flanders WD, Hannon WH, Gunter EW, Spencer CA, Braverman LE. Serum TSH, T(4), and thyroid antibodies in the United States population (1988 to 1994): National Health and Nutrition Examination Survey (NHANES III). J Clin Endocrinol Metab. 2002;87(2):489–99.
3. Kratzsch J, Fiedler GM, Leichtle A, Brugel M, Buchbinder S, Otto L, Sabri O, Matthes G, Thiery J. New reference intervals for thyrotropin and thyroid hormones based on National Academy of Clinical Biochemistry criteria and regular ultrasonography of the thyroid. Clin Chem. 2005;51(8):1480–6.
4. Knudsen N, Bulow I, Jorgensen T, Laurberg P, Ovesen L, Perrild H. Comparative study of thyroid function and types of thyroid dysfunction in two areas in Denmark with slightly different iodine status. Eur J Endocrinol. 2000;143(4):485–91.
5. Spencer CA, Hollowell JG, Kazarosyan M, Braverman LE. National Health and Nutrition Examination Survey III thyroid-stimulating hormone (TSH)-thyroperoxidase antibody relationships demonstrate that TSH upper reference limits may be skewed by occult thyroid dysfunction. J Clin Endocrinol Metab. 2007;92(11):4236–40.
6. Caturegli P, De Remigis A, Rose NR. Hashimoto thyroiditis: clinical and diagnostic criteria. Autoimmun Rev. 2014;13(4–5):391–7.
7. Asvold BO, Bjoro T, Platou C, Vatten LJ. Thyroid function and the risk of coronary heart disease: 12-year follow-up of the HUNT study in Norway. Clin Endocrinol (Oxf). 2012;77(6):911–7.
8. Almeida C, Brasil MA, Costa AJ, Reis FA, Reuters V, Teixeira P, Ferreira M, Marques AM, Melo BA, Teixeira LB, et al. Subclinical hypothyroidism: psychiatric disorders and symptoms. Rev Bras Psiquiatr. 2007;29(2):157–9.
9. Canaris GJ, Manowitz NR, Mayor G, Ridgway EC. The Colorado thyroid disease prevalence study. Arch Intern Med. 2000;160(4):526–34.
10. Brabant G, Beck-Peccoz P, Jarzab B, Laurberg P, Orgiazzi J, Szabolcs I, Weetman AP, Wiersinga WM. Is there a need to redefine the upper normal limit of TSH? Eur J Endocrinol. 2006;154(5):633–7.
11. Wartofsky L, Dickey RA. The evidence for a narrower thyrotropin reference range is compelling. J Clin Endocrinol Metab. 2005;90(9):5483–8.
12. Colagiuri S, Lee CM, Wong TY, Balkau B, Shaw JE, Borch-Johnsen K, Group D-CW. Glycemic thresholds for diabetes-specific retinopathy: implications for diagnostic criteria for diabetes. Diabetes Care. 2011; 34(1):145–50.
13. Wilson PW, D'Agostino RB, Levy D, Belanger AM, Silbershatz H, Kannel WB. Prediction of coronary heart disease using risk factor categories. Circulation. 1998;97(18):1837–47.
14. Czajkowski M, Gill R, Rempala G. Model selection in logistic joinpoint regression with applications to analyzing cohort mortality patterns. Stat Med. 2008;27(9):1508–26.
15. Chan AO, Iu YP, Shek CC. The reference interval of thyroid-stimulating hormone in Hong Kong Chinese. J Clin Pathol. 2011;64(5):433–6.
16. Surks MI, Boucai L. Age- and race-based serum thyrotropin reference limits. J Clin Endocrinol Metab. 2010;95(2):496–502.
17. Asvold BO, Bjoro T, Vatten LJ. Associations of TSH levels within the reference range with future blood pressure and lipid concentrations: 11-year follow-up of the HUNT study. Eur J Endocrinol. 2013;169(1): 73–82.
18. Svare A, Nilsen TI, Bjoro T, Asvold BO, Langhammer A. Serum TSH related to measures of body mass: longitudinal data from the HUNT Study, Norway. Clin Endocrinol (Oxf). 2011;74(6):769–75.
19. Wang F, Tan Y, Wang C, Zhang X, Zhao Y, Song X, Zhang B, Guan Q, Xu J, Zhang J, et al. Thyroid-stimulating hormone levels within the reference range are associated with serum lipid profiles independent of thyroid hormones. J Clin Endocrinol Metab. 2012;97(8):2724–31.

Successful every-other-day liothyronine therapy for severe resistance to thyroid hormone beta with a novel *THRB* mutation

Yoshihiro Maruo*, Asami Mori, Yoriko Morioka, Chihiro Sawai, Yu Mimura, Katsuyuki Matui and Yoshihiro Takeuchi

Abstract

Background: Resistance to thyroid hormone beta (RTHβ) is a rare and usually dominantly inherited syndrome caused by mutations of the thyroid hormone receptor β gene (*THRB*). In severe cases, it is rarely challenging to control manifestations using daily therapeutic replacement of thyroid hormone.

Case presentation: The present case study concerns an 8-year-old Japanese girl with a severe phenotype of RTH (TSH, fT3, and fT4 were 34.0 mU/L, >25.0 pg/mL and, >8.0 ng/dL, respectively), caused by a novel heterozygous frameshift mutation in exon 10 of the thyroid hormone receptor beta gene (*THRB*), c.1347-1357 del actcttccccc : p.E449DfsX11. RTH was detected at the neonatal screening program. At 4 years of age, the patient continued to suffer from mental retardation, hyperactivity, insomnia, and reduced resting energy expenditure (REE), despite daily thyroxine (L-T4) therapy. Every-other-day high-dose liothyronine (L-T3) therapy improved her symptoms and increased her REE, without thyrotoxicosis.

Conclusion: In a case of severe RTH, every-other-day L-T3 administration enhanced REE and psychomotor development, without promoting symptoms of thyrotoxicosis. Every-other-day L-T3 administration may be an effective strategy for the treatment of severe RTH.

Keywords: Congenital hypothyroidism, Resistance to thyroid hormone, Thyroid hormone receptor β, Liothyronine

Background

Resistance to thyroid hormone beta (RTHβ, #MIM 188570) is a rare syndrome characterized by reduced responsiveness of some target tissues to thyroid hormone. RTHβ is usually inherited as an autosomal dominant trait, and is primarily caused by a mutation of the thyroid hormone receptor β gene (*THRB*) [1]. *THRB* is located on chromosome 17 and consists of 10 exons. More than 100 mutations have been reported; with the exception of 1 family, all mutations are located on exons 7–10 [2]. The mutant receptors are able to interfere with the function of the wild-type receptor, known as a dominant-negative effect. As such, heterozygous carriers often suffer from RTHβ. The symptoms of RTHβ are variable depending on the type of mutation. Many patients show a mild phenotype, and typically, treatment is not required. Heterozygous mutations resulting in truncated THRB cause a severe phenotype. Specifically, THRB lacking the last 20–28 amino acid residues causes mental retardation, visual and auditory deficits, and short stature [3]. Patients with biallelic mutations of *THRB* also develop a severe phenotype [4, 5]. Most children with RTHβ experience attention-deficit hyperactivity disorder (ADHD) [6]. In children with RTHβ and ADHD, particularly those who exhibit hyperactivity, liothyronine (L-T3), in supra-physiological doses, may be beneficial in reducing hyperactivity and impulsivity [7].

We report a severe case of RTHβ in an 8-year-old girl, in whom we detected a novel heterozygous deletion

* Correspondence: maruo@belle.shiga-med.ac.jp
The sequence data for nine novel THRB alleles have been submitted to the DDBJ/EMBL/GenBank databases under the accession numbers AB779708 (c.1347_1357 del actcttccccc, p.E449DfsX11).
Department of Pediatrics, Shiga University of Medical Science, Tsukinowa, Seta, Otsu 520-2192, Japan

mutation of *THRB*, which generates a truncated protein. The patient experienced mental retardation, hyperactivity, and insomnia, despite treatment with thyroxine (L-T4) therapy. Using every-other-day L-T3 therapy in large doses improved her symptoms without thyrotoxicosis.

Case presentation

The ethics committee of the Shiga University of Medical Science approved the study. The patient is the first child of the family, born to non-consanguineous parents without a family history of thyroid disease. Informed consent was obtained from the patient's parents.

At 20 days of age, the patient's serum TSH level increased to 198 μU/mL at neonatal screening. At 26 days of age, she visited our outpatient clinic exhibiting failure to thrive, persistent jaundice, and umbilical herniation. The patient's serum TSH, fT3, fT4, total T3, total T4, and TG values were 34.0 mU/L, >25.0 pg/mL, >8.0 ng/dL, 6.20 ng/mL, >24.9 μg/dL, and >800 ng/mL, respectively. She had no signs of heat intolerance, tachycardia, or hyperactivity. Thyroid gland enlargement and delayed bone maturation were noted. Pituitary size, as assessed with magnetic resonance imaging, indicated slight anterior lobe hyperplasia. TRH stimulation tests showed an excessive response (peak TSH: 92 μU/ml). The resting energy expenditure (REE), which was measured using AE300S (Minato Medical Science, Japan) by indirect calorimetry [REE (kcal/day) = 5.616 x VO_2 (ml/min) + 1.584 x VCO_2 (ml/min)] [8], was one-third of the normal values typical for her age. No anti-thyroid antibodies were detected. Based on these results, the patient was diagnosed with RTH. The patient was treated with L-T4 replacement starting at 2 weeks of age (7.5 μg/kg/day). After initiating replacement, TSH levels reduced to normal and her weight gain and REE improved (Fig. 1).

At 2 years of age, the patient showed normal growth (height and weight). However, she developed mental retardation [developmental quotient (DQ): 70–60 (postural-motor region 52, cognitive-adaptive region 63, language-social region 68) (the Kyoto Scale of Psychological Development new edition 2001)] and a learning disability associated with ADHD. At 4 years of age, the patient's DQ reduced to 50 and she showed symptoms of hyperactivity and insomnia. Her bone age was delayed about 1.5 years behind her chronological age, and REE decreased to 78 % of 4-years-girl. To enhance the patient's psychomotor development and REE, we chose to increase the L-T4 dose. However, considering the consistently high fT3, secondary to L-T4 therapy which could worsen insomnia, hyperactivity, and ADHD, the therapy was changed to single every-other-day large doses of L-T3 (75 μg). After start of L-T3 every-other-day replacement in one year, her DQ increased to 60 (Fig. 1). The patient's insomnia and hyperactivity also improved. At the time of publication, the patient is 8 years, 11 months old, with a height of 131.6 cm (+0.28 SD). Her recent TSH, fT3, fT4, and TG were 2.92 μIU/mL, 18.5 pg/mL, 6.21 ng/dL, and 85.9 ng/

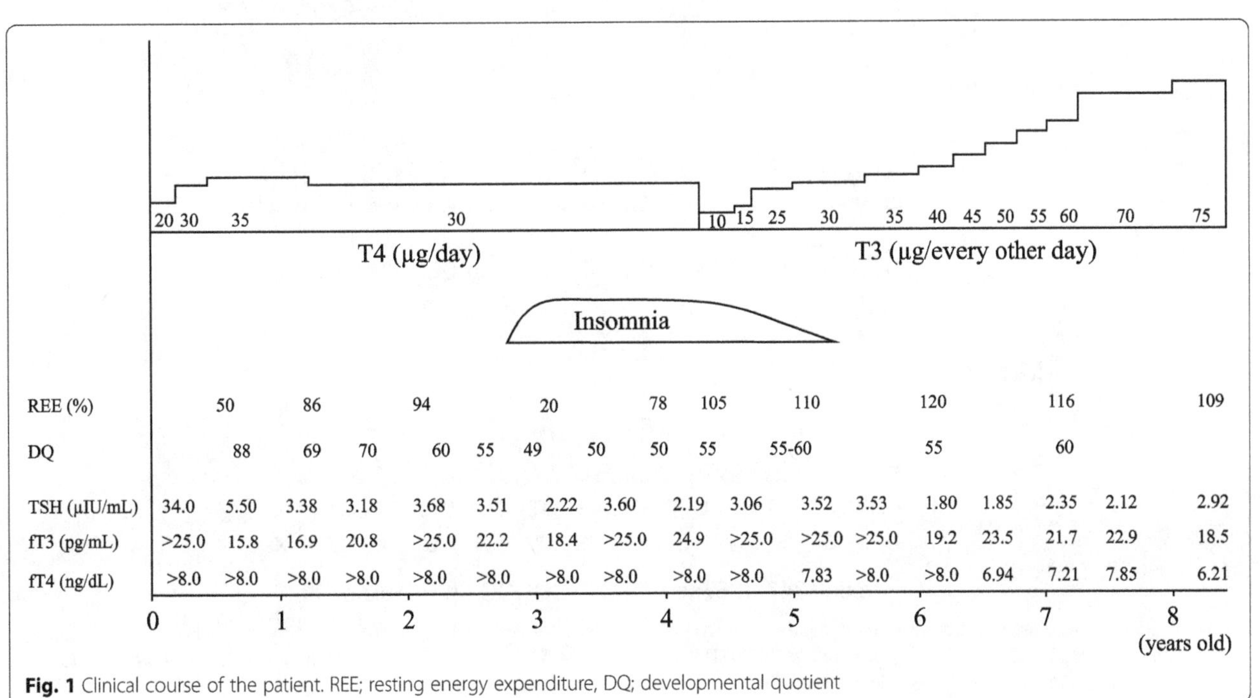

Fig. 1 Clinical course of the patient. REE; resting energy expenditure, DQ; developmental quotient

mL, respectively. REE was 109.3 % of the predicted values for an 8-year-old girl (Fig. 1).

Laboratory testing and sequence analysis

TSH was measured using a fluorescent enzyme immunoassay method (TOSHO, Tokyo, Japan). fT4 and fT3 were measured with a fluorescent enzyme immunoassay (TOSHO, Tokyo, Japan). Thyroglobulin was measured by an immunoradiometric assay (EIKEN CHEMICAL, Tokyo, Japan).

Blood samples were obtained from the patient and her parents. Genomic DNA was isolated from leukocytes by the standard protocol. *THRB* exons were amplified by polymerase chain reaction using a previously reported protocol [9]. The sequences of the amplified DNA fragments were determined directly using a BigDye® Terminators v1.1 Cycle Sequencing Kit (Applied Biosystems, CA) and an ABI PRISM 3130xl Genetic Analyzer (Applied Biosystems, CA).

Homology models of wild type and mutant THRB were predicted using a molecular operating environment (MOE; Chemical Computing Group Inc., Montreal, Quebec, Canada). The query amino acid sequence of human THRB came from GenPret (Accession number P10828). Thyroid receptor alpha (PDB code 1NAVA) was selected as a template structure by alignment of amino acid sequences in the MOE protein database [10].

Results

Gene analysis

We detected a novel deletion mutation in exon 10 of *THRB* (Fig. 2). The 11 bases of nucleotide sequence, "actcttccccc" at 1347_1357 were deleted. This deletion leads to a frameshift, producing a stop at codon 459: c.1347_1357 del actcttccccc (p.E449DfsX11) (Fig. 1). Moreover, this mutation introduces changes in the amino acid sequence from 449–461 "ELFPPLFLEVFED" to 449–459 "DFVLGSVRGLD", and causes two amino acids in the T3 binding domain to be shorter, when compared with wild type THRB. The patient's parents did not show any mutations on *THRB*.

Comparison of the conformation of wild type with p.E449DfsX11 THRB

We used MOE to predict model 3D structures of wild type and p.E449DfsX11 THRB. The p.E449DfsX11 THRB has one different α-helix (amino acid number 450–451) at the C-terminal (Fig. 3). The deletion mutation with amino acid replacement causes significant changes to the tertiary structure of THRB.

Discussion

Usually, patients with RTH are euthyroid and do not require treatment with thyroid hormone. However, in severe cases, to prevent goiter development, daily L-T4

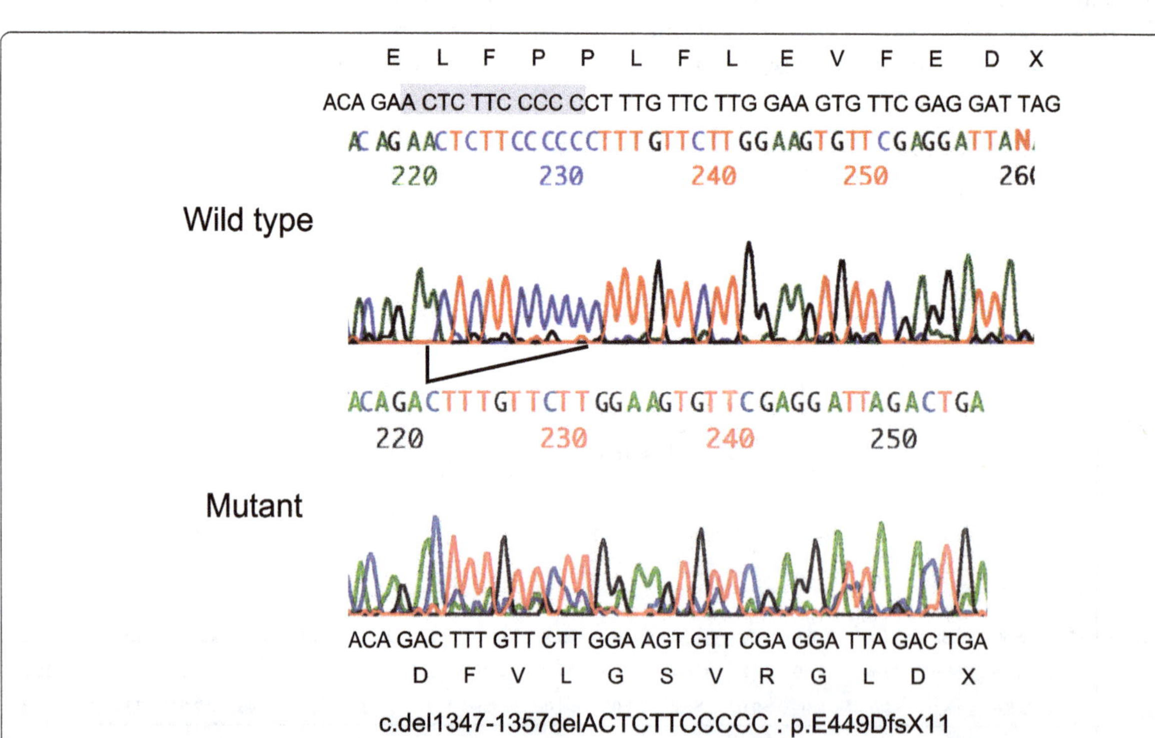

Fig. 2 THRB nucleotide sequences amplified from the genomic DNA of the patient. The mutation, a deletion of "actcttccccc" at position 1347_1357 in THRB cDNA, changed the amino acid sequence from 449–461 "ELFPPLFLEVFED" to 449–459 "DFVLGSVRGLD" and made two amino acids in the T3 binding domain shorter, when compared with wild type THRB

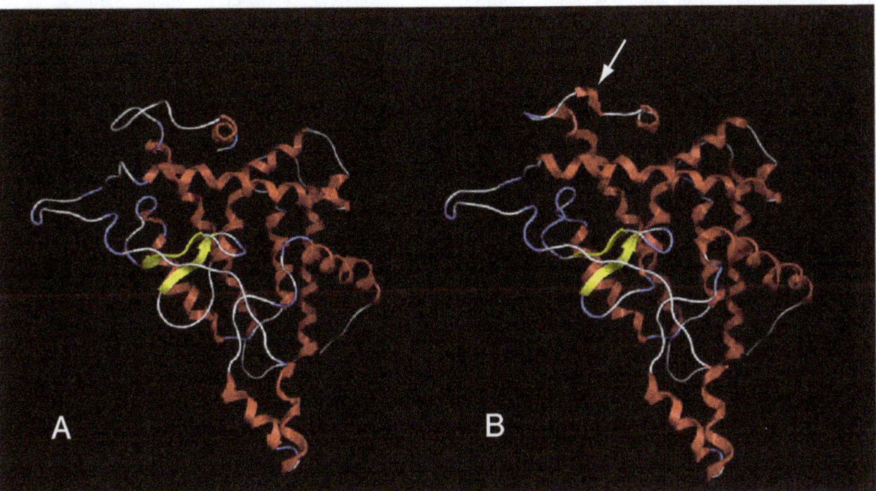

Fig. 3 Ribbon diagrams of the predicted THRB structure from wild type (**a**) and p.E449DfsX11 mutant protein (**b**). The figures were produced with homology-based modeling using MOE. Red ribbons represent α-helices, and yellow arrows indicate the β-sheet. The mutated THRB has one different α-helix (amino acid number 450–451) (arrows)

or L-T3 therapeutic replacement is necessary. It is rarely challenging to control manifestations by using daily therapeutic replacement of L-T4 or L-T3. Every-other-day L-T3 replacement has shown to be effective for treating uncontrolled large goiters in patients with severe RTH, without symptoms of thyrotoxicosis or severely elevated TSH [11, 12]. However, effects on psychological and mental improvement have not been reported. Supra-physiological doses of L-T3 can reduce hyperactivity and impulsivity [7]. However, for patients with severe RTH, such as the present case, extreme elevations in T3 level might worsen psychological and mental development. Daily L-T4 supplementation also induces consistently high T3 levels, which may worsen insomnia, hyperactivity, and ADHD. To suppress TSH levels and prevent consistently high T3 levels, every-other-day L-T3 replacement might be an effective. For RTHβ, treatment of β blocker and 3,5,3'-triiodothyroacetic acid (TRIAC) was also considered as well as L-thyroxine if necessary. Usually REE of patients with RTHβ increases. However decline of REE in our patient suggested that she is in state of hypothyroidism physically. The treatment with L-T3 was chosen. Her mutated THRB might strongly interfere function of the wild THRB. Severe reduction of THRB function might induce low REE.

The novel mutation, c.1347-1357 del actcttccccc, generates a premature stop codon at 459 with an altered C-terminal amino acid sequence (p.E449DfsX11) (Fig. 1). These changes in the 3-dimensional structure of C-terminal might cause severe RTH (Fig. 2). These changes might cause severe RTH in patient with the heterozygous mutation (p.E449DfsX11).

Conclusions

For severe RTH, every-other-day L-T3 therapy may be an effective therapy to improve REE and psychomotor development, without inducing symptoms of thyrotoxicosis.

Consent

The parents of the patient have given their consent for the Case reports to be published.

Abbreviations

RTH: resistance to thyroid hormone; THRB: thyroid hormone receptor β; L-T3: liothyronine; L-T4: thyroxine; TG: thyroglobulin.

Competing interests

The authors do not have competing interests.

Authors' contributions

YM carried out the molecular genetic studies of the patient, counseled the patient and their family, participated in sequence alignment and drafted manuscript. AM treated the patient. YM carried out the molecular genetic studies of the patient and participated in sequence alignment. CS evaluated the development of the patient. YM treated the patient and helped to drafted manuscript. KM analyzed the 3D model of THRB. YT evaluated the development of the patient and helped to draft the manuscript. All authors read and approved the final manuscript.

Acknowledgments

We thank M Suzaki of the Central Research Laboratory, Shiga University of Medical Science, for technical assistance. This work was partly supported by grants-in-aid for scientific research from the Ministry of Education, Science, and Culture of Japan (15 K09710).

References

1. Refetoff S, Bassett JH, Beck-Peccoz P, Bernal J, Brent G, Chatterjee K, et al. Classification and proposed nomenclature for inherited defects of thyroid hormone action, cell transport, and metabolism. Thyroid. 2014;24:407–9.
2. Refetoff S, Weiss RE, Usala SJ. The syndromes of resistance to thyroid hormome. Endocr Rev. 1993;14:348–99.

3. Wu SY, Cohen RN, Simsek E, Senses DA, Yar NE, Noel J, et al. A Novel thyroid hormone receptor-β mutation that fails to bind nuclear receptor corepressor in apatien as an apparent cause of severe, predominantly a pituitary resistance to thyroid hormome. J Clin Endocrinol Metab. 2006;19:1887–95.
4. Ono S, Schwartz ID, Mueller O, Root AW, Usala SJ, Beruc BB. Homozygosity for a dominant negative thyroid hormone receptor gene responsible for generalized resistance to thyroid hormone. J Clin Endocrinol Metab. 1991;73:990–4.
5. Ferrara AM, Onigata K, Ercan O, Woodhead H, Weiss RE, Refetoff S. Homozygous thyroid hormone receptor β-gene mutations in resistance to thyroid hormone: three new cases and review of the literature. J Clin Endocrinol Metab. 2012;97:1328–36.
6. Hauser P, Zametkin AJ, Martinez P, Vitiello B, Matochik JA, Mixson AJ, et al. Attention deficit-hyperactivity disorder in people with generalized resistance to thyroid hormone. N Engl J Med. 1993;328:997–1001.
7. Weiss RE, Stein MA, Refetoff S. Behavioral effects of liothyronine (L-T3) in children with attention deficit hyperactivity disorder in the presence and absence of resistance to thyroid hormone. Thyroid. 1997;7:389–93.
8. Kato J, Koike A, Hoshimoto-Iwamoto M, Nagayama O, Sakurada K, Sato A. Yet al. Relation between oscillatory breathing and cardiopulmonary function during exercise in cardiac patients. Circ J. 2013;77:661–6.
9. Lam CW, On-kei Chan A, Tong SF, Shek CC, Cheung Tui S. DNA-based diagnosis of thyroid hormone resisitance syndrome. Clinica Chimica Acta. 2005;358:55–9.
10. Maruo Y, Verma IC, Matsui K, Takahashi H, Mimura Y. Conformational change of UGT1A1 by a novel missense mutation (p.L131P) causing Crigler-Najjar syndrome type I. J Pediatr Gastroenterol Nutr. 2008;46:308–11.
11. Anselmo J, Refetoff S. Regression of a large goiter in a patient with resistance to thyroid hormone by every other day treatment with triiodothyronine. Thyroid. 2004;14:71–4.
12. Canadas KT, Rivkees SA, Udelsman R, Breuer CK. Resistance to thyroid hormone associated with a novel mutation of the thyroid β receptor gene in a four-year-old female. Int J Pediatr Endocrinol. 2011;2011:3.

Radioiodine treatment for graves' disease

Erin Fanning[1,2*], Warrick J. Inder[1,2*] and Emily Mackenzie[1,3]

Abstract

Background: Radioactive iodine (I^{131}) is a common definitive treatment for Graves' Disease. Potential complications include worsening, or new development of Graves' eye disease and development of a radiation thyroiditis. The purpose of the present study was to assess outcomes of patients treated with I^{131} in an Australian tertiary centre over 10 years.

Methods: Data from 101 consecutive patients treated with I^{131} for a diagnosis of Graves' disease between 2005 to 2015 was collected and reviewed retrospectively. Baseline TSH receptor antibody titre, pre-treatment free thyroxine (FT4), technetium scan uptake, initial treatment, duration of treatment, reason for definitive therapy, complications, and time to remission (defined as euthyroidism or hypothyroidism after 12 months) were recorded.

Results: Of the 92 patients with adequate outcome data, 73 (79.3%) patients achieved remission with a single dose of I^{131}. Of the remaining 19 patients, 12 had a second dose and became hypothyroid. TSH receptor antibody titre at diagnosis was significantly lower in the group that achieved remission with the first dose compared with those who did not ($P = 0.0071$). There was no difference in technetium uptake, I^{131} dose, duration of therapy or pre-treatment free thyroxine (FT4). I^{131} was complicated by development of eye disease in 3 patients and 1 (of 11 with pre-existing eye disease) had worsening eye disease. A clinically apparent flare of hyperthyroidism following I^{131} was evident in 8 patients (8.6%).

Conclusion: Radioiodine is an effective therapy for Graves' Disease with few complications. The majority of patients achieve remission with a single dose. Those who require a second dose are more likely to have higher TSH receptor antibody titres at diagnosis. To the best of our knowledge, this is the first study to report outcomes from radioiodine treatment for Graves' disease in an Australian population.

Keywords: Graves' disease, radioiodine., I^{131}., Graves' disease treatment.

Background

Graves' disease is the most common cause of adult hyperthyroidism in the developed world.

[1, 2]. It is an autoimmune condition caused by stimulating antibodies acting as an agonist on the thyrotropin (TSH) receptor on thyroid follicular cells [3]. Though it can occur at any age it is most commonly diagnosed in women aged 40–60 years [2]. Treatment options include antithyroid drugs, radioiodine therapy (I^{131}) and surgery.

Radioiodine is a safe and effective definitive treatment for Graves' disease. In Australia, it is generally used as second line therapy for relapsed or persistent disease. I^{131} is taken up by the thyroid gland and incorporated into thyroid hormone, releasing beta particles that cause ionising damage and tissue necrosis. This results in eventual ablation of functional thyroid tissue [1, 2]. On average it takes between 6 to 18 weeks before a euthyroid or hypothyroid state is achieved following I^{131} treatment [2]. Following a single dose of radioiodine, around 15–25% of patients remain hyperthyroid and require additional treatment [1–5]. Hypothyroidism eventually develops in 80–90% of patients. Previous studies have reported factors relating to success of radioiodine including gender (lower remission rates in males) [6], more severe hyperthyroidism [7], thyroid size [8], serum TSH receptor antibody titres [9, 10] and thyroid uptake on radionuclide scans [11].

* Correspondence: e.fanning@uq.edu.au; warrick.inder@health.qld.gov.au
[1]Department of Diabetes and Endocrinology, Princess Alexandra Hospital, Brisbane, Queensland, Australia

Potential complications of I^{131} therapy include worsening of Graves' ophthalmopathy and development of a radiation thyroiditis. I^{131} causes an exacerbation or new occurrence of Graves' eye disease in 15–20% of patients [1, 11–14]. TSH receptors are found on orbital fibroblasts and are the likely autoimmune target in Graves' ophthalmopathy. The risk can be mitigated by glucocorticoid prophylaxis in patients with mild disease or patients with multiple risk factors [14, 15]. Early and prompt treatment of hypothyroidism also can prevent the progression of eye disease. Radiation thyroiditis occurs in 1% of patients following radioiodine therapy [2]; the usual onset is within 2 weeks after I^{131} therapy and can be associated with neck tenderness and swelling.

There has been no Australian data regarding the outcome of radioiodine for Graves' disease previously reported. The aim of this study was to assess the final thyroid status of patients treated with I^{131}, including the prevalence and predictors of treatment failure and complications of treatment, in a tertiary endocrinology centre over ten years.

Methods

Data on consecutive patients treated with I^{131} therapy between 2005 to June 2015 at the Princess Alexandra Hospital (Brisbane, Australia) were retrospectively collected and reviewed. Ethics approval was obtained from the Metro South Human Research Ethics Committee. Consent to participate was not a requirement since this study was considered an audit of practice. Patients were identified from the hospital medical imaging database of all patients who received I^{131} treatment over that time. Those with a confirmed diagnosis of Graves' disease who received follow up in the hospital outpatient clinic were included. Diagnosis of Graves' hyperthyroidism was by a suppressed serum TSH (< 0.05 mU/L), along with elevated serum free thyroxine (FT4) and free triiodothyronine (FT3) in association with raised serum TSH receptor antibody titre or a radionuclide scan compatible with Graves' disease. Patients with other causes of hyperthyroidism (e.g. toxic multinodular goitre, single toxic adenoma) and patients referred from and followed up in other centres were excluded due to lack of data.

Baseline assessment and follow up data were obtained through the computer-based outpatient program 'Practix' and supplemented, as required, by patients' paper charts. Pathology was performed by two private Pathology providers (Sullivan and Nicolaides Pathology, Taringa, Queensland, Australia, or Queensland Medical Laboratories, Murarrie, Queensland, Australia) or the public hospital provider Pathology Queensland, Herston, Queensland, Australia according to patient preference. Parameters including baseline TSH receptor antibody titre, technetium scan uptake, baseline pre-treatment FT4, initial treatment, duration of treatment, complications of medical therapy, reason for definitive therapy, complications of radioiodine treatment, presence of eye disease before and after radioiodine, use of prophylactic glucocorticoids, smoking status and time to hypothyroidism were recorded. The presence and severity of eye disease was assessed individually by the treating physician. The detailed eye examination generally included assessment for conjunctival inflammation, chemosis, periorbital oedema, proptosis, eye movement abnormalities or diplopia and any evidence of visual loss. Clinical severity was graded as mild, moderate or severe. Treatment failure was defined as persistent hyperthyroidism at 12 months post I^{131} requiring either long-term thionamide therapy, a repeat dose of I^{131} or thyroidectomy.

I^{131} (sodium iodide powder in prefilled capsules) was administered orally in the Department of Nuclear Medicine at the Princess Alexandra Hospital. A fixed dose (administered activity) of 500 MBq is currently used. In earlier years of the study, this had been 450 MBq and some patients received a lower dose due to the practice of an individual nuclear medicine physician. Antithyroid drugs were ceased 3–5 days prior to and recommenced 5 days following I^{131} treatment as needed. All female patients of childbearing age underwent a pregnancy test (serum beta hCG) prior to proceeding with therapy. Patients were subsequently followed up with thyroid function tests 4–6 weekly after treatment [2]. Remission was defined as hypothyroidism or euthyroidism within 12 months of a single dose RAI.

Continuous data failed parametric assumptions and therefore are presented as median and 95% confidence intervals (CI). Categorical variables are presented as simple proportions (%). A Mann Whitney U test was used to compare continuous baseline variables between groups. A P value of < 0.05 was considered significant. All data analysis was performed using Graphpad Prism 7.03.

Results

One hundred and one eligible patients were identified, 74 (73%) of whom were female. The initial medical therapy was carbimazole in 93 (92%) patients, 6 used PTU (6%) and 2 (2%) patients did not receive medical therapy prior to undergoing I^{131}. During the course of treatment, 17 patients changed therapy from carbimazole to PTU and 1 patient was changed from PTU to carbimazole. An adverse reaction to the antithyroid drug was reported in 29 (28.7%) patients; 19 secondary to carbimazole and 10 due to PTU. The primary indication for definitive treatment was disease relapse following a trial withdrawal of antithyroid drug therapy in 41 patients, a poor response to medical therapy in 29 patients due and intolerance/complications of treatment in 18 patients

(Table 1). The most common adverse reaction to medical therapy was a rash in 8 patients, followed by neutropaenia (neutrophils $< 1.0 \times 10^9$/L) in 6 patients. LFT derangement was reported in 3 patients taking PTU and 1 patient taking carbimazole.

Baseline characteristics are presented in Table 2. Pre-existing eye disease was present in 11 patients; four of these were documented as mild/inactive. The median duration of medical therapy was 24 months prior to receiving radioiodine therapy. The range was 3 weeks to 12 years. A few outliers received a very long duration of medical therapy. The reasons for this included previous lack of ongoing specialist input or prior hesitance on behalf of the patient to undergo definitive therapy. The median TSH receptor antibody titre at diagnosis was 8 IU/L (range 0–240). Fifteen (15%) patients were documented to be smokers. Of the 11 patients who had documented eye disease prior to radioiodine therapy, 7 received prophylactic corticosteroids. The administered activity of I^{131} was between 311 and 580 MBq (mean 495.7 MBq).

Regarding outcomes of radioiodine therapy, 92 patients had adequate follow up data for inclusion (Fig. 1). Remission following a single dose of I^{131} was achieved in 73 (79.3%) patients. Of the 19 patients who did not achieve remission, 12 had a second dose and became hypothyroid, 2 underwent surgery and 5 had persisting hyperthyroidism requiring medical therapy. Of the patients who achieved remission with a single dose of I^{131}, 64 patients became hypothyroid (87.6%) and 9 patients (12.3%) remained euthyroid. The median time from I^{131} administration to hypothyroidism was 4 months [3, 4].

TSH receptor antibody titre at diagnosis was significantly lower in the group that achieved remission with the first dose compared to those who did not ($P = 0.0205$). There was no difference in technetium uptake, I^{131} administered activity, duration of medical therapy, pre-treatment FT4 or duration of disease (Table 3).

Table 1 Reasons for definitive therapy

Reason for definitive therapy	Number
Relapse	41
Poor response/unable to wean medication	29
Intolerant/complications of medical therapy	18
Patient compliance	4
Carbimazole unavailable	2
Remote location	2
Patient preference	2
Likely to require multiple contrast loads	1
Hepatitis C on interferon	2
Cardiovascular comorbidities	4

Table 2 Baseline characteristics

Baseline Characteristics	
Pre-existing eye disease	11 (4 documented as mild/inactive)
Duration of Medical Treatment (months)	24 (3 weeks to 12 years)
Technetium uptake (%)	4.3 (0.8–66)
TSH receptor antibody (IU/L)	8 (0–240)
Smoker (documented)	15
Glucocorticoid cover with pre-existing eye disease	7

Data are expressed as median (range)

Radioiodine therapy was complicated by new onset of eye disease in 3 (3.3%) patients (Table 4). In each of these patients, the eye disease was documented as mild and did not require any treatment. Of the 11 patients with pre-existing eye disease, one developed worsening of their eye disease which was severe and eventually required surgical decompression, long term glucocorticoid therapy and radiotherapy. This patient was documented as having inactive eye disease prior to therapy and therefore did not receive prophylactic glucocorticoids. A clinically significant flare of hyperthyroidism following radioiodine was evident in 8 patients (8.6%).

Discussion

This study assessed the outcomes of patients treated with I^{131} for Graves' disease at an Australian tertiary hospital over 10 years. We found that 79% of patients achieved remission with a single dose of I^{131}. Of the patients who did not achieve remission with the first dose of radioiodine, all those treated with a second dose became hypothyroid. Individuals who did not achieve remission with a single dose were more likely to have higher TSH receptor antibody titres at diagnosis. There was a low rate of complications associated with radioiodine. Only 4.3% of patients developed new-onset or worsening of eye disease and 8.6% developed a transient flare of clinically significant hyperthyroidism. To our knowledge, this is the first study that has reported outcomes of I^{131} therapy for Graves' disease from an Australian centre.

The remission rate following I^{131} in our study is similar to previously published studies. Metso et al. reported a remission rate of 74% with a single dose of I^{131} for treatment of Graves' disease in a prospective cohort study in Finland [4]. Zantut-Wittmann et al. reported a 37.8% rate of persistent hyperthyroidism 12 months following radioiodine therapy [5]. A fixed dose of 370 MBq was used in this study, in comparison to our centre where the mean administered activity was higher at 495.7 MBq. Some studies have reported higher remission rates of up to 93% [7, 16], however these included

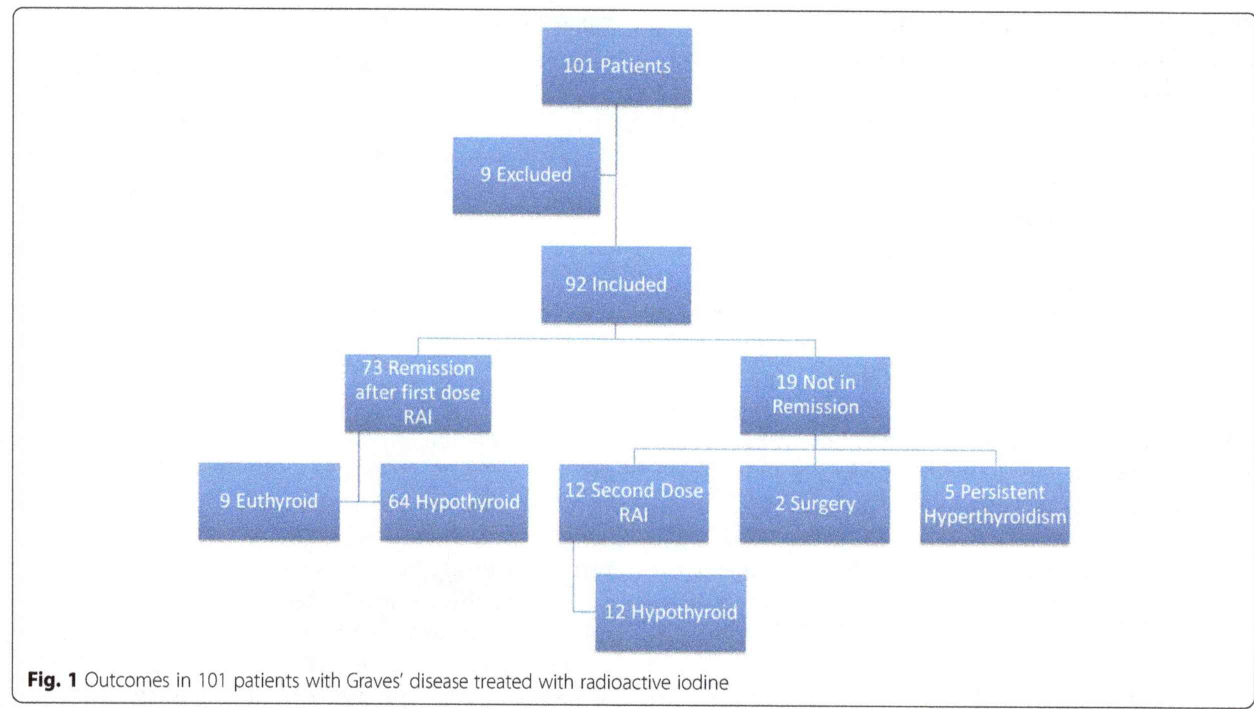

Fig. 1 Outcomes in 101 patients with Graves' disease treated with radioactive iodine

patients treated with I^{131} as first-line therapy. In our centre, patients usually undergo an initial trial of anti-thyroid medication; most are referred for I^{131} in the event of relapse or treatment failure and thus are likely to have more resistant disease.

Consistent with other studies, we found a significant difference in TSH receptor antibody titre at diagnosis comparing patients who achieved remission with a single dose of I^{131} to those who remained hyperthyroid. Murakami et al. found that TSH receptor antibody activity immediately before radioiodine therapy was significantly higher in patients who did not achieve remission with a single dose of I^{131} compared to those who did [9]. Chiovato et al. also found that pre-treatment TSH receptor antibody titres were significantly higher in patients who remained hyperthyroid post I^{131} than in those that became hypothyroid or euthyroid [10]. Our study assessed the TSH receptor antibody titre at diagnosis, rather than pre-treatment as it was consistently available. Based on the above findings, the measurement of TSH receptor antibody titres at the onset of disease and prior to definitive treatment may be a useful tool to help predict patients who may be less likely to achieve remission with a single dose of radioiodine. This can assist with counselling patients prior to treatment. Nearly all patients in our study received antithyroid drugs prior to treatment as is standard management for Graves' disease in Australia. Prolonged treatment with antithyroid drugs reduces the serum TSH receptor antibody level [17]. Given that almost all patients were pre-treated with antithyroid drugs in our study it was not possible to look at the relative impact of the TSH receptor antibody titre at diagnosis and after a long period of antithyroid drug treatment on the success of radioiodine therapy, however this may be a direction for future research.

Table 3 Factors potentially implicated in response to radioiodine treatment

	Remission (n = 73)	No Remission (n = 19)	P
TSH receptor antibody (IU/L)[a]	7.2 (4.5–9)	18 (5.4–68)	0.02
Technetium Uptake (%)	4.3 (3.1–5.2)	3.5 (1.8–7.1)	0.35
I^{131} administered activity (MBq)	500 (500–511)	501 (499–505)	0.58
Duration of medical therapy (months)	21 (12–24)	36 (6–48)	0.31
Duration of disease (years)	3 (2–4)	3 (1–4)	0.88
Pre-Treatment FT4 (pmol/L)	34 (27–39.9)	28.9 (19.6–42)	0.33

Data expressed as median (95% CI)
Remission is defined as hypothyroidism or euthyroidism within 12 months of a single dose RAI
[a]TSH receptor antibody titre at diagnosis

Table 4 Complications of radioiodine

Complication	Number (%)
Worsening of pre-existing eye disease	1 (1.1%)
Severe eye disease requiring decompression	1 (1.1%)
Worsening of eye disease despite prophylactic glucocorticoids	0
Flare of clinically significant hyperthyroidism	8 (8.6%)
New onset eye disease	3 (3.3%)
Failure to achieve remission with single dose of RAI	19 (20.7%)

There was no difference in Technetium uptake, duration of disease, duration of medical therapy, severity of disease (measured by pre-treatment FT4) or administered activity of I^{131} between patients who achieved remission and those who did not. In contrast, Zantut-Whitmann et al. found that patients with a [^{99m}Tc] pertechnetate uptake of ≥12.5% had a 4.1 times increased risk of persistent hyperthyroidism [4]. The authors of this study also reported that thyroid mass < 53.7 g had an 8.9 fold higher probability of treatment success [11]. The relationship between thyroid volume and treatment success has also been reported in other studies, with a larger thyroid volume prior to I^{131} being associated with a reduced chance of treatment success [10, 18]. Data regarding thyroid volume was not included in this study as it was not consistently available.

Radioiodine is associated with the development or worsening of thyroid eye disease in about 15–20% of patients [3, 13, 14, 19]. Traisk et al. assessed the incidence of Graves' ophthalmopathy in patients randomised to either 18 months of medical treatment, or I^{131} therapy. Worsening or development of new-onset eye disease was significantly more common in the I^{131} group (38.7%) compared with the medical treatment group (21.3%) [13]. Bartalena et al. found that radioiodine treatment was often followed by an exacerbation of eye disease in at least half of patients with pre-existing ophthalmopathy [15].

In our cohort, only four patients developed new-onset or worsening of pre-existing eye disease (4.3%), of whom three developed new-onset eye disease. The eye disease was documented to be mild in each case and did not require any treatment. Of these patients, one was a smoker and another was documented to be an ex-smoker. The occurrence of new or worsening eye disease was lower in our cohort than previously reported. This may be explained by several factors including: i) a low rate of pre-existing eye disease (11 patients; 11%); ii) careful patient selection excluding patients with more significant eye disease for I^{131}; and, iii) the use of prophylactic glucocorticoids. The one patient who subsequently developed severe eye disease was a smoker and was documented to have mild, inactive disease prior to therapy and thus did not receive prophylactic glucocorticoids. The TSH receptor antibody titre of this patient was below the mean at 14 U/L.

Other risk factors for the development or progression of ophthalmopathy following radioiodine such as smoking, high levels of pre-treatment serum T3 and post radioiodine hypothyroidism were not examined in the present study due to the low number of patients affected.

Prophylactic glucocorticoids have been shown to be highly effective in reducing the risk of thyroid eye disease in patients treated with I^{131} [15, 16, 19]. In a systematic review, no patients with mild eye disease treated with prophylactic glucocorticoids prior to I^{131} developed worsening of their pre-existing eye disease [20]. Consistent with this, none of the seven patients in our study treated with prophylactic glucocorticoids for pre-existing mild eye disease developed any exacerbation.

It is important to recognise several limitations of this study. Firstly, this is a retrospective study based on chart review. Data for variables such as TSH receptor antibody status were not taken at a consistent time point for each patient and some data (e.g., smoking status), were inconsistently reported. The presence or absence of ophthalmopathy was dependent upon accurate assessment and documentation by the treating clinician and therefore, transient or mild ophthalmopathy may have been missed. This may partly explain the lower rates of new onset or worsening eye disease in our group compared to other studies. The assessment and clinical grading of eye disease is likely to have been variable between clinicians. TSH receptor antibody assays have changed over the included study period and were measured by three different laboratories.

Conclusion

In conclusion, the first published Australian series has confirmed radioiodine is a safe and effective definitive treatment for Graves' Disease. Most patients become hypothyroid following a single dose of I^{131}, with a single dose of radioiodine resulting in long-term remission from Graves' disease in 79%. Of the patients who remained hyperthyroid after the first dose of radioiodine, all those treated with a second dose achieved remission. With careful patient selection, there was a low rate of complications associated with I^{131} therapy.

Abbreviations

FT4: Free thyroxine; TSH: Thyroid stimulating hormone

Acknowledgements

Not applicable.

Funding

No funding was received for this research.

Authors' contributions
EF, WI and EM designed the study. EF collected the data, performed the primary analysis and wrote the first draft of the manuscript. EF, WI and EM edited and approved the final manuscript.

Competing interests
The authors declare they have no competing interests.

Author details
[1]Department of Diabetes and Endocrinology, Princess Alexandra Hospital, Brisbane, Queensland, Australia. [2]Faculty of Medicine, the University of Queensland, Brisbane, Queensland, Australia. [3]Nuclear Medicine, Department of Radiology, Princess Alexandra Hospital, Brisbane, Queensland, Australia.

References

1. Burch HB, Cooper DS. Management of Graves Disease A Review. JAMA. 2016;314:2544–54.
2. Ross DS. Radioiodine therapy for hyperthyroidism. N Engl J Med. 2011; 364:542–50.
3. Metso S, Jaatinen P, Huhtala H, Luukkaala T, Oksala H, Salmi J. Long-term follow-up study of radioiodine treatment of hyperthyroidism. Clin Endocrinol. 2004;61:641–8.
4. Zantut-Wittmann DE, Ramos CD, Santos AO, Lima MMO, Panzan AD, Facuri FVO, et al. High pre-therapy [99mTc]pertechnetate thyroid uptake, thyroid size and thyrostatic drugs: predictive factors of failure in [131I]iodide therapy in Graves' disease. Nucl Med Commun. 2005;26:957–63.
5. Topliss DJ, Eastman CJ. Diagnosis and management of hyperthyroidism and hypothyroidism. Med J Aust. 2004;180:541–2.
6. Allahabadia A, Daykin J, Sheppard MC, Gough SCL, Franklyn JA. Radioiodine treatment of hyperthyroidism—prognostic factors for outcome. J Clin Endocrinol Metab. 2001;86:3611–7.
7. Lewis A, Rea T, Atkinson B, Bell P, Courtney H, McCance D, et al. Outcome of131I therapy in hyperthyroidism using a 550MBq fixed dose regimen. Ulster Med J. 2013;82:85–8.
8. Yang D, Xue J, Ma W, Liu F, Fan Y, Rong J, et al. Prognostic factor analysis in 325 patients with graves' disease treated with radioiodine therapy. Nucl Med Commun. 2018;39:16–21.
9. Murakami Y, Takamatsu J, Sakane S, Kuma K, Ohsawa N. Changes in thyroid volume in response to radioactive iodine for graves' hyperthyroidism correlated with activity of thyroid-stimulating antibody and treatment outcome. J Clin Endocrinol Metab. 1996;81:3257–60.
10. Chiovato L, Fiore E, Vitti P, Rocchi R, Rago T, Dokic D, et al. Outcome of thyroid function in graves' patients treated with radioiodine: role of thyroid-stimulating and thyrotropin-blocking antibodies and of radioiodine-induced thyroid damage. J Clin Endocrinol Metab. 1998;83:40–6.
11. Liu M, Jing D, Hu J, Yin S. Predictive factors of outcomes in personalized radioactive iodine (131I) treatment for graves' disease. Am J Med Sci. 2014; 348:288–93.
12. Bartalena L. Diagnosis and management of graves disease: a global overview. Nat Rev Endocrinol. 2013;9:724–34.
13. Träisk F, Tallstedt L, Abraham-Nordling M, Andersson T, Berg G, Calissendorff J, et al. Thyroid-associated Ophthalmopathy after treatment for graves' hyperthyroidism with Antithyroid drugs or Iodine-131. J Clin Endocrinol Metab. 2009;94:3700–7.
14. Tallstedt L, Lundell G, Torring O, Wallin G, Ljunggren JG, Blomgren H, Taube A, the TSG. Occurrence of opthalmopathy after treatment for graves' hyperthyroidism. N Engl J Med. 1992;326:1733–8.
15. Bartalena L, Marcocci C, Bogazzi F, Panicucci M, Lepri A, Pinchera A. Use of corticosteroids to prevent progresion of graves' opthalmopathy after radioiodine therapy for hyperthyroidism. N Engl J Med. 1989;321:1349–52.
16. Subramanian M, Baby MK, Seshadri KG. The effect of prior antithyroid drug use on delaying remission in high uptake graves' disease following radioiodine ablation. Endocr Connect. 2016;5:34–40.
17. Laurberg P. TSH-receptor autoimmunity in graves ' disease after therapy with anti-thyroid drugs , surgery , or radioiodine : a 5-year prospective randomized study. Eur J Endocrinol. 2008;158:69–75.
18. Sridama V, McCormick M, Kaplan E, Fauchet RDL. Long-term follow-up study of compensated low-dose I131 therapy for graves' disease. N Engl J Med. 1984;311:426–32.
19. Bartalena L, Marcocci C, Bogazzi F, Manetti L, Tanda ML, Dell'Unto E, et al. Relation between therapy for hyperthyroidism and the course of graves' Ophthalmopathy. N Engl J Med. 1998;338:73–8.
20. Acharya SH, Avenell A, Philip S, Burr J, Bevan JS, Abraham P. Radioiodine therapy (RAI) for graves' disease (GD) and the effect on ophthalmopathy: a systematic review. Clin Endocrinol. 2008;69:943–50.

MST-4 and TRAF-6 expression in the peripheral blood mononuclear cells of patients with Graves' disease and its significance

Ai Guo, Yan Tan, Chun Liu* and Xiaoya Zheng

Abstract

Background: MST-4 and TRAF-6 are involved in the regulation of inflammatory and immune responses. However, whether they participate in the pathogenesis of Graves' disease (GD) has not yet been reported. Therefore, the purpose of this study was to investigate the expression of MST-4 and TRAF-6 in the peripheral blood of patients with GD to understand their role in the pathogenesis of GD.

Methods: Thirty newly diagnosed GD patients, 24 GD patients in remission (eGD) and 30 normal controls (NC) were recruited. Thyroid function and autoantibody levels were determined using a chemiluminescence immunoassay. Peripheral blood mononuclear cells (PBMCs) were extracted, and MST-4 and TRAF-6 mRNA and protein levels were determined using real-time PCR and Western blotting, respectively.

Results: 1. Thyroid function in the GD group was significantly different from that in the eGD and NC groups ($P < 0.05$); however, there was no difference in thyroid function between the eGD group and the NC group ($P > 0.05$). The autoantibody levels in the NC group were significantly different from those in the GD and eGD groups ($P < 0.05$); however, the difference in the levels between the GD group and eGD group was not statistically significant ($P > 0.05$). 2. The MST-4 and TRAF-6 mRNA and protein levels in the GD group were significantly lower than those in the NC group ($P < 0.05$); however, there were no differences in mRNA and protein levels between the GD group and the eGD group or between the eGD group and the NC group ($P > 0.05$). 3. The correlation between the MST-4 and TRAF-6 mRNA and protein levels was not significant. However, there was a significant correlation between the TRAF-6 mRNA and TPO Ab levels in the eGD group and between the TRAF-6 mRNA and TR Ab levels in the NC group.

Conclusion: The MST-4 and TRAF-6 mRNA and protein levels were lower in the GD group than in the NC group, suggesting that MST-4 and TRAF-6 may be important in the pathogenesis of GD. Whether MST-4 influences the innate immune response through TRAF-6 and thus regulates the imbalance in downstream effector T cells requires further study. Investigating the expression of MST-4 and TRAF-6 in GD can provide a new perspective and targets for further study of the upstream mechanism responsible for effector T cell imbalance.

Keywords: Graves' disease, Innate immunity, TLRs

* Correspondence: liuchun200157@163.com
Department of Endocrinology, The First Affiliated Hospital of Chongqing Medical University, No.1 Youyi Street, Yuzhong District, Chongqing 400016, China

Background

Graves' disease (GD) is an organ-specific autoimmune disease that causes the level of thyroid hormone to increase. The pathogenesis of GD is still unclear; therefore, there is no effective treatment for it. The immune system plays an important role in GD, and studies have shown that imbalances in the function of effector $CD4^+$ T cells (Th1, Th2, Th17 and Treg, among others) lead to the production of autoantibodies and inflammatory cytokines, which promote the disease [1–3]. However, the mechanisms underlying the imbalance in effector CD4+ T cells are unclear.

TNFR-associated factor 6 (TRAF-6), a member of the TRAF family of proteins, consists of 530 amino acids and has a molecular weight of 60 kDa. It consists of TRAF-N domains, which have a coiled-coil structure, and a conserved TRAF-C domain [4]. Because of its unique receptor-binding specificity, TRAF-6 is critical for the tumor necrosis factor receptor family (TNFR), the interleukin-1 receptor (IL-1R), the toll-like receptor (TLR) signaling pathways [5], CD40 [6] and other signaling pathways. Therefore, TRAF-6 has shown conserved function in activation of the regulation of immunity, apoptosis, stress response, inflammation and bone metabolism [7, 8], etc.

Innate immunity, an organism's first line of defense against pathogens, is the foundation for and initiator of adaptive immunity. Toll-like receptors (TLRs), a receptor family, are the bridge connecting the innate and adaptive immune systems [9]. In the TLR signaling pathway, TRAF-6 is a central adapter molecule. When a TLR ligand binds to the TIR domain, the intracellular domain (TIR) interacts with myeloid differentiation factor 88 (MyD88). MyD88 initiates the phosphorylation of IRAK (IL-1R-associated kinase) proteins, which results in activation of the E3 ubiquitin ligase activity of TRAF-6. Subsequently, TRAF-6 catalyzes the K63-mediated ubiquitination of substrates, including TRAF-6 itself, IKKc/NEMO (NF-kB essential modulator) and the mitogen-activated protein (MAP) kinase TAK1 (TGF-β-activated kinase 1). These events are upstream of the activation of the IKKs, which comprise two kinases, IKKa and IKKb, and the catalytically inactive IKKc regulatory subunit. Together, these IKK proteins coordinate the degradation of I-kB, releasing NF-kB to translocate into the nucleus and induce the transcription of target genes [10].

The mammalian Ste20 family is a large class of serine / threonine protein kinases. The GCKs are a subfamily of the mammalian Ste20-like kinase family. The GCKs can be further subdivided into GCK-I to GCK-VIII [11]. Mammalian Ste20-like kinase 4 (MST-4) is a member of the GCKIII subfamily. MST-4 consists of 416 amino acids and has a molecular weight of 46 kDa. The gene is located on chromosome Xq26. MST-4 consists of a C-terminal regulatory domain and an N-terminal kinase domain [12]. It is widely expressed at various levels in many tissues, such as high expression in the placenta, moderate expression in the brain, heart, lungs, liver, muscle, kidney, and pancreas and low expression in skeletal muscle. MST-4 plays a role in promoting the growth of cells, cell polarization and orientation of the Golgi apparatus.

The latest research suggests that MST-4 has an important regulatory function in innate immunity. In the TLR signaling pathway, MST-4 directly associates with and phosphorylates TRAF-6, impairing its oligomerization and ubiquitination activity, which can lead to the abnormal function of downstream signaling molecules. As a result, MST-4 inhibits the activation of inflammatory pathways, regulating the production of downstream inflammatory mediators [13]. Thus, the abnormal expression of MST-4 may be involved in autoimmune diseases. This study provides a new perspective for the study of immune- and inflammatory-related diseases.

In summary, MST-4 and TRAF-6 are involved in the regulation of inflammatory and immune responses. However, whether they participate in the pathogenesis of GD has not yet been reported. Therefore, the purpose of this study was to investigate the expression of MST-4 and TRAF-6 in the peripheral blood of patients with GD, to understand their role in the pathogenesis of GD, and to provide a new understanding of the mechanism regulating GD.

Methods

Study subjects

Patients with GD and healthy persons were recruited from the First Affiliated Hospital of Chongqing Medical University from September 2015 - April 2016. The subjects were divided into a GD group, a GD remission (eGD) group and a normal control (NC) group. According to the guidelines for the diagnosis and management of thyroid disease presented by the American Thyroid Association(ATA) and the American Association of Clinical Endocrinologists (AACE) in 2011 [14], the GD group inclusion criteria were as follows: (1) symptoms of elevated metabolism; (2) increased thyroid hormone concentration, and decreased serum TSH concentration; (3) diffuse thyroid enlargement (palpation and B-confirmed) with or without goiter; (4) anterior tibial mucinous edema; (5) eye bulging and other infiltrative ophthalmopathy; (6) positive for TR Ab, TS Ab, TPO Ab, and Tg Ab. For the above criteria, (1)-(3) are a prerequisite for the diagnosis of GD, (4)-(6) are the diagnosis of auxiliary conditions. The GD group included newly diagnosed untreated patients, a total of 30 cases, including 19 females and 11 males. The inclusion criteria for the eGD group were as follows: (1) GD was diagnosed; (2) anti-thyroid drug (methimazole) treatment for ≥ 1 year; (3) a normal level of thyroid function with a maintenance dose of 2.5–10 mg / d. The eGD group included a total of 24 cases, including 18 females and 6 males. The NC group was consisted of 30 healthy age- and sex-matched volunteers as normal controls, including 21 females and 9 males. The exclusion criteria included acute and chronic infections, other autoimmune diseases (systemic lupus erythematosus, rheumatoid arthritis, psoriasis, etc.), tumors, pregnancy, and the recent consumption of iodine-containing foods or drugs.

The study was approved by the First Affiliated Hospital of Chongqing Medical University Ethical Committee. All participants were provided informed consent when being enrolled and fully explained the purpose and procedures of the study. Informed consent was obtained from all participants.

Experimental materials

The following reagents were used in this study: human lymphocyte separation medium (TBD Tianjin Biotech, China); RNAiso Plus, Reverse Transcription and Amplification kit (TaKaRa, Japan); cell lysis buffer for Western, BCA Protein Assay Kit, SDS-PAGE gel preparation kit, Prestained Color Protein Molecular Weight Marker (Beyotime, China); WesternBright ECL reagent (Advansta, USA); rabbit anti-human TRAF-6 and anti-MST-4 antibodies (CST, USA); rabbit anti-human β-actin antibody (Proteintech, China); horseradish peroxidase (HRP)-labeled goat anti-rabbit IgG secondary antibody (Proteintech, China); nonfat dry milk (Bio-Rad, USA); PVDF membrane (Millipore, USA); and thyroid function and autoantibody kits and detection equipment (Beckman Coulter, Inc., USA).

Specimen collection

Twelve milliliters of peripheral blood were collected in EDTA anticoagulation Vacutainers; 2 ml were used for detecting antibodies and thyroid function indicators, while the other 10 ml were used for peripheral blood mononuclear cell (PBMC) extraction.

Detection of thyroid function indicators

The Beckman Coulter UniCel DxI 800 automatic immunoassay analyzer and reagents were used to evaluate thyroid function (FT3, FT4, and TSH) and antibody levels (TRAb, TGAb, and TPOAb). Detection was completed by the hospital endocrine laboratory technicians. The normal reference values for the thyroid function indicators and antibodies used in our hospital are as follows: FT3: 2.5-3.9 pg/ml; FT4: 0.61-1.12 ng/dl; TSH: 0.35-3.5 IU/ml; TG Ab: < 4 IU/ml; TPO Ab: < 9 IU/ml; and TR Ab: 0.3-1.8 IU/L.

Extraction of PBMCs

Ficoll density gradient centrifugation was used to isolate PBMCs. One-third of the total PBMCs (approximately 3–4 × 10^6) were used for the RNA extraction, whereas the remaining 2/3 (approximately 6–8 × 10^6) were used for the total protein extraction.

Total RNA extraction and the determination of MST-4 and TRAF-6 mRNA expression via RT-PCR

The expression of MST-4 and TRAF-6 was measured using RT-PCR. Total RNA was extracted from PBMCs. cDNA was synthesized using an RT Reagent Kit (TaKaRa, Japan). The primer sequences are shown in Table 1. The following program was run for 40 cycles: 95 °C, 30 s; 95 °C, 5 s; 60 °C, 30 s. The reactions contained the following reagent proportions: 5 μl SYBR® Premix Ex Taq II (Tli RNaseH Plus) (2 ×), 1 μl upstream primer, 1 μl downstream primer, 1 μl cDNA, and 2 μl RNase-free dH_2O. The threshold cycle (cycle threshold, Ct) was obtained with a fluorescence quantitative PCR instrument (Bio-Rad, USA). The relative levels of MST-4 and TRAF-6 mRNA were calculated using the 2-ΔΔCt method and were normalized to the corresponding β-actin values.

The expression of MST-4 and TRAF-6 protein

Total cellular protein was extracted from PBMCs using the Reagent kit (Beyotime, China). The protein concentration was measured with a Protein Assay Kit (Beyotime, China). Equal amounts of protein per sample were separated by SDS–PAGE and transferred to a PVDF membrane. The membrane was blocked with 5% nonfat milk in Tris-buffered saline with 0.05% Tween20 (TBST) for 3 h. The membranes were washed 3 times for 10 min each in TBST and incubated with monoclonal rabbit anti-human TRAF-6 (1:1000), monoclonal rabbit anti-human MST-4 (1:1000), and monoclonal rabbit anti-human β-actin antibody (1: 2000), followed by horseradish peroxidase (HRP)-labeled goat anti-rabbit IgG secondary antibody (1:5000). Immunoreactive bands were developed using the WesternBright ECL reagent (Advansta, USA). For the image analysis, the films were scanned and analyzed using a chemiluminescence system (VILBER FUSION FX5, France).

Table 1 Primer sequences used for the real-time PCR

Primer	Sequences	bp
MST-4	F 5′ TGAGGAAGCCGAAGATGAAATAG 3′ R 5′ CCAGCTCGAAGAAGATCCAGTG 3′	170
TRAF-6	F 5′ GGATTCTACACTGGCAAACCCG 3′ R 5′ CCAAGGGAGGTGGCTGTCATA 3′	137
β-actin	F 5′ CCACGAAACTACCTTCAACTCC 3′ R 5′ GTGATCTCCTTCTGCATCCTGT 3′	132

Data analysis

Statistical analysis was performed with SPSS software (IBM, Armonk, NY, version 19.0). The results were expressed as x ± s. One-way analysis of variance combined with the Bonferroni test was used for statistical analysis of the data. Correlation between variables was determined with the Pearson correlation coefficient; P-values less than 0.05 were considered statistically significant.

Results

Thyroid function and autoantibody levels

The levels of the indicators of thyroid function (FT3 and FT4) were higher, whereas TSH was lower in the NC group than in the eGD group, and these differences were statistically significant ($P < 0.001$); however, the differences between the eGD group and the NC group were not statistically significant ($P > 0.05$). The level of autoantibodies (TR Ab, TG Ab, and TPO Ab) differed significantly between the GD group and the NC group and between the eGD group and the NC group ($P = 0.000$), but the difference between the eGD group and NC group was not statistically significant ($P > 0.05$), as shown in Table 2.

The expression of MST-4 and TRAF-6 mRNA in the PBMCs of each group

The expression of MST-4 and TRAF-6 mRNA in the GD group was lower than that in the NC group; these differences were statistically significant ($P < 0.05$, $P = 0.024$, $P = 0.019$); However, the differences were not statistically significant between the GD group and the eGD group or between the eGD group and the NC group ($P > 0.05$), as shown in Table 3, Figs. 1 and 2.

The levels of MST-4 and TRAF-6 protein in the PBMCs of each group

The levels of MST-4 and TRAF-6 protein were lower in the GD group than those in the NC group, and these differences were statistically significant ($P < 0.05$, $P = 0.0051$, $P = 0.0047$). However, the differences were not statistically significant between the GD group and the eGD group or between the eGD group and the NC group ($P > 0.05$), as shown in Table 4, Figs. 3, 4, and 5.

Table 2 The levels of indicators of thyroid function and autoantibodies among the three groups ($\bar{x} \pm s$)

	GD group	eGD group	NC group
Age (years)	39.00 ± 19.22	37.13 ± 1 1.78	39.97 ± 13.73
FT3 (pg/ml)	10.87 ± 7.85①②	3.19 ± 0.28	3.14 ± 0.37
FT4 (ng/dl)	3.28 ± 1.71 ①②	0.90 ± 0.13	0.78 ± 0.20
uTSH (μIU/ml)	0.03 ± 0.02①②	1.57 ± 0.73	1.90 ± 0.83
TRAb (ng/ml)	11.30 ± 8.80①	7.90 ± 2.64①	0.64 ± 0.34
TPOAb (IU/ml)	109.50 ± 108.04①	104.84 ± 143.37①	1.16 ± 1.10
TGAb(IU/L)	56.95 ± 56.15①	45.77 ± 76.53①	0.2 ± 0.14
Total (F/M)	30 (19/11)	24 (18/6)	30 (21/9)

①$P < 0.05$ compared with the normal group; ②$P < 0.05$ compared with the eGD group

Table 3 Expression of MST-4 and TRAF-6 mRNA ($\bar{x} \pm s$)

	GD group	eGD group	NC group
MST-4	0.86 ± 0.19①	0.99 ± 0.29	1.03 ± 0.27
TRAF-6	0.81 ± 0.28①	0.90 ± 0.40	1.03 ± 0.26

①$P < 0.05$ compared with the normal group

Correlation analysis

The expression of MST-4 mRNA was not significantly correlated with the level of TRAF-6 mRNA, thyroid function, or the level of autoantibodies in any of the groups. However, the expression of TRAF-6 mRNA was positively correlated with thyroid function and the level of TPO Ab in the eGD group ($r = 0.4291$, $P = 0.0364$) and negatively correlated with the level of TR Ab in the NC group ($r = -0.4085$, $P = 0.025$). There was no significant correlation between the MST-4 or TRAF-6 protein levels and thyroid function or autoantibody levels in any group ($P > 0.05$).

Discussion

MST-4 has been found to participate in a variety of biological functions in cells since it was identified in 2001. Studies have shown that MST-4 promotes cell proliferation to influence the development of neoplastic disease [15–17]. In addition, MST-4 can activate the LKB 1-STRAD-MO25 complex, which is involved in cell polarization [18]. MST-4 can also interact with cerebral cavernous malformations (CCM3) to participate in cell migration and orientation of the Golgi [19]. However, whether MST-4 regulates the immune response was unclear. The other members of the GCK family play important roles in the innate and adaptive immune responses, but each has a different regulatory mechanism. The GCK-1 family member, MAP4K2, is involved in

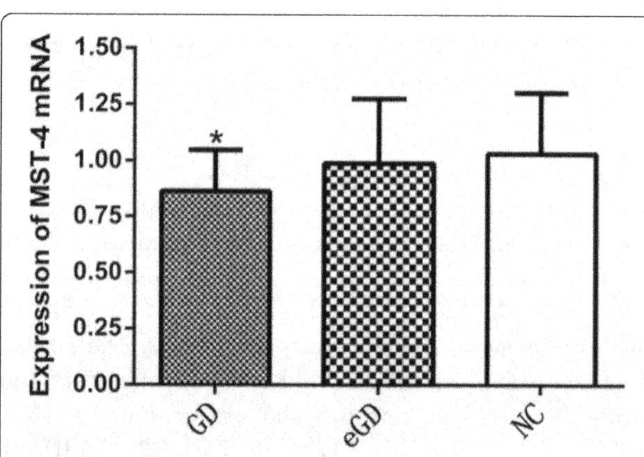

Fig. 1 Expression of MST-4 mRNA in PBMCs *Compared with the normal group

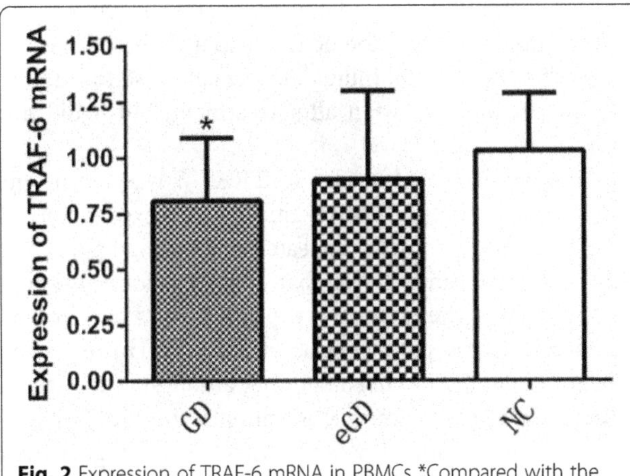

Fig. 2 Expression of TRAF-6 mRNA in PBMCs *Compared with the normal group

pathogen-associated molecular pattern (PAMP) signaling pathways and plays a role in the JNK and p38 pathways [20]. The GCK-II member MST1 is involved in negative regulation of T cell proliferation [21] and plays a key role in lymphocyte chemotaxis and thymocyte emigration [22, 23]. The GCK-VI member Ste20-like proline / alanine-rich kinase (SPAK) is involved in the TCR / CD28-induced activation of the transcription factor AP-1 [24]. The GCK-VII member TAO2 can activate the p38 signaling pathway to regulate the expression of inflammatory cytokines via extracellular signal-regulated kinase kinase 3 (MEK3) and MEK6 [25].

There are still few recent studies about the role of GCK-III family members in the immune mechanism. Therefore, the Chinese group Zhou et al. [21] was the first to explore the role of the MST-4 in the innate immune response in 2015. An analysis of clinical samples from patients with sepsis caused by infection revealed decreased MST-4 levels. In vivo and in vitro experiments revealed that the expression of MST-4 responded dynamically to LPS stimulation and that the phosphorylation of TRAF-6 affected its activity, which caused the signaling information not to be delivered and suppressed the production of the pro-inflammatory cytokines IL-6 and TNF-α. Therefore, MST-4 can participate in the regulation of TLR signaling pathways. Furthermore, mouse models of septic shock were used to further investigate MST-4 function. It was found that MST-4 knockdown could cause a more severe inflammatory response. The study revealed that MST-4 played a similar role in inhibiting an excessive immune response to protect the

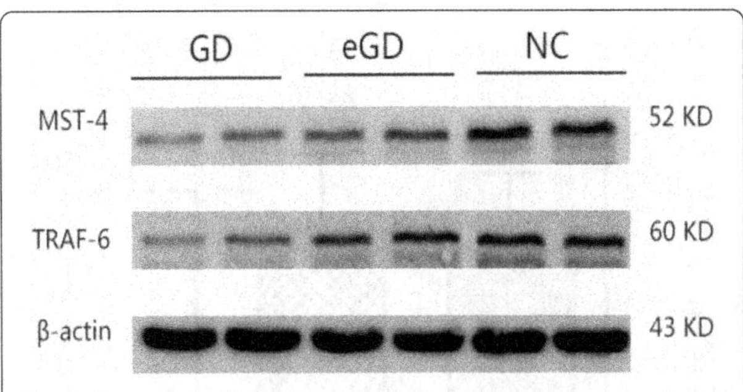

Fig. 3 Expression of MST-4 and TRAF-6 protein, as detected using Western blotting

body. Thus, MST-4 provided a new perspective for the study of immune and inflammatory-related diseases [13].

The imbalance in effector T cells at the level of adaptive immunity plays an important role in GD, but the pathogenesis of innate immunity in GD is poorly understood. Studies have found that polymorphisms in and abnormal expression of TLR receptor genes [26–28] and alterations in the functional activity of antigen-presenting cells (DCs) are important in GD [29, 30] and in other autoimmune diseases, which suggested the functional activation of immune cells (DCs, monocytes, macrophages, etc.). The activation of the TLR signaling pathway influences the proliferation and differentiation of downstream CD4+ effector T cells, augmenting the immune and inflammatory responses and leading to the onset of GD. However, the innate immune mechanism underlying GD still is not entirely clear, and it is necessary to further explore the mechanism of the disease and find a better explanation for the adaptive immune imbalance. Therefore, we need a better understanding of the molecules and related mechanisms involved in regulating the TLR signaling pathway in innate immunity, and we must study the regulatory mechanisms underlying the imbalance in effector CD4+ T cells. As a novel target, MST-4 provides an opportunity to

Table 4 Expression of MST-4 and TRAF-6 protein ($\overline{x} \pm s$)

	GD group	eGD group	NC group
MST-4	0.14 ± 0.09①	0.17 ± 0.12	0.23 ± 0.12
TRAF-6	0.13 ± 0.07①	0.16 ± 0.06	0.20 ± 0.08

①$P < 0.05$ compared with the normal group

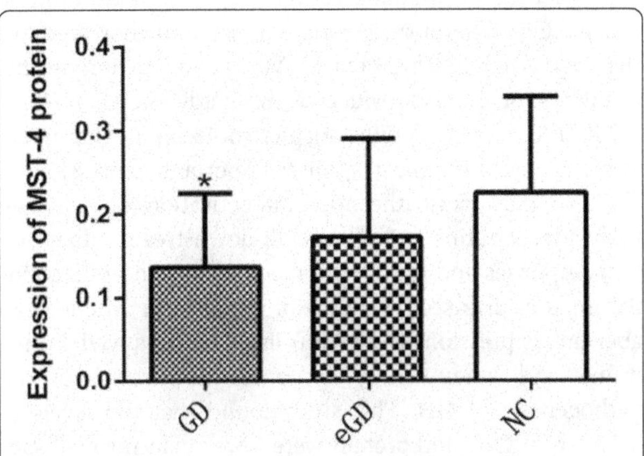

Fig. 4 Expression of MST-4 protein in PBMCs *Compared with the normal group

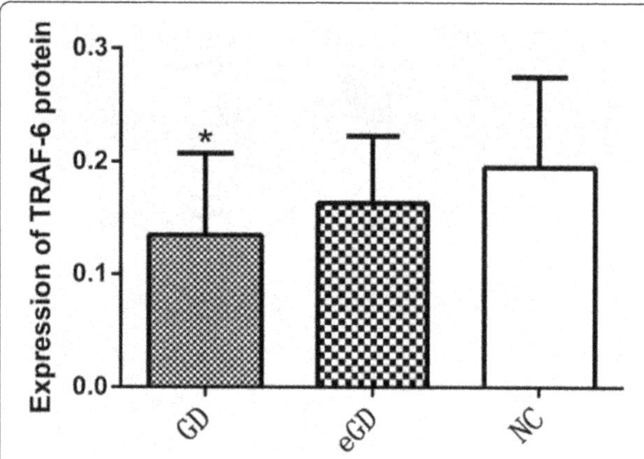

Fig. 5 Expression of TRAF-6 protein in PBMCs *Compared with the normal group

further our understanding of the role of innate immunity in the pathogenesis of GD.

In this study, we first found that the expression of MST-4 mRNA and protein in the GD group was lower than that in the NC group, which was consistent with the results observed in sepsis due to infection [13]. This result indicated that the expression of MST-4 is abnormal in GD. However, the expression of MST-4 was not significantly different between the GD group and the eGD group, or between the eGD group and the NC group, suggesting that the immune inflammatory statue in the eGD group is probably between that of the GD group and the normal controls, which contributed to the above results. However, further study is required to determine whether MST-4 aberrantly regulates TRAF-6 in TLR signaling pathways, promotes the aberrant activation of TLR signaling pathways, activates antigen-presenting cells (APCs), and stimulates downstream effector T cell proliferation and differentiation, further promoting the onset of GD. The present study was the first to explore the expression of MST-4, decreases in which may lead to abnormal innate immune responses, in the autoimmune disease GD. Therefore, a foundation for further study of the regulatory mechanisms of MST-4 in the innate immune response was provided by this study in GD.

TRAF-6 is an important adapter molecule in the innate and adaptive immune responses. Aberrant expression of TRAF-6 may cause the aberrant activation of signaling pathways, resulting in activation of downstream inflammatory responses and the development of immune-related inflammatory diseases. Therefore, it was unclear whether the aberrant expression of TRAF-6 in GD is involved in immune and inflammatory responses and regulates the pathogenesis of GD. This study found that the levels of TRAF-6 mRNA and protein were lower than normal, suggesting that TRAF-6 may have a role in the pathogenesis of GD. However, there were no significant differences in the expression of TRAF-6 between the GD group and the eGD group or between the eGD group and the NC group, suggesting that the immune inflammatory status in the eGD group was remission after treatment, but it did not return to the normal level.

In this study, the decrease in TRAF-6 was consistent with other findings. For example, the expression of TRAF-6 in patients with untreated ankylosing spondylitis (AS) was significantly lower than that in a control group, suggesting that the abnormal expression of TRAF-6 may play a role in the pathogenesis of AS [31]. However, the expression of TRAF-6 in some other autoimmune diseases exhibits the opposite trend. For example, the TRAF-6 level in the synovial tissue of patients with RA was higher than that in the synovial tissue of patients with osteoarthritis (OA), suggesting that TRAF-6 mediates the inflammatory response involved in synovial inflammation and joint destruction in RA [32]. A study demonstrated that two members of the TRAF family, TRAF4 and TRAF-6, were activated in patients with inflammatory bowel disease (IBD) and that both TRAF4 and TRAF-6 showed potential diagnostic value in differential diagnosis [33]. The protein levels of the TLRs, TRAF-6, MyD88, and NF-κB were significantly increased in the adipose tissue of patients with type 2 diabetes [34].

The down-regulation of TRAF-6 in GD may be associated with the presence of other proteins inhibiting TRAF-6 signal transduction. For example, heat shock protein 70 (HSP70) can associate with the C-terminal TRAF domain, prevent its ubiquitination, and inhibit NF-κB activation [35]. Suppression of cytokine signaling-3 (SOCS-3) inhibited TRAF-6 ubiquitination to prevent TRAF-6 and TAK1 interactions [36]. Multifunctional proteins in the β-arrestin family can form a complex with TRAF-6 to prevent TRAF-6 ubiquitination and signal transduction. A zinc finger-like protein (ZCCHCll) also inhibited TRAF-6 signaling [37]. Thus, the decreased expression of TRAF-6 in GD might affect both the regulatory role of MST-4 and the combined effects of various effector protein molecules. The expression of TRAF-6 may be associated with the dynamics of the disease: when the immune system is activated, both the inflammatory response and the related inhibitory factors increase, which requires balancing of the immune and inflammatory responses in order for the body to avoid excessive induction of an immune response.

Studies have shown that TRAF-6 is also essential in immune tolerance. Previous studies have also demonstrated that knocking out TRAF-6 in mouse T cells can cause inflammation in multiple organs and mononuclear cell infiltration into the intestine, liver, lung, and kidney. Higher levels of IL-4 and IL-5 are produced by TRAF-6-deficient T cells, and these mice develop an inflammatory disease mediated by activated Th2 cells. In addition, the serum IgG1, IgE, IgM and anti-DNA autoantibody levels were significantly elevated in TRAF-6-specific T cell-deficient mice, resulting in an enhanced humoral immune response. Therefore, TRAF-6-deficient T cells can affect immune homeostasis, and autoimmune disease can appear [38]. Studies have further found that Treg-specific TRAF-6 knockout (CKO) mice may develop allergic skin diseases, arthritis, swollen lymph nodes and a hyper immunoglobulin E phenotype. Although TRAF-6-knockout Tregs had similar inhibitory activity to wild-type Tregs in vitro, the reduced number of Foxp3-positive cells suggests that TRAF-6 knockout cannot suppress the development of colitis in mice with lymphopenia. These data suggest that TRAF-6 plays an important role in the regulation of T cells, primarily by maintaining Foxp3 regulatory T cells and inhibiting pathogenic Th2-type conversion [39]. In addition, TRAF-6 deficiency may lead to immune tolerance imbalance. Considering that GD is an autoimmune disease, there may be an imbalance in immune tolerance. Thus, in GD, a decreased level of TRAF-6 may also be associated with an imbalance of immune tolerance. However, further study is required to determine whether TRAF-6 participates in the abnormal regulation of Treg cells and promotes the development of GD.

Phosphorylated TRAF-6 (mediated by MST-4) primarily takes part in the immune response. Therefore, total protein and phosphorylated TRAF-6 levels should be detected. Typically, phosphorylation-specific antibodies cannot detect total protein levels, and total protein antibodies can detect all forms of the protein, including the phosphorylated and non-phosphorylated forms. This study examined the expression of total TRAF-6 protein, but not phosphorylated TRAF-6, mainly because phospho-TRAF-6-specific antibodies suitable for Western blot are not currently available commercially. Thus, we did not evaluate phosphorylated TRAF-6. A co-immunoprecipitation assay can measure phosphorylated TRAF-6, but due to the limited amount of peripheral blood samples, we failed to detect phosphorylation of TRAF-6. In this study, the level of total TRAF-6 protein was decreased, suggesting that the phosphorylation of TRAF-6 may also be lower. Although there was no correlation between MST-4 and TRAF-6 levels, this did not completely eliminate the possibility that MST-4 might play a regulatory role in the phosphorylation of TRAF-6 and that the reduction in TRAF-6 levels occurred due to the influence of other regulatory molecules. Therefore, we must study the relationship between MST-4 and phosphorylated TRAF-6 further and analyze whether altered MST-4 expression has a direct effect on TRAF-6 phosphorylation.

This study has some shortcomings, such as the relatively small number of samples collected for each group; thus, the role of MST-4 and TRAF-6 in the pathogenesis of GD must be studied in a large sample to verify these data. It is well known that GD is an organ-specific autoimmune disease. Therefore, it is important to comprehensively evaluate the influence of MST-4 and TRAF-6 in the thyroid gland to fully understand the effects of MST-4 and TRAF-6 in GD. The PBMCs in this study consisted of various types of cells, including lymphocytes (approximately 70 to 90% of PBMCs), monocytes, (approximately 10 to 30%), and dendritic cells (approximately 1 to 2%). Therefore, the expression level determined may be the combined effect of a number of factors. Studying the role of MST-4 in the regulation of TRAF-6 requires the investigation of a relatively specific cell population to eliminate confounding factors.

Conclusion

This study showed that the expression of MST-4 and TRAF-6 was decreased in GD, suggesting the involvement of these molecules in the pathogenesis of GD. However, whether MST-4 had an effect on the interaction between the innate immune response and TRAF-6 in GD and the mechanism responsible for the imbalance in downstream effector T cells require further study. The present study explored the expression of MST-4 and TRAF-6 in GD and provided a new perspective and targets for further study of the upstream mechanism underlying the effector T cell imbalance, which plays a key role in GD pathogenesis. This research provides a new direction for studying the pathogenesis of GD and a new target for the effective diagnosis and treatment of GD pathogenesis.

Abbreviations

AACE: The American Association of Clinical Endocrinologists; ATA: The American Thyroid Association; FT3: Free triiodothyronine; FT4: Free thyroxine; GD: Graves' disease; MST-4: Mammalian Ste20-like kinase 4; Tg Ab: Thyroglobulin antibody; TLR: Toll-like receptor; TPO Ab: Thyroid peroxidase antibody; TR Ab: Thyrotropin receptor antibody; TRAF-6: TNFR-associated factor 6; uTSH: Ultra-sensitive thyrotropin

Acknowledgements

We thank the teachers in the Laboratory of Lipid & Glucose Metabolism, the First Affiliated Hospital of Chongqing Medical University, Chongqing, China for technical support, and we gratefully acknowledge the nurses who helped to collect blood samples at The First Affiliated Hospital of Chongqing Medical University, Chongqing, China.

Funding

This work was supported by grants from 2015 Thyroid Research Project of Young Doctors and National Key Clinical Specialties Construction Program of China (2011).

Authors' contributions

AG conceived and designed the study, performed the data analyses and drafted the manuscript. YT helped in the design of the study, data collection, data analyses and drafting of the manuscript. CL and XZ participated in the design of the study, and the coordination and critical revision of the manuscript. All of the authors read and approved the final manuscript.

Competing interests

The authors declare that they have no competing interests.

References

1. Li H, Wang T. The autoimmunity in Graves's disease. Front Biosci (Landmark Ed). 2013;18:782–7. doi:10.2741/4141.
2. Esfahanian F, Naimi E, Doroodgar F, Jadali Z. Th1/Th2 cytokines in patients with Graves' disease with or without ophthalmopathy. Iran J Allergy Asthma Immunol. 2013;12:168–75.
3. Lv M, Shen J, Li Z, Zhao D, Chen Z, Wan H, et al. [Role of Treg/Th17 cells and related cytokines in Graves' ophthalmopathy]. Nan Fang Yi Ke Da Xue Xue Bao. 2014;34:1809–13.
4. Rothe M, Wong SC, Henzel WJ, Goeddel DV. A novel family of putative signal transducers associated with the cytoplasmic domain of the 75 kDa tumor necrosis factor receptor. Cell. 1994;78:681–92. doi:10.1016/0092-8674(94)90532-0.
5. Kobayashi T, Walsh MC, Choi Y. The role of TRAF6 in signal transduction and the immune response. Microbes Infect. 2004;6:1333–8. doi:10.1016/j.micinf.2004.09.001.
6. Hostager BS. Roles of TRAF6 in CD40 signaling. Immunol Res. 2007;39:105–14. doi:10.1007/s12026-007-0082-3.
7. Ye H, Arron JR, Lamothe B, Cirilli M, Kobayashi T, Shevde NK, et al. Distinct molecular mechanism for initiating TRAF6 signalling. Nature. 2002;418:443–7. doi:10.1038/nature00888.
8. Walsh MC, Lee J, Choi Y. Tumor necrosis factor receptor- associated factor 6 (TRAF6) regulation of development, function, and homeostasis of the immune system. Immunol Rev. 2015;266:72–92. doi:10.1111/imr.12302.
9. Mohammad Hosseini A, Majidi J, Baradaran B, Yousefi M. Toll-like receptors in the pathogenesis of autoimmune diseases. Adv Pharm Bull. 2015;5:605–14. 10.15171/apb.2015.082.
10. Deng L, Wang C, Spencer E, Yang L, Braun A, You J, et al. Activation of the IkappaB kinase complex by TRAF6 requires a dimeric ubiquitin-conjugating enzyme complex and a unique polyubiquitin chain. Cell. 2000;103:351–61. doi:10.1016/S0092-8674(00)00126-4.
11. Dan I, Watanabe NM, Kusumi A. The Ste20 group kinases as regulators of MAP kinase cascades. Trends Cell Biol. 2001;11:220–30. doi:10.1016/S0962-8924(01)01980-8.
12. Qian Z, Lin C, Espinosa R, LeBeau M, Rosner MR. Cloning and characterization of MST4, a novel Ste20-like kinase. J Biol Chem. 2001;276:22439–45. doi:10.1074/jbc.M009323200.
13. Jiao S, Zhang Z, Li C, Huang M, Shi Z, Wang Y, et al. The kinase MST4 limits inflammatory responses through direct phosphorylation of the adaptor TRAF6. Nat Immunol. 2015;16:246–57. doi:10.1038/ni.3097.
14. Bahn Chair RS, Burch HB, Cooper DS, Garber JR, Greenlee MC, Klein I, et al. Hyperthyroidism and other causes of thyrotoxicosis: management guidelines of the American Thyroid Association and American Association of Clinical Endocrinologists. Thyroid. 2011;21:593–646. doi:10.1089/thy.2010.0417.
15. Xiong W, Knox AJ, Xu M, Kiseljak-Vassiliades K, Colgan SP, Brodsky KS, et al. Mammalian Ste20-like kinase 4 promotes pituitary cell proliferation and survival under hypoxia. Mol Endocrinol. 2015;29:460–72. doi:10.1210/me.2014-1332.
16. Sung V, Luo W, Qian D, Lee I, Jallal B, Gishizky M. The Ste20 kinase MST4 plays a role in prostate cancer progression. Cancer Res. 2003;63:3356–63.
17. Lin ZH, Wang L, Zhang JB, Liu Y, Li XQ, Guo L, et al. MST4 promotes hepatocellular carcinoma epithelial-mesenchymal transition and metastasis via activation of the p-ERK pathway. Int J Oncol. 2014;45:629–40. doi:10.3892/ijo.2014.2455.
18. ten Klooster JP, Jansen M, Yuan J, Oorschot V, Begthel H, Di Giacomo V, et al. Mst4 and Ezrin induce brush borders downstream of the LKB1/strad/Mo25 polarization complex. Dev Cell. 2009;16:551–62. doi:10.1016/j.devcel.2009.01.016.
19. Fidalgo M, Fraile M, Pires A, Force T, Pombo C, Zalvide J. CCM3/PDCD10 stabilizes GCKIII proteins to promote Golgi assembly and cell orientation. J Cell Sci. 2010;123:1274–84. doi:10.1242/jcs.061341.
20. Zhong J, Gavrilescu LC, Molnár A, Murray L, Garafalo S, Kehrl JH, et al. GCK is essential to systemic inflammation and pattern recognition receptor signaling to JNK and p38. Proc Natl Acad Sci U S A. 2009;106:4372–7. doi:10.1073/pnas.0812642106.
21. Zhou D, Medoff BD, Chen L, Li L, Zhang XF, Praskova M, et al. The Nore1B/Mst1 complex restrains antigen receptor-induced proliferation of naive T cells. Proc Natl Acad Sci U S A. 2008;105:20321–6. doi:10.1073/pnas.0810773105.
22. Dong Y, Du X, Ye J, Han M, Xu T, Zhuang Y, et al. A cell-intrinsic role for Mst1 in regulating thymocyte egress. J Immunol. 2009;183:3865–72. doi:10.4049/jimmunol.0900678.
23. Katagiri K, Katakai T, Ebisuno Y, Ueda Y, Okada T, Kinashi T. Mst1 controls lymphocyte trafficking and interstitial motility within lymph nodes. EMBO J. 2009;28:1319–31. doi:10.1038/emboj.2009.82.
24. Li Y, Hu J, Vita R, Sun B, Tabata H, Altman A. SPAK kinase is a substrate and target of PKCtheta in T-cell receptor-induced AP-1 activation pathway. EMBO J. 2004;23:1112–22. doi:10.1038/sj.emboj.7600125.
25. Chen Z, Cobb MH. Regulation of stress-responsive mitogen-activated protein (MAP) kinase pathways by TAO2. J Biol Chem. 2001;276:16070–5. doi:10.1074/jbc.M100681200.
26. Li XF, Li Q, Chen ZJ, Liu C. Change of serum heat shock protein 70 in Graves disease and its significance. Chinese General Practice. 2012;18:2028–30 (In Chinese).
27. Peng SQ, Li CY, Yu XH, Liu X, Jing T. The expression of toll-like receptors in peripheral blood mononuclear cells of patients with autoimmune thyroid disease and their clinical significances. In: The 13th Annual Meeting of Chinese Society of Endocrinology. 2014. In Chinese.
28. Liao WL, Chen RH, Lin HJ, Liu YH, Chen WC, Tsai Y, et al. Toll-like receptor gene polymorphisms are associated with susceptibility to Graves' ophthalmopathy in Taiwan males. BMC Med Genet. 2010;11:154. doi:10.1186/1471-2350-11-154.
29. He K, Hu Y, Mao X. Abnormal proportions of immune regulatory cells and their subsets in peripheral blood of patients with Graves' disease. Xi Bao Yu Fen Zi Mian Yi Xue Za Zhi. 2014;30:1190–3.
30. Hassan I, Brendel C, Zielke A, Burchert A, Danila R. Immune regulatory plasmacytoid dendritic cells selectively accumulate in perithyroidal lymph nodes of patients with Graves disease: implications for the understanding of autoimmunity. Rev Med Chir Soc Med Nat Iasi. 2013;117:46–51.
31. He XL, Li XP, Tao JH, Chen ZQ, Li XM. The expression of miR-146a TRAF6 IRAK-1 in the peripheral blood mononuclear cells of patients with ankylosing spondylitis. In: The 17th conference of the Chinese Rheumatology Association. 2012. In Chinese.
32. Zhu LJ, Dai L, Mo YQ, Zheng DH, Zhang BY. The expression of TRAF6 patients with rheumatoid arthritis synovial and significance. In: The 8th Rheumatism Academic Conference Integrated of Traditional and Western Medicine. 2010. In Chinese.
33. Shen J, Qiao Y, Ran Z, Wang T. Different activation of TRAF4 and TRAF6 in inflammatory bowel disease. Mediators Inflamm. 2013;2013:647936. doi:10.1155/2013/647936.
34. Creely SJ, McTernan PG, Kusminski CM, Fisher FM, Da Silva NF, Khanolkar M, et al. Lipopolysaccharide activates an innate immune system response in human adipose tissue in obesity and type 2 diabetes. Am J Physiol Endocrinol Metab. 2007;292:E740–7. doi:10.1152/ajpendo.00302.2006.
35. Chen H, Wu Y, Zhang Y, Jin L, Luo L, Xue B, et al. Hsp70 inhibits lipopolysaccharide-induced NF-kappaB activation by interacting with TRAF6 and inhibiting its ubiquitination. FEBS Lett. 2006;580:3145–52. doi:10.1016/j.febslet.2006.04.066.
36. Frobøse H, Rønn SG, Heding PE, Mendoza H, Cohen P, Mandrup-Poulsen T, et al. Suppressor of cytokine signaling-3 inhibits interleukin-1 signaling by targeting the TRAF-6/TAK1 complex. Mol Endocrinol. 2006;20:1587–96. doi:10.1210/me.2005-0301.
37. Minoda Y, Saeki K, Aki D, Takaki H, Sanada T, Koga K, et al. A novel zinc finger protein, ZCCHC11, interacts with TIFA and modulates TLR signaling. Biochem Biophys Res Commun. 2006;344:1023–30. doi:10.1016/j.bbrc.2006.04.006.
38. King CG, Kobayashi T, Cejas PJ, Kim T, Yoon K, Kim GK, et al. TRAF6 is a T cell-intrinsic negative regulator required for the maintenance of immune homeostasis. Nat Med. 2006;12:1088–92. doi:10.1038/nm1449.
39. Muto G, Kotani H, Kondo T, Morita R, Tsuruta S, Kobayashi T, et al. TRAF6 is essential for maintenance of regulatory T cells that suppress Th2 type autoimmunity. PLoS One. 2013;8:e74639. doi:10.1371/journal.pone.0074639.

Permissions

All chapters in this book were first published in ED, by BioMed Central; hereby published with permission under the Creative Commons Attribution License or equivalent. Every chapter published in this book has been scrutinized by our experts. Their significance has been extensively debated. The topics covered herein carry significant findings which will fuel the growth of the discipline. They may even be implemented as practical applications or may be referred to as a beginning point for another development.

The contributors of this book come from diverse backgrounds, making this book a truly international effort. This book will bring forth new frontiers with its revolutionizing research information and detailed analysis of the nascent developments around the world.

We would like to thank all the contributing authors for lending their expertise to make the book truly unique. They have played a crucial role in the development of this book. Without their invaluable contributions this book wouldn't have been possible. They have made vital efforts to compile up to date information on the varied aspects of this subject to make this book a valuable addition to the collection of many professionals and students.

This book was conceptualized with the vision of imparting up-to-date information and advanced data in this field. To ensure the same, a matchless editorial board was set up. Every individual on the board went through rigorous rounds of assessment to prove their worth. After which they invested a large part of their time researching and compiling the most relevant data for our readers.

The editorial board has been involved in producing this book since its inception. They have spent rigorous hours researching and exploring the diverse topics which have resulted in the successful publishing of this book. They have passed on their knowledge of decades through this book. To expedite this challenging task, the publisher supported the team at every step. A small team of assistant editors was also appointed to further simplify the editing procedure and attain best results for the readers.

Apart from the editorial board, the designing team has also invested a significant amount of their time in understanding the subject and creating the most relevant covers. They scrutinized every image to scout for the most suitable representation of the subject and create an appropriate cover for the book.

The publishing team has been an ardent support to the editorial, designing and production team. Their endless efforts to recruit the best for this project, has resulted in the accomplishment of this book. They are a veteran in the field of academics and their pool of knowledge is as vast as their experience in printing. Their expertise and guidance has proved useful at every step. Their uncompromising quality standards have made this book an exceptional effort. Their encouragement from time to time has been an inspiration for everyone.

The publisher and the editorial board hope that this book will prove to be a valuable piece of knowledge for researchers, students, practitioners and scholars across the globe.

List of Contributors

Marcus M Cranston
Keesler Medical Center, Keesler AFB, Mississippi, USA

Margaret AK Ryan
Naval Hospital, Camp Pendleton, California, USA

Tyler C Smith and Carter J Sevick
Naval Health Research Center, San Diego, California, USA

Stephanie K Brodine
San Diego State University, San Diego, California, USA

Monica Vincenzi and Giacomo Venturi
Department of Life and Reproduction Sciences, University of Verona, Piazzale Scuro 10, 37126 Verona, Italy

Marta Camilot, Francesca Teofoli, Rossella Gaudino, Attilio Boner and Franco Antoniazzi
Department of Life and Reproduction Sciences, University of Verona, Piazzale Scuro 10, 37126 Verona, Italy
Azienda Ospedaliera Universitaria Integrata di Verona, Verona, Italy

Eleonora Ferrarini, Giuseppina De Marco, Patrizia Agretti, Antonio Dimida and Massimo Tonacchera
Department of Endocrinology, Centro di Eccellenza AmbiSEN, University of Pisa, Pisa, Italy

Paolo Cavarzere
Azienda Ospedaliera Universitaria Integrata di Verona, Verona, Italy

Shunyao Liao and Yaming Liang
Diabetes and Endocrinology Center, Sichuan Academy of Medical Science, Sichuan Provincial People's Hospital, Chengdu 610072, China

Jiyuan Huang, Wenzhong Song and Zhenlin Tang
Department of Thyroid Disease and Nuclear Medicine, Sichuan Academy of Medical Science, Sichuan Provincial People's Hospital, Chengdu 610072, China

Yunqiang Liu
Department of Medical Genetics and Division of Morbid Genomics, State Key Laboratory of Biotherapy, West China Hospital, Sichuan University, Chengdu 610041, China

Shaoping Deng
Diabetes and Endocrinology Center, Sichuan Academy of Medical Science, Sichuan Provincial People's Hospital, Chengdu 610072, China
Department of Surgery, Harvard Medical School, Massachusetts General Hospital, Boston, MA, USA

Dandan Dong and Gang Xu
Department of Pathology, Sichuan Academy of Medical Science, Sichuan Provincial People's Hospital, Chengdu 610072, China

Alessandro P Delitala
Department of Biomedical Science, University of Sassari, Sassari, Viale San Pietro 8, 07100 Sassari, Italy

Gianpaolo Vidili, Alessandra Manca, Giuseppe Delitala and Giuseppe Fanciulli
Department of Clinical and Experimental Medicine, University of Sassari, Azienda Ospedaliera Universitaria, Sassari, Italy

Upinder Dial
Department of Pathology, University of Sassari, Azienda Ospedaliera Universitaria, Sassari, Italy

Maciej Owecki, Nadia Sawicka-Gutaj, Jakub Fischbach and Marek Ruchała
Department of Endocrinology, Metabolism and Internal Medicine, Poznan University of Medical Sciences, Przybyszewskiego St. 49, 60-355 Poznań, Poland

Jolanta Dorszewska, Anna Oczkowska, Michał K Owecki and Wojciech Kozubski
Department of Neurology, Poznan University of Medical Sciences, Przybyszewskiego St. 49, 60-355 Poznań, Poland

Michał Michalak
Department of Informatics and Statistics, Poznan University of Medical Sciences, Dąbrowskiego St. 79, 60-529 Poznań, Poland

Maira L Mendonça, Francisco A Pereira, Marcello H Nogueira-Barbosa, Lucas M Monsignore, Sara R Teixeira and Lea MZ Maciel
Department of Internal Medicine, School of Medicine of Ribeirão Preto, University of São Paulo, São Paulo, Brazil

Plauto CA Watanabe
Department of Radiology, School of Dentistry of Ribeirão Preto, University of São Paulo, São Paulo, Brazil

Francisco JA de Paula
Department of Internal Medicine, School of Medicine of Ribeirão Preto, University of São Paulo, São Paulo, Brazil
Department of Internal Medicine, School of Medicine of Ribeirão Preto, University of São Paulo, Av. Bandeirantes 3900, Ribeirão Preto, SP 14049-900, Brazil

Roberto F Casal, Mimi N Phan, D Ray Lazarus and Juan Iribarren
Section of Pulmonary and Critical Care Medicine, Baylor College of Medicine, Michael E. DeBakey VA Medical Center, 2002 Holcombe Blvd. Pulmonary Section 111i, Houston, TX 77030, USA

Keerthana Keshava and Horiana Grosu
Division of Pulmonary and Critical Care Medicine, New York Methodist Hospital, Brooklyn, NY, USA

Jose M Garcia
Division of Endocrinology, Diabetes and Metabolism, Baylor College of Medicine, Houston, TX, USA

Daniel G Rosen
Department of Pathology and Immunology, Baylor College of Medicine, Houston, TX, USA

Carmen Sorina Martin, Carmen Gabriela Barbu, Anca Elena Sirbu and Simona Vasilica Fica
Endocrinology Department, Carol Davila University of Medicine and Pharmacy, Elias University Hospital, 17 Marasti Blvd, sector 1, 011461 Bucharest, Romania

Luminita Nicoleta Ionescu
Cardiology Department, Elias University Hospital, 17 Marasti Blvd, sector 1, Bucharest, Romania

Ioana Maria Lambrescu
Endocrinology Department, Elias University Hospital, 17 Marasti Blvd, sector 1, Bucharest, Romania

Ioana Smarandita Lacau
Radiology Department, Hiperdia, 17 Marasti Blvd, sector 1, Bucharest, Romania

Doina Ruxandra Dimulescu
Cardiology Department, Carol Davila University of Medicine and Pharmacy, Elias University Hospital, 17 Marasti Blvd, sector 1, Bucharest, Romania

Chiara Sabbadin, Valentina Camozzi, Caterina Mian and Decio Armanini
Department of Medicine-Endocrinology, University of Padua, Via Ospedale 105, 35128 Padua, Italy

Gabriella Donà and Luciana Bordin
Department of Molecular Medicine-Biological Chemistry, University of Padua, Padua, Italy

Maurizio Iacobone
Minimally Invasive Endocrine Surgery Unit, Department of Surgery, Oncology and Gastroenterology, University of Padua, Padua, Italy

Eun Ae Cho, Jee Hee Yoon and Ho-Cheol Kang
Department of Internal Medicine, Chonnam National University Medical School, Gwangju, South Korea

Hee Kyung Kim
Department of Internal Medicine, Chonnam National University Medical School, Gwangju, South Korea
Department of Internal Medicine, Chonnam National University Hwasun Hospital, Chonnam National University Medical School, 322 Seoyang-ro, Hwasun-eup, Hwasun-gun, Jeonnam 519-763, South Korea

Merima Oruci
Surgical Oncology clinic, Institute for Oncology and Radiology of Serbia, Pasterova 14, Belgrade 11000, Serbia
Institute for Oncology and Radiology of Serbia, Pasterova 14, Belgrade 11000, Serbia

Yasuhiro Ito
Department of Surgery, Kuma Hospital, 8-2-35, Shimoyamate-dori, Chuo-ku, Kobe 650-0011, Japan

Marko Buta and Igor Djurisic
Surgical Oncology clinic, Institute for Oncology and Radiology of Serbia, Pasterova 14, Belgrade 11000, Serbia

Ziv Radisavljevic
Department of Clinical Research, Brigham and Women's Hospital, Harvard Medical School, Boston, MA, USA

Gordana Pupic
Department of Pathology, Institute for Oncology and Radiology of Serbia, Pasterova 14, Belgrade 11000, Serbia

Radan Dzodic
Surgical Oncology clinic, Institute for Oncology and Radiology of Serbia, Pasterova 14, Belgrade 11000, Serbia
University of Belgrade School of Medicine, Belgrade 11000, Serbia

Victoria Mendoza-Zubieta, Gloria A Gonzalez-Villaseñor, Guadalupe Vargas-Ortega, Baldomero Gonzalez, Mario A Molina-Ayala and Aldo Ferreira-Hermosillo
Endocrinology Departament Hospital de Especialidades Centro Médico Nacional Siglo XXI, Instituto Mexicano del Seguro Social (IMSS), Cuauhtemoc N° 330, Colonia Doctores, México City, DF, Mexico

Claudia Ramirez-Renteria and Moises Mercado
Endocrinology Experimental Investigation Unit Hospital de Especialidades Centro Médico Nacional Siglo XXI, Instituto Mexicano del Seguro Social (IMSS), Cuauhtemoc N° 330, Colonia Doctores, México City, DF, Mexico

Lian-Xi Li
Department of Endocrinology and Metabolism, Shanghai Diabetes Institute; Shanghai Clinical Center for Diabetes; Shanghai key Laboratory of Diabetes Mellitus, Shanghai Jiao Tong University Affiliated Sixth People's Hospital, 600 Yishan Road, Shanghai 200233, China

Xing Wu and Bing Hu
Department of Ultrasonography, Shanghai Jiao Tong University Affiliated Sixth People's Hospital, 600 Yishan Road, Shanghai 200233, China

Hui-Zhen Zhang
Department of Pathology, Shanghai Jiao Tong University Affiliated Sixth People's Hospital, 600 Yishan Road, Shanghai 200233, China

Han-Kui Lu
Department of Nuclear Medicine, Shanghai Jiao Tong University Affiliated Sixth People's Hospital, 600 Yishan Road, Shanghai 200233, China

Jian Zhang
Department of Clinical Laboratory, Jinshan Hospital of Fudan University, Shanghai 201508, China

Wan Xia Xiao
Internal Medicine Department, Xi'an Aviation Group Hospital, Xi'an 710021, China

Yuan Feng Zhu
Endocrinology Department, Jinshan Hospital, Fudan University, 1508 Longhang Road, Shanghai 201508, China
Endocrinology Department, Weinan Central Hospital, Weinan, Shaanxi 714000, China

Fatuma Said Muhali, Ling Xiao, Wen Juan Jiang, Xiao Hong Shi, Lian Hua Zhou and Jin An Zhang
Endocrinology Department, Jinshan Hospital, Fudan University, 1508 Longhang Road, Shanghai 201508, China

Manju Mamtani, Hemant Kulkarni, Thomas D Dyer, Laura Almasy, Michael C Mahaney, Ravindranath Duggirala, Anthony G Comuzzie, John Blangero and Joanne E Curran
Department of Genetics, Texas Biomedical Research Institute, 7620 NW Loop 410, San Antonio, TX, USA

Paul B Samollow
Department of Veterinary Integrative Biosciences, College of Veterinary Medicine and Biomedical Sciences, Texas A&M University, College Station, TX, USA

Naji J Aljohani
Faculty of Medicine, King Saud bin Abdulaziz University for Health Sciences, King Fahad Medical City, Riyadh, Saudi Arabia
Prince Mutaib Chair for Biomarkers of Osteoporosis, King Saud University, Riyadh, Saudi Arabia

Nasser M Al-Daghri, Majed S Alokail, Sobhy Yakout and Shaun Sabico
Biochemistry Department, Biomarkers Research Program, College of Science, King Saud University, Riyadh, Saudi Arabia
Prince Mutaib Chair for Biomarkers of Osteoporosis, King Saud University, Riyadh, Saudi Arabia

Omar S Al-Attas
Biochemistry Department, Biomarkers Research Program, College of Science, King Saud University, Riyadh, Saudi Arabia
Prince Mutaib Chair for Biomarkers of Osteoporosis, King Saud University, Riyadh, Saudi Arabia
Center of Excellence in Biotechnology Research Center, King Saud University, Riyadh, Saudi Arabia

Khalid M Alkhrafy
Biochemistry Department, Biomarkers Research Program, College of Science, King Saud University, Riyadh, Saudi Arabia
Prince Mutaib Chair for Biomarkers of Osteoporosis, King Saud University, Riyadh, Saudi Arabia
Clinical Pharmacy Department, College of Pharmacy, King Saud University, Riyadh, Saudi Arabia

Abdulaziz Al-Othman
Biochemistry Department, Biomarkers Research Program, College of Science, King Saud University, Riyadh, Saudi Arabia
College of Applied Medical Sciences, King Saud University, Riyadh, KSA, Saudi Arabia

Abdulaziz F Alkabba, Ahmed S Al-Ghamdi, Mussa Almalki and Badurudeen Mahmood Buhary
Faculty of Medicine, King Saud bin Abdulaziz University for Health Sciences, King Fahad Medical City, Riyadh, Saudi Arabia

Tullaya Sitasuwan, Thavatchai Peerapatdit and Nuntakorn Thongtang
Division of Endocrinology and Metabolism, Faculty of Medicine Siriraj Hospital, Mahidol University, Bangkok 10700, Thailand

Suchanan Hanamornroongruang
Department of Pathology, Faculty of Medicine Siriraj Hospital, Mahidol University, Bangkok 10700, Thailand

Johan O. Paulsson
Department of Oncology-Pathology, Karolinska Institutet, Stockholm, Sweden

Jan Zedenius
Department of Molecular Medicine and Surgery, Karolinska Institutet, Stockholm, Sweden
Department of Breast and Endocrine Surgery, Karolinska University Hospital, Stockholm, Sweden

C. Christofer Juhlin
Department of Oncology-Pathology, Karolinska Institutet, Stockholm, Sweden
Department of Pathology and Cytology, Karolinska University Hospital, Stockholm, Sweden

Nigel Glynn, Mark J. Hannon, Sarah Lewis, Patrick Hillery, Mohammed Al-Mousa, Christopher J. Thompson, Diarmuid Smith and Amar Agha
Department of Endocrinology, Beaumont Hospital and RCSI Medical School, Dublin 9, Ireland

Arnold D. K. Hill
Department of Surgery, Beaumont Hospital and RCSI Medical School, Dublin 9, Ireland

Frank Keeling and Martina Morrin
Department Radiology, Beaumont Hospital and RCSI Medical School, Dublin 9, Ireland

Derval Royston and Mary Leader
Department of Pathology, Beaumont Hospital and RCSI Medical School, Dublin 9, Ireland

Aoife Garrahy and Amar Agha
Department of Endocrinology, Beaumont Hospital, Dublin, Ireland

David Hogan and James Paul O'Neill
Department of Otolaryngology, Head and Neck Surgery, Beaumont Hospital, Dublin, Ireland

Shuo Zhang, Yang Wang, Sisi Zhong, Xingtong Liu, Yazhuo Huang, Sijie Fang, Ai Zhuang, Yinwei Li, Jing Sun, Huifang Zhou and Xianqun Fan
Department of Ophthalmology, Ninth People's Hospital, Shanghai Jiao Tong University School of Medicine, No. 639 ZhiZaoJu Road, Shanghai 200011, China

Geoffrey Omuse, Ali Kassim and Francis Kiigu
Department of Pathology, Aga Khan University Hospital, Nairobi, Kenya

Syeda Ra'ana Hussain and Mary Limbe
Department of Paediatrics, Aga Khan University Hospital, Nairobi, Kenya

Haiyang Zhou, Xinhuan Liang, Yingfen Qing, Bihui Meng, Jia Zhou, Song Huang, Shurong Lu, Zhenxing Huang, Haiyan Yang, Yan Ma and Zuojie Luo
The Department of Endocrinology, The First Affiliated Hospital of Guangxi Medical University, Nanning 530021, China

Bruce H. R. Wolffenbuttel, Hanneke J. C. M. Wouters, Sandra N. Slagter, Robert P. van Waateringe, Jana V. van Vliet-Ostaptchouk, Thera P. Links and Melanie M. van der Klauw
Department of Endocrinology, University of Groningen, University Medical Center Groningen, HPC AA31, 9700 RB Groningen, The Netherlands

Anneke C. Muller Kobold
Department of Clinical Chemistry, University of Groningen, University Medical Center Groningen, HPC AA31, 9700 RB Groningen, The Netherlands

Stella Bernardi and Bruno Fabris
Department of Medical Surgical and Health Sciences, Università degli Studi di Trieste, Cattinara Teaching Hospital, Strada di Fiume 447, 34149 Trieste, Italy
Endocrinology Unit - Azienda Sanitaria Universitaria Integrata Trieste, Cattinara Teaching Hospital, Strada di Fiume 447, 34149 Trieste, Italy

Andrea Michelli
Department of Medical Surgical and Health Sciences, Università degli Studi di Trieste, Cattinara Teaching Hospital, Strada di Fiume 447, 34149 Trieste, Italy

Deborah Bonazza and Fabrizio Zanconati
Department of Medical Surgical and Health Sciences, Università degli Studi di Trieste, Cattinara Teaching Hospital, Strada di Fiume 447, 34149 Trieste, Italy
Pathology Unit - Azienda Sanitaria Universitaria Integrata Trieste, Cattinara Teaching Hospital, Strada di Fiume 447, 34149 Trieste, Italy

Veronica Calabrò
Endocrinology Unit - Azienda Sanitaria Universitaria Integrata Trieste, Cattinara Teaching Hospital, Strada di Fiume 447, 34149 Trieste, Italy

Gabriele Pozzato
Department of Medical Surgical and Health Sciences, Università degli Studi di Trieste, Cattinara Teaching Hospital, Strada di Fiume 447, 34149 Trieste, Italy
Haematology Unit - Azienda Sanitaria Universitaria Integrata Trieste, Cattinara Teaching Hospital, Strada di Fiume 447, 34149 Trieste, Italy

Yu Li, Dong-Ning Chen and Jing Cui
Physical Examination Department, Beijing Tongren Hospital, Capital Medical University, Beijing 100730, China

Zhong Xin, Guang-Ran Yang and Jin-Kui Yang
Department of Endocrinology, Beijing Key Laboratory of Diabetes Research and Care, Beijing Tongren Hospital, Capital Medical University, Beijing 100730, China

Ming-Jia Niu
Department of Endocrinology, First Hospital of Qinghuangdao, Qinghuangdao 066000, China

Yoshihiro Maruo, Asami Mori, Yoriko Morioka, Chihiro Sawai, Yu Mimura, Katsuyuki Matui and Yoshihiro Takeuchi
Department of Pediatrics, Shiga University of Medical Science, Tsukinowa, Seta, Otsu 520-2192, Japan

Erin Fanning and Warrick J. Inder
Department of Diabetes and Endocrinology, Princess Alexandra Hospital, Brisbane, Queensland, Australia
Faculty of Medicine, the University of Queensland, Brisbane, Queensland, Australia

Emily Mackenzie
Department of Diabetes and Endocrinology, Princess Alexandra Hospital, Brisbane, Queensland, Australia
Nuclear Medicine, Department of Radiology, Princess Alexandra Hospital, Brisbane, Queensland, Australia

Ai Guo, Yan Tan, Chun Liu and Xiaoya Zheng
Department of Endocrinology, The First Affiliated Hospital of Chongqing Medical University, No.1 Youyi Street, Yuzhong District, Chongqing 400016, China

Index

U

www.ingramcontent.com/pod-product-compliance
Lightning Source LLC
Chambersburg PA
CBHW082018190326
41458CB00010B/3219

* 9 7 8 1 6 3 9 2 7 1 2 6 9 *